JN260916

Atlas of Developmental Anomalies in Experimental Animals
実験動物発生異常アトラス

Skeletal Anomalies
骨格異常

Edited by Project of the Terminology Committee of the Japanese Teratology Society

日本先天異常学会用語委員会　編集

FOREWORD

The first harmonized terminology (Version 1) of developmental anomalies in experimental animals, which was discussed by members of the International Federation of Teratology Societies including North America, Europe and Japan, had been published in 1997 (Teratology, 55:249-292, 1997; Cong. Anom., 37:165-210,1997). And then, the Japanese version of this terminology was made in the next year (Cong. Anom., 38:153-237, 1998).

The revised edition (Version 2) of this terminology had been published by the almost same members in 2009 (Cong. Anom., 49(3):123-246, 2009; Birth Defects Research (Part B), 86:227-327, 2009; Repro. Toxicol. 28:371-434, 2009). This version is described by simple words and is useful for laboratory technicians.

The Terminology committee of Japanese Teratology Society established "a Database of Congenital Anomalies in Laboratory animals" in the society homepage in 2010 and provided photographs of malformations and variations submitted by many companies in Japan until now. Submitted photographs were reviewed by a terminology project, some members in the committee, and were registered to the database mentioned above.

This textbook, "Atlas of Congenital Anomalies in Experimental Animals" gathered up photographs of skeletal anomalies and their explanations. We already published this series of the Atlas, external and visceral anomalies, in this year. We will expect that these Atlases including this textbook are used by researches that conduct teratological studies and review the data of the reproductive and developmental toxicity.

Smith CL et al. The Mammalian Phenotype Ontology as a tool for annotating, analyzing and comparing phenotypic information. Genome Biol. 6(1): R7, 2005

Kohler S et al. The Human Phenotype Ontology project: linking molecular biology and disease through phenotype data. Nucleic Acids Res. 42:D966, 2014.

はじめに

　1960 年代のサリドマイド薬禍を契機として、化合物の暴露による先天異常発現が問題となり、多くの研究者により実験動物を用いた発生毒性研究が進められました。また、これら研究成果の科学的信憑性を担保するため、催奇形性試験や生殖発生毒性試験に関するガイドラインも各国の規制当局により制定・改訂され、今日に至っています。しかし、実験動物を用いた試験・研究においては、実際に観察する発生異常の診断は、臨床で用いられている先天異常用語を参考にして行っていたのが現状でした。1997 年に日欧米三極の研究者により実験動物での発生用語の統一が図られ、実験動物発生異常用語集 Version 1（Teratology, 55:249-292, 1997; Cong. Anom., 37:165-210,1997）が提示されました。また、翌年には日本語版として、「実験動物発生異常用語集」（Cong. Anom., 38:153-237, 1998）も発表されました。この用語集で用いられている所見名はいわゆる診断用語であり、試験・研究の実務担当者には扱いにくい面もあることから、より簡易な用語を用いた用語集 Version 2 として 2009 年に改訂されました（Cong. Anom., 49(3):123-246, 2009; Birth Defects Research (Part B), 86:227-327, 2009; Repro. Toxicol., 28:371-434, 2009）。

　これを受けて、日本先天異常学会 用語委員会は 2010 年、学会ホームページに「実験動物先天異常データベース」を開設し、Version 2 に規定された用語集の日本語版を掲載すると共に、それらに該当する写真の公開を行っています。これまで多くの企業、施設のご協力により、貴重な異常・変異の写真を提供していただきました。この場を借り、お礼申し上げます。委員会では、審査プロジェクトを組み、メンバーにより写真及びその診断、説明の妥当性を審査し、上記データベースに登録してきました。

　本アトラスは、生殖発生毒性研究を実施される研究者や生殖発生毒性を評価される方々に活用いただける様、上記データベースを基に実験動物の骨格異常の写真及びその説明をまとめたものです。外表異常及び内臓異常については既にアトラス（2015 年 3 月及び 5 月）を出版しており、本アトラスにて、外表・内臓・骨格の全てが公表されることになります。

　また、近年、遺伝子解析技術の飛躍的な発展によって、先天異常学分野全般の研究が加速しています。今後、遺伝子改変動物の表現型の解析を通じた、遺伝子機能の決定、遺伝子変異とヒト遺伝性疾患の患者の症状の関係の研究の一層の展開が期待されます。遺伝子変異データがデジタルデータであるのに対して、表現型のデータはフォーマットの一定しないデータと見なされてきましたが、表現型をデジタル化可能な

コードとして国際標準化しようとする動きが進んでいます。著者らはこの動きに呼応するかたちで、本アトラスに示される表現型に対してコードを示しました（Table 2 参照）。本アトラスが動物の胎児への薬物毒性の研究者のみならず、広く遺伝子改変動物やヒト遺伝性疾患の研究者にとって有用なレファレンスになればと願っています。

協力企業・施設

- アステラス製薬株式会社
- あすか製薬株式会社
- 株式会社新日本科学
- 第一三共株式会社
- 田辺三菱製薬株式会社
- 一般財団法人残留農薬研究所
- 株式会社化合物安全性研究所
- 株式会社ボゾリサーチセンター
- 株式会社 LSI メディエンス
- 大塚製薬株式会社
- 旭化成ファーマ株式会社
- 武田薬品工業株式会社
- 株式会社イナリサーチ

Project members of the Terminology Committee in Japanese Teratology Society

Yojiro Ooshima

Michio Fujiwara (Astellas Pharma Inc.)

Kazuhiro Chihara (Sumitomo Dainippon Pharma Co., Ltd.)

Yuko Izumi (Takeda Pharmaceutical Company Ltd.)

Yoshihiro Katsumata (BoZo Research Center Inc.)

Hiroshi Sumida (Hiroshima International University)

Makoto Ema (AIST)

Kenjiro Kosaki (Keio University)

Advisors

Kohei Shiota (Shiga University of Medical Science)

Kok Wah Hew (Takeda Pharmaceutical Company Ltd., USA)

CONTENTS

Foreword

Table 1 List of Skeletal Anomalies	1
General Comments of Skeletal Anomalies	45
Table 2 Comparative List of This Atlas Findings, Mouse Phenotype, and Human Phenotype	54
Photographs of Normal Fetuses in Rats and Rabbits	61

Photographs of Skeletal Anomalies

1.	Skull	71
2.	Clavicle and Scapula	111
3.	Forelimb	119
4.	Hindlimb	131
5.	Phalanx of fore- and hind-paw	143
6.	Sternebra	153
7.	Rib	167
8.	Vertebral canal and Cervical vertebra	199
9.	Thoracic vertebra	225
10.	Lumbar vertebra	249
11.	Sacral and Caudal vertebrae	265
12.	Pelvic girdle	281

Table 1   List of Skeletal Anomalies

Region / Organ / Structure	Observation		Synonym or *Related Term*	Ver. 1 Code No.	Definition	Note	Photo No.
Skull 頭蓋骨	**Alisphenoid** 蝶形骨翼状突起	Absent　欠損		10407			
		Fused　癒合	*Cartilaginous fusion* 軟骨性癒合	10409			
		Hole　孔		10408		GC 1	
		Large　大型(化)		New			
		Malpositioned　位置異常		New		GC 12	
		Misshapen　形態異常		10411		GC 12	
		Small　小型(化)		10412			
		Supernumerary site　過剰部位		New			
		Incomplete ossification 不完全骨化		10410			
		Increased ossification 骨化亢進		New			
		Unossified　未骨化		10413			
		Unossified area　未骨化領域		New			
Skull 頭蓋骨	**Auditory ossicles** (incus, malleus, stapes) 耳小骨(キヌタ骨、ツチ骨、アブミ骨)	Absent　欠損		10414			
		Fused　癒合	*Cartilaginous fusion* 軟骨性癒合	10415			
		Large　大型(化)		New			
		Malpositioned　位置異常		New		GC 12	
		Misshapen　形態異常		10416		GC 12	
		Small　小型(化)		New			
		Supernumerary　過剰		New			
		Supernumerary site　過剰部位		New			
		Incomplete ossification 不完全骨化		New			
		Increased ossification 骨化亢進		New			
		Unossified　未骨化		10417			
Skull 頭蓋骨	**Basioccipital** 底後頭骨	Absent　欠損		10418			
		Fused　癒合	*Cartilaginous fusion* 軟骨性癒合	10420			**1-1**
		Hole　孔		10419		GC 1	
		Large　大型(化)		New			
		Malpositioned　位置異常		New		GC 12	
		Misshapen　形態異常	*Long, Short* 長大(化)、短小(化)	10422		GC 12	
		Small　小型(化)		10423			

Table 1 List of Skeletal Anomalies

Region / Organ / Structure	Observation		Synonym or *Related Term*	Ver. 1 Code No.	Definition	Note	Photo No.
		Split　分離		New		GC 2	
		Supernumerary　過剰		New			
		Supernumerary site　過剰部位		New			
		Incomplete ossification 不完全骨化		10421			
		Increased ossification 骨化亢進		New			
		Isolated ossification site 分離骨化部位		New			
		Unossified　未骨化		10424			
		Unossified area　未骨化領域		New			
		Unossified line　線状未骨化		New			
Skull 頭蓋骨	**Basisphenoid** (pterygoid processes and craniopharyngeal canal may be described separately) 底蝶形骨(翼状突起および頭蓋咽頭管は区別して記述する場合がある)	Absent　欠損		10425			
		Fused　癒合	*Cartilaginous fusion* 軟骨性癒合	10427			
		Hole　孔		10426		GC 1	
		Large　大型(化)		New			
		Malpositioned　位置異常		New		GC 12	
		Misshapen　形態異常		10429		GC 12	**1-2**
		Small　小型(化)		10430			
		Split　分離		New		GC 2	
		Supernumerary　過剰		New			
		Supernumerary site 過剰部位		New			
		Incomplete ossification 不完全骨化		10428			
		Increased ossification 骨化亢進		New			
		Isolated ossification site 分離骨化部位		New			
		Unossified　未骨化		10431			
		Unossified area　未骨化領域		New			
		Unossified line　線状未骨化		New			
Skull 頭蓋骨	**Exoccipital** (hypoglossal canal may be described separately)	Absent　欠損		10432			
		Fused　癒合	*Cartilaginous fusion* 軟骨性癒合	10434			**1-3**
		Hole　孔		10433		GC 1	

Table 1　List of Skeletal Anomalies

Region / Organ / Structure	Observation		Synonym or *Related Term*	Ver. 1 Code No.	Definition	Note	Photo No.
	外後頭骨(舌下神経管は区別して記述する場合がある)	Large　大型(化)		New			
		Malpositioned　位置異常		New		GC 12	
		Misshapen　形態異常		10436		GC 12	
		Small　小型(化)		10437			
		Supernumerary　過剰		New			
		Supernumerary site　過剰部位		New			
		Incomplete ossification 不完全骨化		10435			
		Increased ossification 骨化亢進		New			
		Isolated ossification site 分離骨化部位		New			
		Unossified　未骨化		10438			
		Unossified area　未骨化領域		New			
Skull 頭蓋骨	**Frontal** (orbital processes may be described separately) 前頭骨(眼窩突起は区別して記述する場合がある)	Absent　欠損		10439			
		Fused　癒合		10441			**1-4**
		Hole　孔		10440		GC 1	
		Large　大型(化)		New			
		Malpositioned　位置異常		New		GC 12	
		Misaligned　配列異常		New			
		Misshapen　形態異常	*Long, Short* 長大(化)、短小(化)	10443		GC 12	**1-5**
		Small　小型(化)		10444			
		Split　分離		New		GC 2	
		Supernumerary　過剰		New			
		Supernumerary site　過剰部位		New			
		Incomplete ossification 不完全骨化		10442			
		Increased ossification 骨化亢進		New			
		Isolated ossification site 分離骨化部位		New			
		Unossified　未骨化		10445			
		Unossified area　未骨化領域		New			
		Unossified line　線状未骨化		New			
Skull 頭蓋骨	**Hyoid body**, greater horn (ala), or lesser	Absent　欠損		10446			
		Bent　弯曲		10447			

Table 1 List of Skeletal Anomalies

Region / Organ / Structure	Observation		Synonym or *Related Term*	Ver. 1 Code No.	Definition	Note	Photo No.
	horn (ala) 舌骨体、大角(翼) あるいは小角(翼) In rat and mouse fetuses, both greater and lesser horns are usually unossified. In the rabbit, ossification is usually present in the greater horns but not in the lesser horns ラットおよびマウスの胎児では、通常、大角、小角ともに骨化していない。ウサギ胎児では、通常、大角は骨化しているが、小角は骨化していない	Fused　癒合	*Cartilaginous fusion* 軟骨性癒合	New			
		Hole　孔		10440		GC 1	
		Large　大型(化)		New			
		Long　長大(化)		New			
		Malpositioned　位置異常		New		GC 12	
		Misshapen　形態異常		10449		GC 12	1-6
		Short　短小(化)		New			
		Small　小型(化)		10450			
		Split　分離	*Interrupted*　不連続	New			1-7
		Supernumerary　過剰		New			
		Supernumerary site　過剰部位		New			
		Bipartite ossification 二分骨化		New			
		Incomplete ossification 不完全骨化		10448			
		Increased ossification 骨化亢進		New			
		Isolated ossification site 分離骨化部位		New			
		Unossified　未骨化		10451			
		Unossified area　未骨化領域		New			
Skull 頭蓋骨	**Interparietal** 頭頂間骨	Absent　欠損		10452			
		Bent　弯曲		New			
		Fused　癒合		10454			
		Hole　孔		10456		GC 1	
		Large　大型(化)		New			
		Malpositioned　位置異常		New		GC 12	
		Misshapen　形態異常		10457		GC 12	
		Small　小型(化)		10458			
		Split　分離		New		GC 2	
		Supernumerary　過剰		New			
		Bipartite ossification 二分骨化		10453			
		Incomplete ossification 不完全骨化		10455			

Table 1 List of Skeletal Anomalies

Region / Organ / Structure	Observation		Synonym or *Related Term*	Ver. 1 Code No.	Definition	Note	Photo No.
		Increased ossification 骨化亢進		New			
		Isolated ossification site 分離骨化部位		New			
		Unilateral ossification 片側(性)骨化		New			
		Unossified 未骨化		10459			
		Unossified area 未骨化領域		New			
		Unossified line 線状未骨化		New			
Skull 頭蓋骨	**Mandible** (processes [dental, coronoid, condyloid, angular], foramen [mental], and symphysis may be described separately 下顎骨(歯突起、筋突起、関節突起、角突起、オトガイ孔および結合)は区別して記述する場合がある)	Absent 欠損		10466			
		Bent 弯曲		New			
		Fused 癒合		10467			**1-8**
		Hole 孔		New		GC 1	
		Large 大型(化)		New			
		Long 長大(化)		New			
		Malpositioned 位置異常		New		GC 12	
		Misaligned 配列異常		New			
		Misshapen 形態異常		10469		GC 12	**1-9**
		Single incisor socket 単一切歯窩	Fused incisor sockets 切歯窩の癒合	New	One incisor socket absent 切歯窩の片側性欠損		
		Short 短小(化)		New			**1-10**
		Small 小型(化)		10470			**1-11**
		Splayed 放散		New	Paired structures diverge from one another 対となる構造物がお互いにずれている		
		Supernumerary 過剰		New			
		Supernumerary site 過剰部位		New			
		Thick 肥厚(化)		New		GC 3	
		Thin 菲薄(化)		New		GC 3	
		Incomplete ossification 不完全骨化		10468			
		Increased ossification 骨化亢進		New			
		Isolated ossification site 分離骨化部位		New			
		Unossified 未骨化		10471			

Table 1 List of Skeletal Anomalies

Region / Organ / Structure	Observation		Synonym or *Related Term*	Ver. 1 Code No.	Definition	Note	Photo No.
		Unossified area　未骨化領域		New			
Skull 頭蓋骨	**Maxilla** (processes [dental, orbital, palatine, zygomatic] and foramina [infra-orbital, palatine] may be described separately) 上顎骨(歯突起、眼窩突起、口蓋突起、頬骨突起および眼窩下孔、口蓋孔は区別して記述する場合がある)	Absent　欠損		10472			
		Fused　癒合		10473			
		Hole　孔		New		GC 1	
		Large　大型(化)		New			
		Long　長大(化)		New			
		Malpositioned　位置異常		New		GC 12	
		Misshapen　形態異常		10475		GC 12	**1-12**
		Short　短小(化)		New			
		Small　小型(化)		10476			**1-13**
		Split　分離	Not fused　未癒合	New			
		Supernumerary　過剰		New			
		Supernumerary site　過剰部位		New			
		Incomplete ossification 不完全骨化		10474			
		Isolated ossification site 分離骨化部位		New			
		Unossified　未骨化		10477			
		Unossified area　未骨化領域		New			
Skull 頭蓋骨	**Nasal** (nasal cartilages, medial and lateral, may be described separately) 鼻骨(鼻軟骨、内側、外側は区別して記述する場合がある)	Absent　欠損		10478			
		Fused　癒合		10479			**1-14**
		Hole　孔		10482		GC 1	
		Large　大型(化)		New			
		Malpositioned　位置異常		New		GC 12	
		Misaligned　配列異常		New			
		Misshapen　形態異常	*Long, Short* 長大(化)、短小(化)	10481		GC 12	**1-15**
		Small　小型(化)		10483			**1-16**
		Split　分離		New		GC 2	
		Supernumerary　過剰		New			
		Supernumerary site　過剰部位		New			
		Incomplete ossification 不完全骨化		10480			
		Increased ossification 骨化亢進		New			

Table 1　List of Skeletal Anomalies

Region / Organ / Structure		Observation	Synonym or *Related Term*	Ver. 1 Code No.	Definition	Note	Photo No.
		Isolated ossification site 分離骨化部位		New			
		Unossified　未骨化		10484			
		Unossified area　未骨化領域		New			
		Unossified line　線状未骨化		New			
Skull 頭蓋骨	**Palatine** 口蓋骨	Absent　欠損		10485			
		Fused　癒合		10486			
		Hole　孔		New		GC 1	
		Large　大型(化)		New			
		Malpositioned　位置異常		New		GC 12	
		Misaligned　配列異常		New			
		Misshapen　形態異常	*Long, Short* 長大(化)、短小(化)	10488		GC 12	
		Small　小型(化)		10489			
		Split　分離	*Cleft palate*; Not fused 口蓋裂、未癒合	10490			
		Supernumerary　過剰		New			
		Supernumerary site　過剰部位		New			
		Incomplete ossification 不完全骨化		10487			
		Isolated ossification site 分離骨化部位		New			
		Unossified　未骨化		10491			
		Unossified area　未骨化領域		New			
Skull 頭蓋骨	**Parietal** 頭頂骨	Absent　欠損		10492			
		Fused　癒合		10493			
		Hole　孔		10496		GC 1	**1-17**
		Large　大型(化)		New			
		Malpositioned　位置異常		New		GC 12	
		Misaligned　配列異常		New			
		Misshapen　形態異常		10495		GC 12	**1-18**
		Small　小型(化)		10497			
		Split　分離		New		GC 2	**1-19**
		Supernumerary　過剰		New			
		Supernumerary site 過剰部位		New			

Table 1 List of Skeletal Anomalies

Region / Organ / Structure	Observation		Synonym or *Related Term*	Ver. 1 Code No.	Definition	Note	Photo No.
		Incomplete ossification 不完全骨化		10494			
		Increased ossification 骨化亢進		New			
		Isolated ossification site 分離骨化部位		New			
		Unossified　未骨化		10498			
		Unossified area　未骨化領域		New			**1-20**
		Unossified line　線状未骨化		New			
Skull 頭蓋骨	**Premaxilla** (processes [nasofrontal, palatine] and palatine foramen may be described separately] 顎間骨(鼻前頭突起、口蓋突起および口蓋孔は区別して記述する場合がある) Bone may be called incisive 切歯骨とよぶ場合がある。 「訳者注：顎前骨とよぶ場合がある」	Absent　欠損		10499			
		Fused　癒合		10500			**1-21**
		Hole　孔		10503		GC 1	
		Large　大型(化)		New			
		Malpositioned　位置異常		New		GC 12	**1-22**
		Misshapen　形態異常	*Long, Short* 長大(化)、短小(化)	10502		GC 12	**1-23**
		Small　小型(化)		10504			**1-24**
		Split　分離	Not fused　未癒合	New			
		Supernumerary　過剰		New			
		Supernumerary site　過剰部位		New			
		Incomplete ossification 不完全骨化		10501			
		Increased ossification 骨化亢進		New			
		Isolated ossification site 分離骨化部位		New			
		Unossified　未骨化		10505			
		Unossified area　未骨化領域		New			
Skull 頭蓋骨	**Presphenoid** (orbitosphenoid and optic foramen may be described separately) 前蝶形骨(眼窩蝶形骨および視神経孔は区別して記述する場合がある)	Absent　欠損		10506			
		Fused　癒合	*Cartilaginous fusion* 軟骨性癒合	10507			
		Hole　孔		10510		GC 1	
		Large　大型(化)		New			
		Malpositioned　位置異常		New		GC 12	
		Misshapen　形態異常		10509		GC 12	
		Small　小型(化)		10511			
		Split　分離		New		GC 2	

Table 1 List of Skeletal Anomalies

Region / Organ / Structure		Observation	Synonym or *Related Term*	Ver. 1 Code No.	Definition	Note	Photo No.
		Supernumerary site　過剰部位		New			
		Incomplete ossification 不完全骨化		10508			
		Increased ossification 骨化亢進		New			
		Isolated　ossification site 分離骨化部位		New			
		Unossified　未骨化		10512			
		Unossified area　未骨化領域		New			
Skull 頭蓋骨	**Supraoccipital** 上後頭骨	Absent　欠損		10520			
		Bent　弯曲	*Protruding*　突出	New			
		Fused　癒合	*Cartilaginous fusion* 軟骨性癒合	10522			
		Hole　孔		10526		GC 1	
		Large　大型(化)		New			
		Malpositioned　位置異常		New		GC 12	
		Misshapen　形態異常		10524		GC 12	
		Small　小型(化)		10525			
		Split　分離		New		GC 2	
		Supernumerary　過剰		New			
		Supernumerary site　過剰部位		New			
		Bipartite ossification　二分骨化		10521			
		Incomplete ossification 不完全骨化		10523			
		Increased ossification 骨化亢進		New			
		Isolated ossification site 分離骨化部位		New			
		Unilateral ossification 片側(性)骨化		New			
		Unossified　未骨化		10527			
		Unossified area　未骨化領域		New			
		Unossified line　線状未骨化		New			
Skull 頭蓋骨	**Tympanic annulus** 鼓室輪	Absent　欠損		10528			**1-25**
		Fused　癒合	*Cartilaginous fusion* 軟骨性癒合	10529			
		Interrupted　不連続		New			
		Large　大型(化)		New			

Table 1 List of Skeletal Anomalies

Region / Organ / Structure	Observation		Synonym or Related Term	Ver. 1 Code No.	Definition	Note	Photo No.
		Malpositioned 位置異常		New		GC 12	**1-26**
		Misshapen 形態異常		10531		GC 12	
		Small 小型(化)		10532			
		Supernumerary 過剰		New			
		Supernumerary site 過剰部位		New			
		Incomplete ossification 不完全骨化		10530			
		Increased ossification 骨化亢進		New			
		Isolated ossification site 分離骨化部位		New			
		Unossified 未骨化		10533			
Skull 頭蓋骨	Zygomatic arch (maxillary process, squamosal process, and zygomatic [jugal, malar, zygoma] may be described separately) 頬骨弓、上顎骨の頬骨突起、側頭骨の頬骨突起、頬骨 (jugal, malar, zygoma(訳者注：何れも日本語訳は頬骨))は区別して記述する場合がある)	Absent 欠損		10540			
		Fused 癒合		10541		GC 13	**1-27**
		Large 大型(化)		New			
		Long 長大(化)		New			
		Malpositioned 位置異常		New		GC 12	
		Misshapen 形態異常		10543		GC 12	**1-28**
		Short 短小(化)		New			
		Small 小型(化)		10544			
		Supernumerary 過剰		New			
		Supernumerary site 過剰部位		New			
		Incomplete ossification 不完全骨化		10542			
		Increased ossification 骨化亢進		New			
		Isolated ossification site 分離骨化部位		New			
		Unossified 未骨化		10545			
		Unossified area 未骨化領域		New			
		Unossified line 線状未骨化		New			
Skull, fontenelles 頭蓋骨、泉門	Fontanellar bone 泉門骨		Bone island, Isolated bone, Supernumerary bone 島状骨、遊離骨、過剰骨	New	Any supernumerary bone occurring in a fontanelle 泉門の中にみられる過剰骨		
Skull, fontenelles	Fontanelle 泉門	Absent 欠損		New			
		Large 大型(化)	*Wide* 拡張(化)	10405			**1-29**

Table 1 List of Skeletal Anomalies

Region / Organ / Structure	Observation		Synonym or *Related Term*	Ver. 1 Code No.	Definition	Note	Photo No.
頭蓋骨、泉門		Malpositioned　位置異常		New		GC 12	
		Misshapen　形態異常		New		GC 12	
		Small　小型(化)		New			
Skull, sutures 頭蓋骨、縫合線	Sutural bone 縫合骨		Bone island, Isolated bone, Supernumerary bone, Suture bone 島状骨、遊離骨、過剰骨、縫合骨	New	Any supernumerary bone occurring in a cranial suture 頭蓋縫合の中にみられる過剰骨		**1-30**
Skull, sutures 頭蓋骨、縫合線	Suture 縫合線	Fused　癒合		New	Premature closure of a cranial suture with fusion of bone 頭蓋骨の癒合を伴う頭蓋縫合の成熟前閉鎖		
		Large　大型(化)		New			
		Malpositioned　位置異常		New		GC 12	
		Supernumerary　過剰		New			
		Wide　拡張(化)	*Large　大型(化)*	New			
Clavicle 鎖骨	Clavicle 鎖骨	Absent　欠損		10546			
		Bent　弯曲		10547			**2-1**
		Fused　癒合	*Cartilaginous fusion 軟骨性癒合*	New			
		Large　大型(化)		New			
		Long　長大(化)		New			
		Malpositioned　位置異常		New		GC 12	
		Misshapen　形態異常		10549		GC 12	**2-2**
		Short　短小(化)		New			
		Small　小型(化)		10550			
		Supernumerary　過剰		New			
		Supernumerary site　過剰部位		New			
		Thick　肥厚(化)		10551		GC 3	**2-3**
		Thin　菲薄(化)		New		GC 3	
		Incomplete ossification 不完全骨化		10548			
		Increased ossification 骨化亢進		New			
		Isolated　ossification site 分離骨化部位		New			

Table 1 List of Skeletal Anomalies

Region / Organ / Structure		Observation	Synonym or *Related Term*	Ver. 1 Code No.	Definition	Note	Photo No.
		Unossified　未骨化		10552			
Scapula 肩甲骨	Scapula (blade, spine, and processes [coracoid, acromion, metacromion] may be described separately) 肩甲骨（扁平部、棘および烏口突起、肩峰、鈎上突起は区別して記述する場合がある）	Absent　欠損		10553			
		Bent　弯曲		10554			2-4
		Branched　分岐		New			
		Fused　癒合	*Cartilaginous fusion* 軟骨性癒合	New			
		Large　大型(化)		New			
		Long　長大(化)		New			
		Malpositioned　位置異常		New		GC 12	
		Misshapen　形態異常		10556		GC 12	2-5
		Short　短小(化)		New			
		Small　小型(化)		New			2-6
		Supernumerary　過剰		New			
		Supernumerary site　過剰部位		New			
		Thick　肥厚(化)		10557		GC 3	
		Thin　菲薄(化)		New		GC 3	
		Incomplete ossification 不完全骨化		10555			
		Increased ossification 骨化亢進		New			
		Isolated ossification site 分離骨化部位		New			
		Unossified　未骨化		10558			
Forelimb 前肢	Humerus (deltoid tuberosity and proximal and distal epiphyses may be described separately) 上腕骨（三角筋粗面、近位および遠位端は区別して記述する場合がある）	Absent　欠損		10559			
		Bent　弯曲		10560			
		Fused　癒合	*Cartilaginous fusion* 軟骨性癒合	10561			
		Long　長大(化)		New			
		Malpositioned　位置異常		10563		GC 12	
		Misshapen　形態異常		10564		GC 12	3-1
		Short　短小(化)		10565			3-2
		Supernumerary　過剰		New			
		Supernumerary site　過剰部位		New			
		Thick　肥厚(化)		10566		GC 3	
		Thin　菲薄(化)		New		GC 3	

Table 1   List of Skeletal Anomalies

Region / Organ / Structure	Observation	Synonym or *Related Term*	Ver. 1 Code No.	Definition	Note	Photo No.
	Distal ossification site 遠位端骨化部位	Epiphyseal ossification site 骨端骨化部位	New	Ossification site(s) in the cartilaginous distal region of the bone 上腕骨の遠位端軟骨部における骨化部位		
	Incomplete ossification 不完全骨化		10562			
	Increased ossification 骨化亢進		New			
	Isolated ossification site 分離骨化部位		New		GC 15	
	Proximal ossification site 近位端骨化部位	Epiphyseal ossification site 骨端骨化部位	New	Ossification site(s) in the cartilaginous proximal region of the bone 上腕骨の近位端軟骨部における骨化部位		
	Unossified　未骨化		10567			
Forelimb 前肢	**Radius** (proximal and distal epiphyses may be described separately) 橈骨(近位および遠位端は区別して記述する場合がある)	Absent　欠損	Radial hemimelia 橈側半肢	10568			**3-3**
		Bent　弯曲		10569			**3-4**
		Fused　癒合	*Cartilaginous fusion 軟骨性癒合*	10570			
		Long　長大(化)		New			
		Malpositioned　位置異常		10572		GC 12	
		Misshapen　形態異常		10573		GC 12	**3-5**
		Short　短小(化)		10574			**3-6**
		Supernumerary　過剰		New			
		Supernumerary site　過剰部位		New			
		Thick　肥厚(化)		10575		GC 3	
		Thin　菲薄(化)		New		GC 3	
	Distal ossification site 遠位端骨化部位	Epiphyseal ossification site 骨端骨化部位	New	Ossification site(s) in the cartilaginous distal region of the bone 橈骨の遠位端軟骨部における骨化部位		
	Incomplete ossification 不完全骨化		10571			

Table 1 List of Skeletal Anomalies

Region / Organ / Structure	Observation		Synonym or *Related Term*	Ver. 1 Code No.	Definition	Note	Photo No.
		Increased ossification 骨化亢進		New			
		Isolated ossification site 分離骨化部位		New		GC 15	
		Proximal ossification site 近位端骨化部位	Epiphyseal ossification site 骨端骨化部位	New	Ossification site(s) in the cartilaginous proximal region of the bone 橈骨の近位端軟骨部における骨化部位		
		Unossified 未骨化		10576			
Forelimb 前肢	**Ulna** (olecranon process and proximal and distal epiphyses may be described separately) 尺骨(肘頭突起、近位および遠位端は区別して記述する場合がある)	Absent 欠損	Ulnar hemimelia 尺側半肢	10577			**3-7**
		Bent 弯曲		10578			**3-8**
		Fused 癒合	*Cartilaginous fusion 軟骨性癒合*	10579			
		Long 長大(化)		New			
		Malpositioned 位置異常		10581		GC 12	
		Misshapen 形態異常		10582		GC 12	
		Short 短小(化)		10583			
		Supernumerary 過剰		New			
		Supernumerary site 過剰部位		New			
		Thick 肥厚(化)		10584		GC 3	
		Thin 菲薄(化)		New		GC 3	
		Distal ossification site 遠位端骨化部位	Epiphyseal ossification site 骨端骨化部位	New	Ossification site(s) in the cartilaginous distal region of the bone 尺骨の遠位端軟骨部における骨化部位		
		Incomplete ossification 不完全骨化		10580			
		Increased ossification 骨化亢進		New			
		Isolated ossification site 分離骨化部位		New		GC 15	

Table 1　List of Skeletal Anomalies

Region / Organ / Structure		Observation	Synonym or *Related Term*	Ver. 1 Code No.	Definition	Note	Photo No.
		Proximal ossification site 近位端骨化部位	Epiphyseal ossification site 骨端骨化部位	New	Ossification site(s) in the cartilaginous proximal region of the bone 尺骨の近位端軟骨部における骨化部位		
		Unossified　未骨化		10585			
Forelimb 前肢	**Carpal bone** 手根骨	Absent　欠損		10586			
		Bent　弯曲		New			
	In the rat, mouse, and rabbit, carpal bones are not usually ossified ラット、マウスおよびウサギ(訳者注：胎児)では、通常、手根骨は骨化していない	Fused　癒合	*Cartilaginous fusion 軟骨性癒合*	10587			
		Large　大型(化)	*Long, Thick 長大(化)、肥厚(化)*	New			
		Malpositioned　位置異常		10589		GC 12	
		Misshapen　形態異常		10590		GC 12	
		Small　小型(化)	*Short, Thin 短小(化)、菲薄(化)*	10591			
		Supernumerary　過剰		10592			
		Supernumerary site　過剰部位		New			
		Incomplete ossification 不完全骨化		10588			
		Increased ossification 骨化亢進		New			
		Unossified　未骨化		10593			
Forelimb 前肢	**Metacarpal** 中手骨	Absent　欠損		10594			
		Bent　弯曲		New			
		Fused　癒合	*Cartilaginous fusion 軟骨性癒合*	10595			
		Large　大型(化)		New			
		Long　長大(化)		New			
		Malpositioned　位置異常		10597		GC 12	
		Misshapen　形態異常		10598		GC 12	
		Short　短小(化)		New			
		Small　小型(化)		10599			
		Supernumerary　過剰		10600			
		Supernumerary site　過剰部位		New			
		Thick　肥厚(化)		New			
		Thin　菲薄(化)		New			

Table 1   List of Skeletal Anomalies

Region / Organ / Structure	Observation		Synonym or *Related Term*	Ver. 1 Code No.	Definition	Note	Photo No.
		Incomplete ossification 不完全骨化		10596			
		Increased ossification 骨化亢進		New			
		Isolated ossification site 分離骨化部位		New			
		Unossified　未骨化		10601			
Forelimb 前肢	**Forepaw phalanx** 指節骨	Absent　欠損	*Aphalangia*　無指	10602			**5-1**
		Bent　弯曲		New			
		Fused　癒合	*Cartilaginous fusion* 軟骨性癒合	10603			**5-2**
		Large　大型(化)		New			
		Long　長大(化)		New			
		Malpositioned　位置異常		10605		GC 12	
		Misshapen　形態異常		10606		GC 12	
		Short　短小(化)		New			
		Small　小型(化)		10607			
		Supernumerary　過剰		10608			**5-3**
		Supernumerary site　過剰部位		New			
		Thick　肥厚(化)		10609			
		Thin　菲薄(化)		New			
		Incomplete ossification 不完全骨化		10604			
		Increased ossification 骨化亢進		New			
		Isolated ossification site 分離骨化部位		New			
		Unossified　未骨化		10610			
Sternebra 胸骨分節	**Sternebra** (sternebra 1 may be called the manubrium; sternebra 6 may be called the xiphoid process) **胸骨分節**(第1胸骨分節は胸骨柄、第	Absent　欠損		10611		GC 4	
		Asymmetric　非対称		New			
		Bent　弯曲		New			
		Branched　分岐		New		GC 16	
		Fused　癒合		10614		GC 14	**6-1**
		Hemisternebra　半胸骨分節		New	Absent sternebral hemicenter 片側の胸骨分節の欠損		
		Long　長大(化)		New		GC 17	

Table 1 List of Skeletal Anomalies

Region / Organ / Structure		Observation	Synonym or *Related Term*	Ver. 1 Code No.	Definition	Note	Photo No.
	6胸骨分節は剣状突起とよぶ場合がある)	Malpositioned 位置異常		10616		GC 12	
		Misaligned 配列異常		10617	Misaligned sternebral hemicenters and costal cartilages 左右の胸骨分節および肋軟骨の配列異常	GC 18	**6-2**
		Misshapen 形態異常	*Assymetric* 非対称	10618		GC 12	**6-3**
		Short 短小(化)	*Small* 小型(化)	New		GC 19	
		Split 分離		New			**6-4**
		Supernumerary 過剰		New		GC 20	
		Supernumerary site 過剰部位		New		GC 21	
		Wide 拡張(化)		New			
		Asymmetric ossification 非対称骨化		New	Non-equivalent proportions when bisected by a longitudinal plane; Alizarin red stain uptake greater in one hemicenter than the other 長軸方向に分割した場合に、対称でない；一方の胸骨分節のアリザリンレッド染色性が他方よりも強い		**6-5**
		Bipartite ossification 二分骨化		10612			**6-6**
		Dumbbell ossification ダンベル状骨化		New			
		Incomplete ossification 不完全骨化	*Fragmented ossification* 断片骨化	10615			
		Increased ossification 骨化亢進		New		GC 21	
		Isolated ossification site 分離骨化部位		10613		GC 21	
		Misaligned ossification sites 骨化部位配列異常		New	Ossification sites misaligned, but misalignment of costal cartilages not confirmed 肋軟骨の配列異常を伴わない骨化部位の配列異常		

Table 1 List of Skeletal Anomalies

Region / Organ / Structure	Observation		Synonym or *Related Term*	Ver. 1 Code No.	Definition	Note	Photo No.
		Misshapen ossification site 骨化部位形態異常		New		GC 12	
		Unilateral ossification 片側(性)骨化		New			6-7
		Unossified 未骨化		10620			
Sternebra 胸骨分節	Intersternebral cartilage 胸骨分節間軟骨	Discontinuous 不連続		New			
		Long 長大(化)		New			
		Misshapen 形態異常		New		GC 12	
		Short 短小(化)		New			
		Split 分離		New	Split cartilage between sternebrae 胸骨分節間の軟骨の分離	GC 22	
		Wide 拡張(化)		New			
Sternebra 胸骨分節	Xiphoid cartilage 剣状軟骨	Branched 分岐		New			
		Hole 孔		New			
		Misshapen 形態異常	*Long, short, wide* 長大(化)、短小(化)、拡張(化)	New		GC 12	
		Split 分離		New			6-8
		Supernumerary 過剰		New			
Sternum 胸骨	Sternum (omosternum may be described separately) 胸骨(肩鎖骨は区別して記述する場合がある)	Bent 弯曲		New			
		Long 長大(化)		New			
		Misshapen 形態異常		New		GC 12	6-9
		Shifted 転位	Malpositioned 位置異常	New	Sternebrae located one or more positions higher or lower, relative to ribs/vertebrae 胸骨分節が肋骨/椎骨に対して1つ以上前方あるいは後方に位置すること	GC 12	
		Short 短小(化)		New			
		Split 分離	Sternoschisis 胸骨裂	10619			6-10
		Supernumerary 過剰		New			
		Wide 拡張(化)		New			

Table 1　List of Skeletal Anomalies

Region / Organ / Structure		Observation	Synonym or *Related Term*	Ver. 1 Code No.	Definition	Note	Photo No.
		Supernumerary ossification site　過剰骨化部位		New		GC 23	**6-11**
Rib　肋骨	**Rib** (tubercle may be described separately)　肋骨(結節は区別して記述する場合がある)	Absent　欠損	'N" only, Reduced number　N個のみ、数の減少	10621		GC 4	**7-1**
		Bent　弯曲		10622	Shaped like an angle　折れ曲がっている		
		Branched　分岐		10623	A rib that partially (distally or proximally) divides into two or more ribs　2つ以上に(近位または遠位部が)分かれた肋骨		**7-2**
		Detached　分離	Non-articulated　関節結合していない	10626	Rib, not at cervicothoracic or thoracolumbar border, not articulated with vertebral column　頚胸部あるいは胸腰部の境界部に位置せず、脊柱と関節結合していない肋骨		**7-3**
		Fused　癒合	*Cartilaginous fusion*　軟骨性癒合	10629			**7-4**
		Intercostal　肋間	Supernumerary non-articulated　過剰で関節結合していない	10632	An additional rib-like structure between two other ribs, not articulated with vertebral column　肋骨間に存在する過剰な肋骨様の構造物で、脊柱と関節結合していないもの		**7-5**
		Interrupted　不連続		10627	Absence of cartilage and alizarin red stain uptake in a central region of a rib usually forming two segments　肋骨中心部の軟骨およびアリザリンレッド染色部位の欠損で、通常2つに分かれた部分で構成されている	GC 24	**7-6**
		Long　長大(化)		New		GC 25	

Table 1   List of Skeletal Anomalies

Region / Organ / Structure		Observation	Synonym or *Related Term*	Ver. 1 Code No.	Definition	Note	Photo No.
		Malpositioned　位置異常		10634		GC 12	
		Misaligned　配列異常		10635			**7-7**
		Misshapen　形態異常		10636		GC 12	**7-8**
		Nodulated　結節状	Focal enlargement, Knobby 局所肥大、ノブ状	10633	A rounded protuberance on a rib 肋骨上の円形隆起		**7-9**
		Partially duplicated　部分重複		New			
		Short　短小(化)		10637		GC 26	**7-10**
		Supernumerary articulated 過剰	*Increased number, 'N'* 数の増加、「N」	New	An additional full rib between two other ribs, articulated with vertebral column 肋骨間にあり、脊柱と関節結合している過剰な完全肋骨	GC 5	**7-11**
		Supernumerary site　過剰部位		New			
		Thick　肥厚(化)		10639		GC 3	**7-12**
		Thin　菲薄(化)		New		GC 3	
		Wavy　波状	Kinked　よじれ	10641	Undulation(s) along the length of a rib 肋骨の長軸に沿ったうねり	GC 27	**7-13**
		Incomplete ossification 不完全骨化	*Discontinuous ossification, Interrupted ossification* 不連続骨化	10631			
		Increased ossification 骨化亢進	Long ossified portion 骨化部位の長大(化)	New			
		Isolated ossification site 分離骨化部位		New			
		Unossified　未骨化		10640			
Rib 肋骨	**Costal cartilage** 肋軟骨	Absent　欠損		New			
		Branched　分岐		10624	A rib cartilage that partially (distally or proximally) divides into two or more cartilages 2つ以上に(近位または遠位部が)分かれた肋軟骨		**7-14**

Table 1   List of Skeletal Anomalies

Region / Organ / Structure		Observation	Synonym or *Related Term*	Ver. 1 Code No.	Definition	Note	Photo No.
		Intercostal　肋間	Supernumerary non-articulated　過剰で関節結合していない	New	An additional, cartilaginous rib-like structure between two ribs, not articulated with vertebral column　肋骨間に存在する過剰な肋軟骨様の構造物で、脊柱と関節結合していないもの		
		Interrupted　不連続	Discontinuous　不連続	New			**7-15**
		Fused　癒合		10630			**7-16**
		Fused to sternum　胸骨接続		New		GC 28	
		Not fused to sternum　胸骨不接続		New		GC 29	**7-17**
		Long　長大(化)		New			
		Misaligned　配列異常		New			
		Misshapen　形態異常	*Knobby, Nodulated, Wide*　ノブ状, 結節状、拡張(化)	New		GC 12	
		Partially duplicated　部分重複		New			**7-18**
		Short　短小(化)		New		GC 30	
		Thick　肥厚(化)		New		GC 3	
		Thin　菲薄(化)		New		GC 3	
Supernumerary rib　過剰肋骨	**Cervical**　頸部	Full　完全	Cervical rib (CR), Cervical rib full, Cervical rib long, Long　頸肋、頸部完全肋骨、頸部長大肋骨、長大(化)	New	An extra rib at the cervicothoracic border with length greater than one third of the length of the ossified portion of the first thoracic rib and/or costal cartilage distal　頸胸部の境界にあり、長さが胸部第1肋骨の骨化部分の1/3より長い過剰肋骨で、遠位部に肋軟骨を有することもある	GC 8	**7-19**

Table 1 List of Skeletal Anomalies

Region / Organ / Structure	Observation		Synonym or *Related Term*	Ver. 1 Code No.	Definition	Note	Photo No.
		Short　短小	Cervical ossification site (COS), Cervical rib rudimentary, Cervical rib short, Rudimentary 頸部骨化部位、頸部痕跡肋骨、頸部短小肋骨、痕跡	10625	An extra rib at the cervicothoracic border with the distal extremity rounded, length less than one third of the length of the ossified portion of the first thoracic rib and no costal cartilage distal 頸胸部の境界にあり、長さが胸部第1肋骨の骨化部分の1/3未満の過剰肋骨で、遠位部に肋軟骨がなく先端が円形になっている	GC 9	**7-20**
		Cartilaginous　軟骨性		New		GC 31	
Supernumerary rib 過剰肋骨	Thoracolumbar 胸腰部	Full　完全	Extra thoracic rib, Extra thoracolumbar rib full, Extra thoracolumbar rib long, Long, Lumbar rib (LR), Lumbar rib full, Lumbar rib long 胸部過剰肋骨、胸腰部完全過剰肋骨、胸腰部長大過剰肋骨、長大(化)、腰肋、腰部完全肋骨、腰部長大肋骨	10628	An extra rib at the thoracolumbar border with length greater than one third of the ossified portion of the preceding rib and/or with costal cartilage distal 胸腰部の境界にあり、長さが前方の肋骨の骨化部分の1/3より長い過剰肋骨で、遠位部に肋軟骨を有することもある	GC 10	**7-21**
		Short　短小	Extra thoracolumbar rib rudimentary, Extra thoracolumbar rib short, Lumbar ossification site (LOS), Lumbar rib rudimentary, Lumbar rib short, Rudimentary 胸腰部痕跡過剰肋骨、胸腰部短小過剰肋骨、腰部骨化部位、腰部痕跡肋骨、腰部短小肋骨、痕跡	10638	An extra rib at the thoracolumbar border with the distal extremity rounded, length less than one third of the length of the ossified portion of the preceeding rib and no costal cartilage distal 胸腰部の境界にあり、長さが前方の肋骨の骨化部分の1/3未満の過剰肋骨で、遠位部に肋軟骨がなく先端が円形になっている	GC 11	**7-22**

Table 1　List of Skeletal Anomalies

Region / Organ / Structure		Observation	Synonym or *Related Term*	Ver. 1 Code No.	Definition	Note	Photo No.
		Cartilaginous　軟骨性		New		GC 31	
Supernumerary rib 過剰肋骨	**Supernumerary rib cartilage** 過剰肋軟骨	Branched　分岐		10624	A rib cartilage that partially (distally or proximally) divides into two or more cartilages 2つ以上に(近位または遠位部が)分かれた肋軟骨		
		Fused　癒合		10630			
		Fused to sternum　胸骨接続		New			
		Interrupted　不連続	Discontinuous 不連続	New			
		Long　長大		New			
		Present　存在		New			
Vertebra 椎骨	**Vertebra,** General (Intervertebral discs may be described separately) 椎骨、全般(椎間円板は区別して記述する場合がある)	Absent　欠損	'N' only, 'N' prepelvic, 'N' presacral, *Reduced number* N個のみ、骨盤前「N」、仙椎前「N」、数の減少	10642		GC 4	
		Supernumerary　過剰	*Increased number*, 'N', 'N' prepelvic, 'N' presacral 数の増加、「N」、骨盤前「N」、仙椎前「N」	10643		GC 6	**8-1**
		Supernumerary site　過剰部位		New	An additional cartilaginous or ossified site located along the vertebral column that cannot be clearly identified as an arch or centrum 椎骨に沿って存在する過剰な軟骨あるいは骨化部位で、椎弓や椎体とは明確に特定できないもの		
		Isolated ossification site 分離骨化部位		New			
Vertebra 椎骨	**Vertebral canal** 脊柱管	Absent　欠損	*Occluded*　閉塞	New		GC 32	
		Interrupted　不連続		New			**8-2**
		Large　大型(化)		New			

Table 1　List of Skeletal Anomalies

Region / Organ / Structure	Observation		Synonym or *Related Term*	Ver. 1 Code No.	Definition	Note	Photo No.
		Double　二重	Duplicated　重複	New			**8-3**
		Small　小型(化)	Narrow　狭窄(化)	New			
Vertebra 椎骨	**Atlas, ventral arch** (Atlas = cervical vertebra 1), (ventral tubercle may be described separately) 環椎、腹弓(環椎＝第1頸椎)(腹結節は区別して記述する場合がある)	Absent　欠損		New			**8-4**
		Fused　癒合	*Cartilaginous fusion* 軟骨性癒合	New			**8-5**
		Hemicentric　半椎体		New			
		Large　大型(化)		New			
		Malpositioned　位置異常		New		GC 12	
		Misaligned　配列異常		New			
		Misshapen　形態異常	*Long, Short* 長大(化)、短小(化)	New		GC 12	**8-6**
		Small　小型(化)		New			**8-7**
		Split　分離		New			
		Supernumerary　過剰		New			
		Supernumerary site　過剰部位		New			
		Bipartite ossification　二分骨化		New			
		Incomplete ossification 不完全骨化	*Fragmented ossification* 断片骨化	New			
		Increased ossification 骨化亢進		New			
		Isolated ossification site 分離骨化部位		New			
		Unilateral ossification 片側(性)骨化		New			
		Unossified　未骨化		New			
Vertebra 椎骨	**Cervical arch** (anterior tubercle [ventral plate, lamina ventralis], usually located on vertebra 6, and transverse foramen [vertebraterial canal] may be described separately) 頸椎弓(第6椎骨に	Absent　欠損	'N' only, Reduced number N個のみ、数の減少	10644		GC 4	
		Bent　弯曲		New			
		Branched　分岐		New			
		Fused　癒合	*Cartilaginous fusion* 軟骨性癒合	10645			**8-8**
		Incompletely fused dorsal 背側不完全癒合		New		GC 33	
		Large　大型(化)		New			
		Malpositioned　位置異常		10647		GC 12	
		Misaligned　配列異常		10648			

Table 1 List of Skeletal Anomalies

Region / Organ / Structure		Observation	Synonym or *Related Term*	Ver. 1 Code No.	Definition	Note	Photo No.
	通常位置する前結節 [腹板] および横突孔は区別して記述する場合がある)	Misshapen　形態異常	*Long, Short*　長大(化)、短小(化)	10649		GC 12	**8-9**
		Not fused dorsal　背側未癒合		New		GC 33	
		Small　小型(化)		10650			
		Splayed　放散		New	Paired structures diverge from one another 対となる構造物（椎弓）が開放している（離れる）	GC 34	
		Split　分離	*Interrupted*　不連続	New			**8-10**
		Supernumerary　過剰	*Increased number, 'N'*　数の増加、「N」	10651		GC 6	
		Supernumerary site　過剰部位		New			
		Thick　肥厚(化)	*Wide*　拡張(化)	New			**8-11**
		Thin　菲薄(化)	*Narrow*　狭窄(化)	New			**8-12**
		Incomplete ossification 不完全骨化	*Discontinuous ossification, Interrupted ossification* 不連続骨化	10646			
		Increased ossification 骨化亢進		New		GC 35	
		Isolated ossification site 分離骨化部位		New			**8-13**
		Unossified　未骨化		10652			
Vertebra 椎骨	**Cervical centrum** (odontoid process [dens] of cervical vertebra 2 may be defined separately) 頸椎体(第2頸椎の歯突起は区別して記述する場合がある)	Absent　欠損	*'N' only, Reduced number* N個のみ、数の減少	10653		GC 4	**8-14**
		Dumbbell-shaped　ダンベル状		10656			
		Fused　癒合	*Cartilaginous fusion* 軟骨性癒合	10657			**8-15**
		Hemicentric　半椎体		10659			
		Large　大型(化)		New			
		Malpositioned　位置異常		New		GC 12	
		Misaligned　配列異常		10661			
		Misshapen　形態異常	*Asymmetric*　非対称	10662		GC 12	**8-16**
		Small　小型(化)		New			
		Split　分離		10663			**8-17**

Table 1   List of Skeletal Anomalies

Region / Organ / Structure	Observation		Synonym or *Related Term*	Ver. 1 Code No.	Definition	Note	Photo No.
		Supernumerary　過剰	*Increased number, 'N'*　数の増加、「N」	10664		GC 6	
		Supernumerary site　過剰部位		New			
		Asymmetric ossification 非対称骨化		New	Alizarin red stain uptake greater in one hemicenter than the other 一方の椎体のアリザリンレッド染色性が他方よりも強い		
		Bipartite ossification　二分骨化		10654			
		Dumbbell ossification ダンベル状骨化		10655			**8-18**
		Incomplete ossification 不完全骨化		10660			
		Increased ossification 骨化亢進		New			
		Isolated ossification site 分離骨化部位		New			
		Misshapen ossification site 骨化部位形態異常		New		GC 12	
		Unilateral ossification 片側(性)骨化		New			
		Unossified　未骨化		10666			
Vertebra 椎骨	**Cervical vertebra** (Atlas and Axis may be defined separately) 頸椎(環椎と軸椎は区別して記述する場合がある)	Absent　欠損	*'N' only, Reduced number* N個のみ、数の減少	10667		GC 4	**8-19**
		Hemivertebra　半椎		10668		GC 7	
		Malpositioned　位置異常		10669		GC 12	
		Misaligned　配列異常		New			
		Small　小型(化)		New			
		Supernumerary hemivertebra 過剰半椎		New			
		Supernumerary　過剰	*Increased number, 'N'*　数の増加、「N」	10670		GC 6	
Vertebra 椎骨	**Thoracic arch** (processes [e.g., neural spine, articular processes]	Absent　欠損	*'N' only, Reduced number* N個のみ、数の減少	10671		GC 4	**9-1**
		Bent　弯曲		New			
		Branched　分岐		New			

Table 1 List of Skeletal Anomalies

Region / Organ / Structure		Observation	Synonym or *Related Term*	Ver. 1 Code No.	Definition	Note	Photo No.
	may be described separately) 胸椎弓(突起 [例えば神経棘、関節突起] は区別して記述する場合がある)	Fused 癒合	*Cartilaginous fusion* 軟骨性癒合	10672			**9-2**
		Incompletely fused dorsal 背側不完全癒合		New		GC 33	
		Large 大型(化)		New			**9-3**
		Malpositioned 位置異常		10674		GC 12	
		Misaligned 配列異常		10675			
		Misshapen 形態異常	*Long, Short* 長大(化)、短小(化)	10676		GC 12	**9-4**
		Not fused dorsal 背側未癒合		New		GC 33	
		Small 小型(化)		10677			**9-5**
		Splayed 放散		New	Paired structures diverge from one another 対となる構造物（椎弓）が開放している（離れる）	GC 34	
		Split 分離	*Interrupted* 不連続	New			
		Supernumerary 過剰	*Increased number, 'N'* 数の増加、「N」	10678		GC 6	
		Supernumerary site 過剰部位		New			
		Thick 肥厚(化)	*Wide* 拡張(化)	New			
		Thin 菲薄(化)	*Narrow* 狭窄(化)	New			
		Incomplete ossification 不完全骨化	*Discontinuous ossification, Interrupted ossification* 不連続骨化	10673			
		Increased ossification 骨化亢進		New		GC 35	
		Isolated ossification site 分離骨化部位		New			**9-6**
		Unossified 未骨化		10679			
Vertebra 椎骨	Thoracic centrum 胸椎体	Absent 欠損	*'N' only, Reduced number* N個のみ、数の減少	10680		GC 4	**9-7**
		Dumbbell-shaped ダンベル状		10683			
		Fused 癒合	*Cartilaginous fusion* 軟骨性癒合	10684			**9-8**
		Hemicentric 半椎体		10686			
		Large 大型(化)		New			

Table 1 List of Skeletal Anomalies

Region / Organ / Structure		Observation	Synonym or *Related Term*	Ver. 1 Code No.	Definition	Note	Photo No.
		Malpositioned 位置異常		New		GC 12	
		Misaligned 配列異常		10688			
		Misshapen 形態異常	*Asymmetric* 非対称	10689		GC 12	
		Small 小型(化)		New			**9-9**
		Split 分離		10690			
		Supernumerary 過剰	*Increased number, 'N'* 数の増加、「N」	10691		GC 6	
		Supernumerary site 過剰部位		New			
		Asymmetric ossification 非対称骨化		New	Alizarin red stain uptake greater in one hemicenter than the other 一方の椎体のアリザリンレッド染色性が他方よりも強い		
		Bipartite ossification 二分骨化		10681			**9-10**
		Dumbbell ossification ダンベル状骨化		10682			**9-11**
		Incomplete ossification 不完全骨化		10687			
		Increased ossification 骨化亢進		New			
		Isolated ossification site 分離骨化部位		New			
		Misshapen ossification site 骨化部位形態異常		New		GC 12	
		Unilateral ossification 片側(性)骨化		New			
		Unossified 未骨化		10693			**9-12**
Vertebra 椎骨	**Thoracic vertebra** 胸椎	Absent 欠損	*'N' only, Reduced number* N個のみ、数の減少	10694		GC 4	**9-13**
		Hemivertebra 半椎		10696		GC 7	**9-14**
		Malpositioned 位置異常		10695		GC 12	
		Misaligned 配列異常		New			
		Small 小型(化)		New			
		Supernumerary 過剰	*Increased number, 'N'* 数の増加、「N」	10697		GC 6	

Table 1　List of Skeletal Anomalies

Region / Organ / Structure	Observation		Synonym or *Related Term*	Ver. 1 Code No.	Definition	Note	Photo No.
		Supernumerary hemivertebra 過剰半椎		New			
Vertebra 椎骨	**Lumbar arch** (processes [e.g., neural spine, transverse processes, articular processes] may be described separately) 腰椎弓(突起 [例えば神経棘、横突起、関節突起] は区別して記述する場合がある)	Absent　欠損	*'N' only, Reduced number* *N個のみ、数の減少*	10698		GC 4	
		Bent　弯曲		New			
		Branched　分岐		New			
		Fused　癒合	*Cartilaginous fusion* *軟骨性癒合*	10699			**10-1**
		Incompletely fused dorsal 背側不完全癒合		New		GC 33	
		Large　大型(化)		New			
		Malpositioned　位置異常		10701		GC 12	
		Misaligned　配列異常		10702			
		Misshapen　形態異常	*Long, Short* *長大(化)、短小(化)*	10703		GC 12	**10-2**
		Not fused dorsal　背側未癒合		New		GC 33	
		Small　小型(化)		10704			
		Splayed　放散		New	Paired structures diverge from one another 対となる構造物（椎弓）が開放している（離れる）	GC 34	**10-3**
		Split　分離	*Interrupted*　*不連続*	New			
		Supernumerary　過剰	*Increased number, 'N'* *数の増加、「N」*	10705		GC 6	
		Supernumerary site　過剰部位		New			**10-4**
		Thick　肥厚(化)	*Wide*　*拡張(化)*	New			
		Thin　菲薄(化)	*Narrow*　*狭窄(化)*	New			
		Incomplete ossification 不完全骨化	*Discontinuous ossification, Interrupted ossification* *不連続骨化*	10700			
		Increased ossification 骨化亢進		New		GC 35	**10-5**
		Isolated ossification site 分離骨化部位		New			
		Unossified　未骨化		10706			

Table 1 List of Skeletal Anomalies

Region / Organ / Structure		Observation	Synonym or *Related Term*	Ver. 1 Code No.	Definition	Note	Photo No.
Vertebra 椎骨	**Lumbar centrum** 腰椎体	Absent　欠損	*'N' only, Reduced number* N個のみ、数の減少	10707		GC 4	
		Dumbbell-shaped　ダンベル状		10710			
		Fused　癒合	*Cartilaginous fusion* 軟骨性癒合	10711			**10-6**
		Hemicentric　半椎体		10713			
		Large　大型(化)		New			
		Malpositioned　位置異常		New		GC 12	
		Misaligned　配列異常		10715			**10-7**
		Misshapen　形態異常	*Asymmetric* 非対称	10716		GC 12	
		Small　小型(化)		New			
		Split　分離		10717			
		Supernumerary　過剰	*Increased number, 'N'* 数の増加、「N」	10718		GC 6	
		Supernumerary site　過剰部位		New			
		Asymmetric ossification 非対称骨化		New	Alizarin red stain uptake greater in one hemicenter than the other 一方の椎体のアリザリンレッド染色性が他方よりも強い		
		Bipartite ossification　二分骨化		10708			**10-8**
		Dumbbell ossification ダンベル状骨化		10709			
		Incomplete ossification 不完全骨化		10714			
		Increased ossification 骨化亢進		New			
		Isolated ossification site 分離骨化部位		New			
		Misshapen ossification site 骨化部位形態異常		New		GC 12	
		Unilateral ossification 片側(性)骨化		New			
		Unossified　未骨化		10720			
Vertebra 椎骨	**Lumbar vertebra** 腰椎	Absent　欠損	*'N' only, Reduced number* N個のみ、数の減少	10721		GC 4	**10-9**

Table 1　List of Skeletal Anomalies

Region / Organ / Structure	Observation		Synonym or *Related Term*	Ver. 1 Code No.	Definition	Note	Photo No.
		Hemivertebra　半椎		10722		GC 7	**10-10**
		Malpositioned　位置異常		10723		GC 12	
		Misaligned　配列異常		New			
		Small　小型(化)		New			
		Supernumerary　過剰	*Increased number, 'N'*　数の増加、「N」	10724		GC 6	**10-11**
		Supernumerary hemivertebra　過剰半椎		New			
Vertebra　椎骨	**Sacral arch** (processes [e.g., neural spine, transverse processes, articular processes] may be described separately)　仙椎弓(突起 [例えば神経棘、横突起、関節突起] は区別して記述する場合がある)	Absent　欠損	*'N' only, Reduced number*　N個のみ、数の減少	10725		GC 4	
		Bent　弯曲		New			
		Branched　分岐		New			
		Fused　癒合	*Cartilaginous fusion*　軟骨性癒合	10726			**11-1**
		Incompletely fused dorsal　背側不完全癒合		New		GC 33	
		Large　大型(化)		New			
		Malpositioned　位置異常		10728		GC 12	
		Misaligned　配列異常		10729			
		Misshapen　形態異常	*Long, Short*　長大(化)、短小(化)	10730		GC 12	**11-2**
		Not fused　未癒合		New		GC 36	**11-3**
		Not fused dorsal　背側未癒合		New		GC 33	
		Small　小型(化)		10731			
		Splayed　放散		New	Paired structures diverge from one another　対となる構造物（椎弓）が開放している（離れる）	GC 34	
		Split　分離	*Interrupted*　不連続	New			
		Supernumerary　過剰	*Increased number, 'N'*　数の増加、「N」	10732		GC 6	
		Supernumerary site　過剰部位		New			
		Thick　肥厚(化)	*Wide*　拡張(化)	New			
		Thin　菲薄(化)	*Narrow*　狭窄(化)	New			

Table 1   List of Skeletal Anomalies

Region / Organ / Structure		Observation	Synonym or *Related Term*	Ver. 1 Code No.	Definition	Note	Photo No.
		Incomplete ossification 不完全骨化	*Discontinuous ossification, Interrupted ossification* 不連続骨化	10727			
		Increased ossification 骨化亢進		New		GC 35	
		Isolated ossification site 分離骨化部位		New			
		Unossified　未骨化		10733			
Vertebra 椎骨	**Sacral centrum** 仙椎体	Absent　欠損	'*N*' *only, Reduced number* N個のみ、数の減少	10734		GC 4	
		Dumbbell-shaped　ダンベル状		10737			
		Fused　癒合	*Cartilaginous fusion* 軟骨性癒合	10738			
		Hemicentric　半椎体		10740			
		Large　大型(化)		New			
		Malpositioned　位置異常		New		GC 12	
		Misaligned　配列異常		10742			
		Misshapen　形態異常	*Asymmetric*　非対称	10743		GC 12	
		Small　小型(化)		New			
		Split　分離		10744			
		Supernumerary　過剰	*Increased number*, '*N*' 数の増加、「N」	10745		GC 6	
		Supernumerary site　過剰部位		New			
		Asymmetric ossification 非対称骨化		New	Alizarin red stain uptake greater in one hemicenter than the other 一方の椎体のアリザリンレッド染色性が他方よりも強い		
		Bipartite ossification　二分骨化		10735			
		Dumbbell ossification ダンベル状骨化		10736			
		Incomplete ossification 不完全骨化		10741			
		Increased ossification 骨化亢進		New			
		Isolated ossification site 分離骨化部位		New			

Table 1   List of Skeletal Anomalies

Region / Organ / Structure		Observation	Synonym or *Related Term*	Ver. 1 Code No.	Definition	Note	Photo No.
		Misshapen ossification site 骨化部位形態異常		New		GC 12	
		Unilateral ossification 片側(性)骨化		New			
		Unossified 未骨化		10747			
Vertebra 椎骨	**Sacral vertebra** 仙椎	Absent 欠損	*'N' only, Reduced number* N個のみ、数の減少	10748		GC 4	**11-4**
		Hemivertebra 半椎		10750		GC 7	
		Malpositioned 位置異常		10749		GC 12	
		Misaligned 配列異常		New			
		Small 小型(化)		New			
		Supernumerary 過剰	*Increased number, 'N'* 数の増加、「N」	10751		GC 6	
		Supernumerary hemivertebra 過剰半椎		New			
Vertebra 椎骨	**Caudal arch** (processes [e.g., neural spine] may be described separately) 尾椎弓(突起 [例えば神経棘] は区別して記述する場合がある)	Absent 欠損	*Fewer than 'N', Reduced number* N個より少ない、数の減少	10752			
		Bent 弯曲		New			
		Branched 分岐		New			
		Fused 癒合	*Cartilaginous fusion* 軟骨性癒合	10753			
		Incompletely fused dorsal 背側不完全癒合		New		GC 33	
		Large 大型(化)		New			
		Malpositioned 位置異常		10755		GC 12	
		Misaligned 配列異常		10756			
		Misshapen 形態異常	*Long, Short* 長大(化)、短小(化)	10757		GC 12	
		Not fused dorsal 背側未癒合		New		GC 33	
		Small 小型(化)		10758			
		Splayed 放散		New	Paired structures diverge from one another 対となる構造物（椎弓）が開放している（離れる）	GC 34	

Table 1 List of Skeletal Anomalies

Region / Organ / Structure		Observation	Synonym or *Related Term*	Ver. 1 Code No.	Definition	Note	Photo No.
		Split　分離	*Interrupted*　不連続	New			
		Supernumerary　過剰	*Increased number, More than 'N'*　数の増加、N個より多い	New			
		Supernumerary site　過剰部位		New			
		Thick　肥厚(化)	*Wide*　拡張(化)	New			
		Thin　菲薄(化)	*Narrow*　狭窄(化)	New			
		Incomplete ossification 不完全骨化	*Discontinuous ossification, Interrupted ossification*　不連続骨化	10754			
		Increased ossification 骨化亢進		New			
		Isolated ossification site 分離骨化部位		New			
		Unossified　未骨化		10759			
Vertebra 椎骨	**Caudal centrum** 尾椎体	Absent　欠損	*Fewer than 'N', Reduced number*　N個より少ない、数の減少	10760			
		Fused　癒合	*Cartilaginous fusion*　軟骨性癒合	10763			**11-5**
		Hemicentric　半椎体		10764			
		Large　大型(化)		New			
		Malpositioned　位置異常		New		GC 12	
		Misaligned　配列異常		10766			**11-6**
		Misshapen　形態異常	*Asymmetric*　非対称	10767		GC 12	
		Small　小型(化)		New			
		Split　分離		New			
		Supernumerary　過剰	*Increased number, More than 'N'*　数の増加、N個より多い	New			
		Supernumerary site　過剰部位		New			

Table 1　List of Skeletal Anomalies

Region / Organ / Structure		Observation	Synonym or *Related Term*	Ver. 1 Code No.	Definition	Note	Photo No.
		Asymmetric ossification 非対称骨化		New	Alizarin red stain uptake greater in one hemicenter than the other 一方の椎体のアリザリンレッド染色性が他方よりも強い		
		Bipartite ossification　　二分骨化		10761			
		Dumbbell ossification ダンベル状骨化		10762			
		Incomplete ossification 不完全骨化		10765			**11-7**
		Increased ossification 骨化亢進		New			
		Isolated ossification site 分離骨化部位		New			
		Misshapen ossification site 骨化部位形態異常		New		GC 12	
		Unilateral ossification 片側(性)骨化		New			
		Unossified 未骨化		10768			**11-8**
Vertebra 椎骨	Caudal vertebra 尾椎	Absent　　欠損	*Fewer than 'N', Reduced number* *N個より少ない、数の減少*	10769			**11-9**
		Hemivertebra　　半椎		10770		GC 7	**11-10**
		Malpositioned　　位置異常		New		GC 12	
		Misaligned　　配列異常		New			**11-11**
		Small　　小型(化)		New			
		Supernumerary　　過剰	*Increased number, More than 'N'* *数の増加、N個より多い*	10772			
		Supernumerary hemivertebra 過剰半椎		New			

Table 1 List of Skeletal Anomalies

Region / Organ / Structure		Observation	Synonym or *Related Term*	Ver. 1 Code No.	Definition	Note	Photo No.
Pelvic girdle 後肢帯	**Pelvic girdle** 後肢帯	Malpositioned caudal bilateral 両側(性)尾方位置異常	Caudal shift bilateral, Displaced articulation bilateral [caudal], Misaligned caudal bilateral, *Supernumerary prepelvic vertebra(e)/vertebral arches, Supernumerary presacral vertebra(e)/vertebral arches* 両側(性)尾方移動、両側(性)関節偏位[尾方]、両側(性)尾方配列異常、*骨盤前椎骨/椎弓過剰、仙椎前椎骨/椎弓過剰*	New		GC 37	
		Malpositioned cranial bilateral 両側(性)頭方位置異常	Cranial shift bilateral, Displaced articulation bilateral [cranial], Misaligned cranial bilateral, *Reduced number of prepelvic vertebra(e)/vertebral arches, Reduced number of presacral vertebra(e)/vertebral arches* 両側(性)頭方移動、両側(性)関節偏位[頭方]、両側(性)頭方配列異常、*骨盤前椎骨/椎弓減少、仙椎前椎骨/椎弓減少*	New		GC 37	**12-1**

Table 1 List of Skeletal Anomalies

Region / Organ / Structure		Observation	Synonym or *Related Term*	Ver. 1 Code No.	Definition	Note	Photo No.
		Malpositioned caudal unilateral 片側(性)尾方位置異常	Caudal shift unilateral, Displaced articulation unilateral [caudal], Misaligned caudal unilateral, *Supernumerary prepelvic vertebral arches*, *Supernumerary presacral vertebral arches* 片側(性)尾方移動、片側(性)関節偏位[尾方]、片側(性)尾方配列異常、*骨盤前椎弓過剰、仙椎前椎弓過剰*	New		GC 37	**12-2**
		Malpositioned cranial unilateral 片側(性)頭方位置異常	Cranial shift unilateral, Displaced articulation unilateral [cranial], Misaligned cranial unilateral, *Reduced number of prepelvic vertebral arches, Reduced number of presacral vertebral arches* 片側(性)頭方移動、片側(性)関節偏位[頭方]、片側(性)頭方配列異常、*骨盤前椎弓減少、仙椎前椎弓減少*	New		GC 37	
Pelvic girdle 後肢帯	**Ilium** 腸骨	Absent 欠損		10773			
		Bent 弯曲		10774			
		Fused 癒合	*Cartilaginous fusion* *軟骨性癒合*	10775			
		Large 大型(化)		New			
		Malpositioned 位置異常		10777		GC 12 GC 38	
		Misaligned 配列異常		New		GC 38	
		Misshapen 形態異常	*Long, Short* *長大(化)、短小(化)*	10778		GC 12	
		Small 小型(化)		10779			
		Supernumerary 過剰		New			
		Supernumerary site 過剰部位		New			

Table 1 List of Skeletal Anomalies

Region / Organ / Structure	Observation		Synonym or *Related Term*	Ver. 1 Code No.	Definition	Note	Photo No.
		Thick　肥厚(化)		10780			
		Thin　菲薄(化)		New			
		Incomplete ossification 不完全骨化		10776			
		Increased ossification 骨化亢進		New			
		Isolated　ossification site 分離骨化部位		New			
		Unossified　未骨化		10781			
Pelvic girdle 後肢帯	**Ischium** (Ischial arch may be described separately) 坐骨(坐骨弓は区別して記述する場合がある)	Absent　欠損		10782			
		Bent　弯曲		10783			
		Fused　癒合	*Cartilaginous fusion 軟骨性癒合*	10784			
		Large　大型(化)		New			
		Malpositioned　位置異常		10786		GC 12 GC 38	
		Misaligned　配列異常		New		GC 38	
		Misshapen　形態異常	*Long, Short 長大(化)、短小(化)*	10787		GC 12	
		Small　小型(化)		10788			
		Supernumerary　過剰		New			
		Supernumerary site　過剰部位		New			
		Thick　肥厚(化)		10789			
		Thin　菲薄(化)		New			
		Incomplete ossification 不完全骨化		10785			
		Increased ossification 骨化亢進		New			
		Isolated　ossification site 分離骨化部位		New			
		Unossified　未骨化		10790			
Pelvic girdle 後肢帯	**Pubis** (Pubic symphysis may be described separately) 恥骨(恥骨結合は	Absent　欠損		10791			
		Bent　弯曲		10792			
		Fused　癒合	*Cartilaginous fusion 軟骨性癒合*	New			
		Large　大型(化)		New			

Table 1 List of Skeletal Anomalies

Region / Organ / Structure		Observation	Synonym or *Related Term*	Ver. 1 Code No.	Definition	Note	Photo No.
	区別して記述する場合がある)	Malpositioned 位置異常		10794		GC 12 GC 38	
		Misaligned 配列異常		10795		GC 38	
		Misshapen 形態異常	*Long, Short* *長大(化)、短小(化)*	10796		GC 12	
		Small 小型(化)		10797			
		Supernumerary 過剰		New			
		Supernumerary site 過剰部位		New			
		Thick 肥厚(化)		10798			
		Thin 菲薄(化)		New			
		Incomplete ossification 不完全骨化		10793			
		Increased ossification 骨化亢進		New			
		Isolated ossification site 分離骨化部位		New			
		Unossified 未骨化		10799			
Hindlimb 後肢	**Femur** (proximal and distal epiphyses may be described separately) 大腿骨(近位および遠位端は区別して記述する場合がある)	Absent 欠損		10800			
		Bent 弯曲		10801			**4-1**
		Fused 癒合	*Cartilaginous fusion* *軟骨性癒合*	10802			
		Long 長大(化)		New			
		Malpositioned 位置異常		10804		GC 12	
		Misshapen 形態異常		10805		GC 12	**4-2**
		Short 短小(化)		10806			**4-3**
		Supernumerary 過剰		New			
		Supernumerary site 過剰部位		New			
		Thick 肥厚(化)		10807		GC 3	
		Thin 菲薄(化)		New		GC 3	
		Distal ossification site 遠位端骨化部位	Epiphyseal ossification site 骨端骨化部位	New	Ossification site(s) in the cartilaginous distal region of the bone 大腿骨の遠位端軟骨部における骨化部位		
		Incomplete ossification 不完全骨化		10803			

Table 1　List of Skeletal Anomalies

Region / Organ / Structure		Observation	Synonym or *Related Term*	Ver. 1 Code No.	Definition	Note	Photo No.
		Increased ossification 骨化亢進		New			
		Isolated ossification site 分離骨化部位		New		GC 15	
		Proximal ossification site 近位端骨化部位	Epiphyseal ossification site 骨端骨化部位	New	Ossification site(s) in the cartilaginous proximal region of the bone 大腿骨の近位端軟骨部における骨化部位		
		Unossified 未骨化		10808			
Hindlimb 後肢	**Patella** 膝蓋骨	Absent 欠損		New			
		Large 大型(化)		New			
		Malpositioned 位置異常		New		GC 12	
		Misshapen 形態異常		New		GC 12	
		Small 小型(化)		New			
		Supernumerary 過剰		New			
Hindlimb 後肢	**Fibula** (proximal and distal epiphyses may be described separately) 腓骨(近位および遠位端は区別して記述する場合がある) 「訳者注：ウサギは胎児期に癒合しているが、ラット、マウスは生後発育に伴って癒合する」	Absent 欠損		10809			
		Bent 弯曲		10810			**4-4**
		Fused 癒合	*Cartilaginous fusion* 軟骨性癒合	10811			
		Long 長大(化)		New			
		Malpositioned 位置異常		10813		GC 12	
		Misshapen 形態異常		10814		GC 12	
		Not fused to tibia 脛骨との未癒合		New		GC 39	
		Short 短小(化)		10815			**4-5**
		Supernumerary 過剰		New			
		Supernumerary site 過剰部位		New			
		Thick 肥厚(化)		10816		GC 3	
		Thin 菲薄(化)		New		GC 3	
		Distal ossification site 遠位端骨化部位	Epiphyseal ossification site 骨端骨化部位	New	Ossification site(s) in the cartilaginous distal region of the bone 腓骨の遠位端軟骨部における骨化部位		
		Incomplete ossification 不完全骨化		10812			

Table 1 List of Skeletal Anomalies

Region / Organ / Structure	Observation		Synonym or *Related Term*	Ver. 1 Code No.	Definition	Note	Photo No.
		Increased ossification 骨化亢進		New			
		Isolated ossification site 分離骨化部位		New		GC 15	
		Proximal ossification site 近位端骨化部位	Epiphyseal ossification site 骨端骨化部位	New	Ossification site(s) in the cartilaginous proximal region of the bone 腓骨の近位端軟骨部における骨化部位		
		Unossified　　未骨化		10817			
Hindlimb 後肢	**Tibia** (proximal and distal epiphyses may be described separately) 脛骨(近位および遠位端は区別して記載する場合がある) 「訳者注：ウサギは胎児期に腓骨と癒合しているが、ラット、マウスは生後発育に伴って癒合する」	Absent　　欠損	Tibial hemimelia 脛骨半肢	10818			**4-6**
		Bent　　弯曲		10819			
		Fused　　癒合	*Cartilaginous fusion* 軟骨性癒合	10820			
		Lack of fusion to fibula 腓骨との未癒合		New		GC 40	
		Long　　長大(化)		New			
		Malpositioned　　位置異常		10822		GC 12	
		Misshapen　　形態異常		10823		GC 12	**4-7**
		Short　　短小(化)		10824			**4-8**
		Supernumerary　　過剰		New			
		Supernumerary site　　過剰部位		New			
		Thick　　肥厚(化)		10825		GC 3	**4-9**
		Thin　　菲薄(化)		New		GC 3	
		Distal ossification site 遠位端骨化部位	Epiphyseal ossification site 骨端骨化部位	New	Ossification site(s) in the cartilaginous distal region of the bone 脛骨の遠位端軟骨部における骨化部位		
		Incomplete ossification 不完全骨化		10821			
		Increased ossification 骨化亢進		New			
		Isolated ossification site 分離骨化部位		New		GC 15	

Table 1　List of Skeletal Anomalies

Region / Organ / Structure		Observation	Synonym or *Related Term*	Ver. 1 Code No.	Definition	Note	Photo No.
		Proximal ossification site 近位端骨化部位	Epiphyseal ossification site 骨端骨化部位	New	Ossification site(s) in the cartilaginous proximal region of the bone 脛骨の近位端軟骨部における骨化部位		
		Unossified　未骨化		10826			
Hindlimb 後肢	**Calcaneus** 踵骨	Absent　欠損		10827			
		Bent　弯曲		New			
		Fused　癒合	*Cartilaginous fusion* 軟骨性癒合	10828			
		Large　大型(化)	*Long, Thick* 長大(化)、肥厚(化)	New			
		Malpositioned　位置異常		10830		GC 12	
		Misshapen　形態異常		10831		GC 12	
		Small　小型(化)	*Short, Thin* 短小(化)、菲薄(化)	10832			
		Supernumerary　過剰		10833			
		Supernumerary site　過剰部位		New			
		Incomplete ossification 不完全骨化		10829			
		Increased ossification 骨化亢進		New			
		Isolated ossification site 分離骨化部位		New			
		Unossified　未骨化		10834			
Hindlimb 後肢	**Talus** 距骨	Absent　欠損		10835			
		Bent　弯曲		New			
		Fused　癒合	*Cartilaginous fusion* 軟骨性癒合	10836			
		Large　大型(化)	*Long, Thick* 長大(化)、肥厚(化)	New			
		Malpositioned　位置異常		10838		GC 12	
		Misshapen　形態異常		10839		GC 12	
		Small　小型(化)	*Short, Thin* 短小(化)、菲薄(化)	10840			
		Supernumerary　過剰		New			
		Supernumerary site　過剰部位		New			

Table 1   List of Skeletal Anomalies

Region / Organ / Structure	Observation		Synonym or *Related Term*	Ver. 1 Code No.	Definition	Note	Photo No.
		Isolated ossification site 分離骨化部位		New			
		Unossified 未骨化		10842			
Hindlimb 後肢	**Tarsal bone** (for purpose of this table, excludes calcaneus and talus) 足根骨(踵骨と距骨を含まない)「訳者注：足根骨は、立方骨、中間楔状骨、外側楔状骨、内側楔状骨、舟状骨、脛側足根骨(マウス、ラットのみ)で構成される」	Absent 欠損		10843			
		Bent 弯曲		New			
		Fused 癒合	*Cartilaginous fusion* 軟骨性癒合	10844			
		Large 大型(化)	*Long, Thick* 長大(化)、肥厚(化)	New			
		Malpositioned 位置異常		10846		GC 12	
		Misshapen 形態異常		10847		GC 12	
		Small 小型(化)	*Short, Thin* 短小(化)、菲薄(化)	10848			
		Supernumerary 過剰		10849			
		Incomplete ossification 不完全骨化		10845			
		Increased ossification 骨化亢進		New			
		Unossified 未骨化		10851			
Hindlimb 後肢	**Metatarsal** 中足骨	Absent 欠損		10852			
		Bent 弯曲		New			
		Fused 癒合	*Cartilaginous fusion* 軟骨性癒合	10853			
		Large 大型(化)		New			
		Long 長大(化)		New			
		Malpositioned 位置異常		10855		GC 12	
		Misshapen 形態異常		10856		GC 12	
		Short 短小(化)		New			
		Small 小型(化)		10857			
		Supernumerary 過剰		10858			
		Supernumerary site 過剰部位		New			
		Thick 肥厚(化)		New			
		Thin 菲薄(化)		New			
		Incomplete ossification 不完全骨化		10854			

Table 1 List of Skeletal Anomalies

Region / Organ / Structure		Observation	Synonym or *Related Term*	Ver. 1 Code No.	Definition	Note	Photo No.
		Increased ossification 骨化亢進		New			
		Isolated ossification site 分離骨化部位		New			
		Unossified 未骨化		10859			
Hindlimb 後肢	**Hindpaw phalanx** 趾節骨	Absent 欠損	*Aphalangia* 無趾	10860			**5-4**
		Bent 弯曲		New			
		Fused 癒合	*Cartilaginous fusion* 軟骨性癒合	10861			
		Large 大型(化)		New			
		Long 長大(化)		New			
		Malpositioned 位置異常		10863		GC 12	
		Misshapen 形態異常		10864		GC 12	
		Short 短小(化)		New			
		Small 小型(化)		10865			
		Supernumerary 過剰		10866			**5-5**
		Supernumerary site 過剰部位		New			
		Thick 肥厚(化)		10867			
		Thin 菲薄(化)		New			
		Incomplete ossification 不完全骨化		10862			
		Increased ossification 骨化亢進		New			
		Isolated ossification site 分離骨化部位		New			
		Unossified 未骨化		10868			

General Comments of Skeletal Anomalies

1. Hole in the skull　頭蓋骨における孔

    This finding should not be confused with "Unossified area".

    本所見については、「未骨化領域」と混同しない様に注意して観察する必要がある。

2. Split in the skull　頭蓋骨における分離

    This finding should not be confused with "Unossified line".

    本所見については、「線状未骨化」と混同しない様に注意して観察する必要がある。

3. Thick and Thin　肥厚及び菲薄

    Because these findings may be generalized or localized, their details are recommended to be recorded.

    本所見については、変化が全体に及ぶ場合と局所的な場合があるので、詳細を記録することが望まれる。

4. Absent in ribs, vertebrae, or sternebrae　肋骨、椎骨、あるいは、胸骨分節の欠損

    "*Reduced number*" is proposed as a related term of "Absent" in rib, vertebra, cervical vertebral arch, cervical vertebral body, cervical vertebra, thoracic vertebral arch, thoracic vertebral body, thoracic vertebra, lumbar vertebral arch, lumbar vertebral body, lumbar vertebra, sacral vertebral arch, sacral vertebral body, and sacral vertebra. This related term, "*Reduced number*" is recommended only when complexity of abnormality precludes use of normal numbering system　Where possible, total number of ribs or vertebrae present should be specified.

    Absent sternebra may be associated with reduced number of thoracic vertebra, ribs, and/or fewer costal cartilage(s) that fuse with the sternum.

    本アトラスでは、「欠損」の*関連用語*として「*数の減少*」と言う所見が、肋骨及び椎骨（椎骨、頸椎弓、頸椎体、頸椎、胸椎弓、胸椎体、胸椎、腰椎弓、腰椎体、腰椎、仙椎弓、仙椎体、仙椎）に記載されている。*関連用語*である「*数の減少*」は異常が複雑で正常な番号付けができない場合にのみ推奨される。可能であれば、肋骨総数あるいはそれぞれの椎骨（椎弓、椎体）数を特定することが望まれる。

胸骨分節の欠損は、胸椎数、肋骨数の減少および/あるいは胸骨に接続した肋軟骨数の減少を伴う場合がある。

5. Supernumerary articulated ribs　肋骨過剰

This anomaly is usually associated with supernumerary thoracic vertebra(e)/ hemivertebra(e), vertebral arch(es).　Should not be confused with supernumerary ribs found at the cervicothoracic or thoracolumbar borders (see separate Supernumerary Rib section below).

Related terms, "*Increased number*", is recommended only when complexity of abnormality precludes use of normal numbering system.

本所見は、通常、過剰な胸椎/半椎/椎弓を伴う。頸胸部あるいは胸腰部の境界にある過剰肋骨と混同しない様に注意して観察する（下記の過剰肋骨の項目を参照）。関連用語である「*数の増加*」は、異常が複雑で正常な番号付けができない場合にのみ推奨される。

6. Supernumerary in vertebrae

"*Increased number*" is proposed as a related term of "Supernumerary" in vertebra, cervical vertebral arch, cervical vertebral body, cervical vertebra, thoracic vertebral arch, thoracic vertebral body, thoracic vertebra, lumbar vertebral arch, lumbar vertebral body, lumbar vertebra, sacral vertebral arch, sacral vertebral body, and sacral vertebra. This related term, "*Increased number*" is recommended only when complexity of abnormality precludes use of normal numbering system　Where possible, total number of vertebrae present should be specified.

本アトラスでは、「過剰」の*関連用語*として「*数の増加*」と言う所見が、椎骨（椎骨、頸椎弓、頸椎体、頸椎、胸椎弓、胸椎体、胸椎、腰椎弓、腰椎体、腰椎、仙椎弓、仙椎体、仙椎）に記載されている。*関連用語*である「*数の増加*」は異常が複雑で正常な番号付けができない場合にのみ推奨される。可能であれば、それぞれの椎骨（椎弓、椎体）数を特定することが望まれる。

7. Hemivertebra　半椎

"Absent arch" and "Hemicentrum" may be recorded separately.

椎弓欠損と半椎体は、区別して記述する場合がある。

8. Full cervical supernumerary rib　頸部完全過剰肋骨

This anomaly is usually associated with the last cervical vertebra. If location is elsewhere or more than one supernumerary rib is present, details should be specified. Presence of costal cartilage may be described separately.

本所見は、通常、頸椎最後部に付属する。他の位置にある場合や 2 つ以上の過剰肋骨が存在する場合には、詳細を特定することが望まれる。肋軟骨が存在する場合は、区別して記述する場合がある。

9. Short cervical supernumerary rib　頸部短小過剰肋骨

This anomaly is usually associated with the last cervical vertebra. If location is elsewhere or more than one supernumerary rib is present, details should be specified.

本所見は、通常、頸椎最後部に付属する。他の位置にある場合や 2 つ以上の過剰肋骨が存在する場合には、詳細を特定することが望まれる。

10. Full thoracolumbar supernumerary rib　胸腰部完全過剰肋骨

This anomaly is usually associated with the first lumbar vertebra or supernumerary thoracic vertebra. If location is not at thoracolumbar border or more than one supernumerary rib is present, details should be specified. Presence of costal cartilage may be described separately.

本所見は、通常、第 1 腰椎あるいは過剰胸椎に付属する場合が多い。胸腰部境界以外の位置にある場合や 2 つ以上の過剰肋骨が存在する場合には、詳細を特定することが望まれる。肋軟骨が存在する場合は、区別して記述する場合がある。

11. Short thoracolumbar supernumerary rib　胸腰部短小過剰肋骨

This anomaly is usually associated with the first lumbar vertebra. If location is elsewhere or more than one supernumerary rib is present, details should be specified.

本所見は、通常、第 1 腰椎に付属する。他の位置にある場合や 2 つ以上の過剰肋骨が存在する場合には、詳細を特定することが望ましい。

12. "Malpositioned" and "Misshapen"　「位置異常」と「形態異常」

In these findings, its position or shape (as a figure if possible) is recommended to be recorded.

これら所見では、必要に応じて位置あるいは形態（可能であれば図として）を記録しておくことが推奨される。

13. Fused zygomatic arch　頬骨弓癒合

Position of fusion should be specified (e.g., between maxillary process and zygomatic or between squamosal process and zygomatic).

癒合部位を特定する(例えば、上顎骨の頬骨突起と頬骨、あるいは側頭骨の頬骨突起と頬骨)。

14. Fused sternebra　胸骨分節癒合

Gradation(s) of severity may be described. In the case of severe fusion, involving reduction of the interval between affected sternebrae (and hence, potentially, permanent shortening of the sternum), a severity grading is recommended.

重篤度の程度を記述する場合がある。影響のみられた胸骨分節の間隔の縮小(従って、永続的な胸骨の短小の可能性がある)を含む重度な癒合の場合は、重篤度のグレード分けをすることが推奨される。

15. Isolated ossification site in fore- and hind-limb　前肢及び後肢における分離骨化部位

See also "Proximal ossification site" and "Distal ossification site" in each long bone.

各長骨の近位端骨化部位および遠位端骨化部位を参照すること。

16. Branched sternebra　胸骨分節分岐

Branched sternebra is usually applicable to sternebra 1 and/or 6.

通常、第1及び/あるいは第6胸骨分節で見られる。

17. Long sternebra　　胸骨分節長大（化）

This finding should not be confused with "Increased ossification of sternebra". Interval between costal cartilages should be increased.

胸骨分節の骨化亢進と混同しないこと。肋軟骨の間隔が開大している。

18. Misaligned sternebra　　胸骨分節配列異常

This finding should not be confused with "Misaligned ossification sites".

骨化部位配列異常と混同しないこと。

19. Short sternebra, or Small sternebra　　胸骨分節短小（化）あるいは小型（化）

This finding should not be confused with "Incomplete ossification of sternebra". Interval between costal cartilages should be decreased.

胸骨分節の不完全骨化と混同しないこと。肋軟骨の間隔が狭小している。

20. Supernumerary sternebrae　　胸骨分節過剰

This finding may be associated with "Increased number of thoracic vertebrae and/or ribs". This finding is usually associated with additional vertebrosternal costal cartilage(s).

胸椎数および/あるいは肋骨数の増加を伴う場合がある。通常、過剰な肋軟骨の胸骨接続を伴う。

21. Supernumerary site, Increased ossification and Isolated ossification site of the sternebra　　胸骨分節過剰部位、骨化亢進及び分離骨化部位

See also: Sternum – Supernumerary ossification site.

胸骨の過剰骨化部位を参照。

22. Split intersternebral cartilage　　胸骨分節間軟骨分離

Location of split (in relation to sternebral positions) should be specified.

分離の位置(胸骨分節の位置との関連)を特定すること。

23. Supernumerary ossification site of the sternum　　胸骨過剰骨化部位

    Usually refers to advanced ossification between sternebral centers.
    通常、胸骨分節間の骨化を記述する際に用いる。

24. Interrupted rib　　肋骨不連続

    This finding should not be confused with "Interrupted ossification of ribs".
    肋骨不連続骨化と混同しないこと。

25. Long rib　　肋骨長大（化）

    This finding should not be confused with "Increased ossification of rib".
    肋骨の骨化亢進と混同しないこと。

26. Short rib　　肋骨短小（化）

    This finding should not be confused with "Incomplete ossification of rib".
    肋骨の不完全骨化と混同しないこと。

27. Wavy rib　　波状肋骨

    This finding may be transient in rats.
    ラットでは一過性の変化の場合がある。

28. Costal cartilage fused to sternum　　肋軟骨胸骨接続
    Applies to cervical ribs and 'false' ribs only.
    頸肋および仮肋にのみ適用。

29. Costal cartilage not fused to sternum　　肋軟骨胸骨不連続
    Applies to 'true' ribs only.
    真肋にのみ適用。

30. Short costal cartilage　　肋軟骨短小（化）
    Applies to 'true' ribs and 'false' ribs only.
    真肋および仮肋にのみ適用。

31. Cartilagious cervical supernumerary rib and Cartilagious thoracolumbar supernumerary rib　　軟骨性頸部過剰肋骨及び軟骨性胸腰部過剰肋骨
    Length (e.g., 'full' or 'short') may be specified.
    長さ（例えば、完全または短小）を同定する場合がある。

32. Absent vertebral canal　　脊柱管欠損
    Most likely to be used when describing the entire vertebral column.
    脊柱全体について記述する場合に用いられることが多い。

33. Incompletely fused dorsal and Not fused dorsal　　背側不完全癒合及び背側未癒合
    Refers to cartilaginous dorsal fusion of arches, around vertebral canal.
    脊柱管をとりまく椎弓の背部軟骨癒合を記述する際に用いる。

34. Splayed   放散

   See also "Not fused dorsal".
   背側未癒合を参照。

35. Increased ossification   骨化亢進

   Specific vertebral processes may be specified.
   特定の突起を同定する場合がある。

36. Not fused sacral arch   仙椎弓未癒合

   Refers to lateral fusion of adjacent arches to form sacrum.   In rat, mouse, and rabbit fetuses fusions are normally cartilaginous.
   仙骨を形成する隣接した椎弓の外側癒合について記述する際に用いる。ラット、マウスおよびウサギ胎児において、正常では軟骨は癒合している。

37. Malpositioned caudal bilateral (unilateral), Malpositioned cranial bilateral (unilateral) of the pelvic girdle
      後肢帯の両側性（片側性）尾方位置異常、及び、両側性（片側性）頭方位置異常

   Number (and laterality) of prepelvic vertebrae can be specified. This includes complete girdle (ilium, ischium and pubis).
   骨盤前椎骨数（及び側性）を特定する。肢帯全体(腸骨、坐骨および恥骨)を含む。

38. Malpositioned and Misaligned in the pelvic girdle   後肢帯における位置異常及配列異常

   See other pelvic girdle observations.
   他の後肢帯の所見を参照。

39. Not fused to tibia　　脛骨との未癒合
    Normal in rat and mouse.
    ラット及びマウスでは正常。

40. Lack of fusion to fibula　　腓骨との未癒合
    Rabbit only.
    ウサギのみ。

Table 2 Comparative List of This Atlas Findings, Mouse Phenotype, and Human Phenotype

Photo No.	Atlas Term	MP No.	MP Term	HP No.	HP Term
1-1	Fused basioccipital bone 底後頭骨癒合	0000079	Abnormal basioccipital bone morphology	0012294	Abnormality of the occipital bone
1-2	Misshapen basisphenoid bone 底蝶形骨形態	0000106	Abnormal basisphenoid bone morphology	0002693	Abnormality of the skull base
1-3	Fused exoccipital bone 外後頭骨癒合	0010728	Fusion of atlas and occipital bones	0012294	Abnormality of the occipital bone
1-4	Fused frontal bone 前頭骨癒合	0000107	Abnormal frontal bone morphology	0430000	Abnormality of the frontal bone
		0000081	Premature suture closure	0001363	Craniosynostosis
1-5	Misshapen frontal bone 前頭骨形態異常	0000107	Abnormal frontal bone morphology	0430000	Abnormality of the frontal bone
		0000440	Domed cranium	0000242	Parietal bossing
1-6	Misshapen hyoid body 舌骨体形態異常	0009917	Abnormal hyoid bone body morphology		
1-7	Split hyoid body 舌骨体分離	0009917	Abnormal hyoid bone body morphology		
1-8	Fused mandible 下顎骨癒合	0000458	Abnormal mandible morphology	0000277	Abnormality of the mandible
1-9	Misshapen mandible 下顎骨形態異常	0000458	Abnormal mandible morphology	0000277	Abnormality of the mandible
		0004596	Abnormal mandibular angle morphology	0005446	Obtuse angle of mandible
1-10	Short mandible 下顎骨短小(化)	0000088	Short mandible	0000278	Retrognathia
1-11	Small mandible 下顎骨小型(化)	0004592	Small mandible	0000347	Micrognathia
1-12	Misshapen maxilla 上顎骨形態異常	0000455	Abnormal maxilla morphology	0000326	Abnormality of the maxilla
1-13	Small maxilla 上顎骨小型(化)	0004540	Small maxilla	0000327	Hypoplasia of the maxilla
1-14	Fused nasal bone 鼻骨癒合	0000102	Abnormal nasal bone morphology	0010939	Abnormality of the nasal bone
		0000081	Premature suture closure	0001363	Craniosynostosis
1-15	Misshapen nasal bones 鼻骨形態異常	0000102	Abnormal nasal bone morphology	0010939	Abnormality of the nasal bone
1-16	Small nasal bone 鼻骨小型(化)	0004470	Small nasal bone	0011430	Hypoplasia of fetal nasal bone
1-17	Hole in the parietal bone 頭頂骨孔	0000109	Abnormal parietal bone morphology	0002696	Abnormality of the parietal bone
				0002697	Parietal foramina
1-18	Misshapen parietal bone 頭頂骨形態異常	0000109	Abnormal parietal bone morphology	0002696	Abnormality of the parietal bone
				0000242	Parietal bossing
1-19	Split parietal bone 頭頂骨分離	0000109	Abnormal parietal bone morphology	0002696	Abnormality of the parietal bone
		0003843	Abnormal sagittal suture morphology	0012800	Accessory cranial suture
1-20	Unossified area in the parietal bone 頭頂骨未骨化領域	0003420	Delayed intramembranous bone	0012790	Abnormal intramembranous ossification
				0005474	Decreased calvarial ossification
1-21	Fused premaxilla 顎間骨(切歯骨)癒合	0002820	Abnormal premaxilla morphology	0010758	Abnormality of the premaxilla
1-22	Malpositioned premaxilla 顎間骨(切歯骨)位置異常	0002820	Abnormal premaxilla morphology	0010758	Abnormality of the premaxilla
1-23	Misshapen premaxilla 顎間骨(切歯骨)形態異常	0002820	Abnormal premaxilla morphology	0010758	Abnormality of the premaxilla
1-24	Small premaxilla 顎間骨(切歯骨)小型(化)	0004870	Small premaxilla	0010650	Premaxillary underdevelopment
1-25	Absent tympanic annulus 鼓室輪欠損	0003138	Absent tympanic ring	0009911	Abnormality of the temporal bone
1-26	Malpositioned tympanic annulus 鼓室輪位置	0000030	Abnormal tympanic ring morphology	0009911	Abnormality of the temporal bone

MP: Mouse phenotype
HP: Human phenotype
In some cases, MP and HP terms indicate a more general description for the Atlas term.

Table 2 Comparative List of This Atlas Findings, Mouse Phenotype, and Human Phenotype

Photo No.	Atlas Term	MP No.	MP Term	HP No.	HP Term
1-27	Fused zygomatic arch　頬骨弓癒合	0004469	Abnormal zygomatic arch morphology	0005557	Abnormality of the zygomatic arch
1-28	Misshapen zygomatic arch　頬骨弓形態異常	0004469	Abnormal zygomatic arch morphology	0005557	Abnormality of the zygomatic arch
1-29	Large fontanelle　泉門大型(化)	0000085	Large anterior fontanelle	0000239	Large fontanelles
1-30	Sutural bone　縫合骨			0002645	Wormian bones
2-1	Bent clavicle　鎖骨弯曲	0005298	Abnormal clavicle morphology	0000895	Hooked clavicles
2-2	Misshapen clavicle　鎖骨形態異常	0005298	Abnormal clavicle morphology	0000889	Abnormality of the clavicles
2-3	Thick clavicle　鎖骨肥厚(化)	0005298	Abnormal clavicle morphology	0006599	Medial widening of clavicles
2-4	Bent scapula　肩甲骨弯曲	0000149	Abnormal scapula morphology	0000782	Abnormality of the scapula
				0003691	Scapular winging
2-5	Misshapen scapula　肩甲骨形態異常	0000149	Abnormal scapula morphology	0000782	Abnormality of the scapula
2-6	Small scapula　肩甲骨小型(化)	0004343	Small scapula	0000882	Hypoplastic scapulae
3-1	Misshapen humerus　上腕骨形態異常	0004354	Absent deltoid tuberosity	0003889	Abnormality of the deltoid tuberosities
3-2	Short humerus　上腕骨短小(化)	0004351	Short humerus	0005792	Short humerus
3-3	Absent radius　橈骨欠損	0000553	Absent radius	0003974	Absent radius
3-4	Bent radius　橈骨弯曲	0004374	Bowed radius	0002986	Radial bowing
3-5	Msshapen radius　橈骨形態異常	0000552	Abnormal radius morphology	0045008	Abnormal shape of the radius
3-6	Short radius　橈骨短小(化)	0004355	Short radius	0002984	Hypoplasia of the radius
3-7	Absent ulna　尺骨欠損	0004360	Absent ulna	0003982	Absent ulna
3-8	Bent ulna　尺骨弯曲	0004361	Bowed ulna	0003031	Ulnar bowing
4-1	Bent femur　大腿骨弯曲	0004371	Bowed femur	0002980	Femoral bowing
4-2	Misshapen femur　大腿骨形態異常	0000559	Abnormal femur morphology	0002823	Abnormality of the femur
4-3	Short femur　大腿骨短小(化)	0003109	Short femur	0003097	Short femur
4-4	Bent fibula　腓骨弯曲	0004372	Bowed fibula	0010502	Fibular bowing
4-5	Short fibula　腓骨短小(化)	0002765	Short fibula	0003038	Ffibular hypoplasia
4-6	Absent tibia　脛骨欠損	0002728	Absent tibia	0009556	Absent tibia
4-7	Misshapen tibia　脛骨形態異常	0000558	Abnormal tibia morphology	0002992	Abnomality of the tibia
4-8	Short tibia　脛骨短小(化)	0002764	Short tibia	0005736	Short tibia
4-9	Thick tibia　脛骨肥厚(化)	0008162	Increased diameter of tibia	0002992	Abnomality of the tibia
5-1	Absent forepaw phalanx　指節骨欠損	0005306	Abnormal phalanx morphology	0009658	Aplasia/Hypoplasia of the phalanges of the
		0000565	Oligodactyly	0001180	Oligodactyly (hands)
5-2	Fused forepaw phalanx　指節骨癒合	0008730	Fused phalanges	0010492	Osseous finger syndactyly
		0000564	Syndactyly	0010709	2-4 finger syndactyly
5-3	Supernumerary forepaw phalanx　指節骨過剰	0000413	Polyphalangy	0009997	Duplication of phalanx of hand
		0000562	Polydactyly	0009948	Duplication of the distal phalanx of the 2nd
				0009942	Duplication of thumb phalanx
				0001161	Hand polydactyly

MP: Mouse phenotype
HP: Human phenotype
In some cases, MP and HP terms indicate a more general description for the Atlas term.

Table 2 Comparative List of This Atlas Findings, Mouse Phenotype, and Human Phenotype

Photo No.	Atlas Term	MP No.	MP Term	HP No.	HP Term
5-4	Absent hindpaw phalanx 趾節骨欠損	0005306 0000565	Abnormal phalanx morphology Oligodactyly	0001849	Oligodactyly (feet)
5-5	Supernumerary hindpaw phalanx 趾節骨過剰	0000413 0009743	Polyphalangy Preaxial polydactyly	0010181 0010100 0005873	Duplication of phalanx of toe Complete duplication of hallux phalanx Polydactyly of hallux
6-1	Fused sternebrae 胸骨分節癒合	0010082	Sternebra fusion	0006590	Premature sternal synostosis
6-2	Misaligned sternebrae 胸骨分節配列異常	0012285	Misaligned sternebrae	0000766	Abnormality of the sternum
6-3	Misshapen sternebrae 胸骨分節形態異常	0004322	Abnormal sternebra morphology	0000766	Abnormality of the sternum
6-4	Split sternebra 胸骨分節分離	0004320	Split sternum	0010309	Bifid sternum
6-5	Asymmetric ossification of sternebra 胸骨分節非対称骨化	0008277	Abnormal sternum ossification	0011863	Abnormal sternal ossification
6-6	Bipartite ossification of sternebra 胸骨分節二分骨化	0008277	Abnormal sternum ossification	0011863	Abnormal sternal ossification
6-7	Unilateral ossification of sternebra 胸骨分節片側性骨化	0008277	Abnormal sternum ossification	0011863	Abnormal sternal ossification
6-8	Split xiphoid cartilage 剣状軟骨分離	0004678	Split xiphoid process	0100891	Bifid xiphoid process
6-9	Misshapen sternum 胸骨形態異常				
6-10	Split sternum 胸骨分離	0004320	Split sternum	0010309	Bifid sternum
6-11	Supernumerary ossification site of sternum 胸骨過剰骨化部位	0008277	Abnormal sternum ossification	0011863	Abnormal sternal ossification
7-1	Absent rib 肋骨欠損	0003345	Decreased rib number	0000921	Missing ribs
7-2	Branched rib 肋骨分岐	0000153	Rib bifurcation	0000892	Bifid ribs
7-3	Detached rib 肋骨分離	0008149 0000152	Abnormal rib-vertebral column Absent proximal rib	0006593	Anomalous rib insertion to vertebrae
7-4	Fused rib 肋骨癒合	0000154	Rib fusion	0000902	Rib fusion
7-5	Intercostal rib 肋間肋骨	0000150	Abnormal rib morphology	0000772	Abnormality of the ribs
7-6	Interrupted rib 肋骨不連続	0000150	Abnormal rib morphology	0000772	Abnormality of the ribs
7-7	Misaligned ribs 肋骨配列異常	0004624	Abnormal thoracic cage morphology	0000772	Abnormality of the ribs
7-8	Misshapen rib 肋骨形態異常	0000152	Absent proximal rib	0000772	Abnormality of the ribs
7-9	Nodulated rib 肋骨結節状	0000150	Abnormal rib morphology	0000923	Beaded ribs
7-10	Short rib 肋骨短小(化)	0004672	Short rib	0000773	Short ribs
7-11	Supernumerary articulated rib 肋骨過剰	0000480 0008147	Increased rib number Asymmetric rib-vertebral column	0005815	Supernumerary ribs
7-12	Thick rib 肋骨肥厚(化)	0004676	Wide ribs	0000900	Thickened ribs
7-13	Wavy rib 波状肋骨	0000150	Abnormal rib morphology	0010561	Undulate ribs

MP: Mouse phenotype
HP: Human phenotype
In some cases, MP and HP terms indicate a more general description for the Atlas term.

Table 2 Comparative List of This Atlas Findings, Mouse Phenotype, and Human Phenotype

Photo No.	Atlas Term	MP No.	MP Term	HP No.	HP Term
7-14	Branched costal cartilage 肋軟骨分岐			0000772	Abnormality of the ribs
7-15	Interrupted costal cartilage 肋軟骨不連続	0006432	Abnormal costal cartilage morphology	0000772	Abnormality of the ribs
7-16	Fused costal catilage 肋軟骨癒合	0006432	Abnormal costal cartilage morphology	0000772	Abnormality of the ribs
7-17	Costal cartilage not fused to sternum 肋軟骨胸骨不接続	0008148	Abnormal rib-sternum attachment	0000919	Abnormality of the costochondral junction
7-18	Partially dupulicated costal cartilage 肋軟骨部分重複	0006432	Abnormal costal cartilage morphology	0001547	Abnormality of the rib cage
7-19	Full cervical supernumerary rib 頸部完全過剰肋骨	0008922	Abnormal cervical rib	0000891	Cervical ribs
7-20	Short cervical supernumerary rib 頸部短小過剰肋骨	0008922	Abnormal cervical rib	0000891	Cervical ribs
7-21	Full thoracolumbar supernumerary rib 胸腰部完全過剰肋骨	0000480	Increased rib number	0005815	Supernumerary ribs
7-22	Short thoracolumbar supernumerary rib 胸腰部短小過剰肋骨	0000480	Increased rib number	0005815	Supernumerary ribs
8-1	Supernumerary vertebrae 椎骨過剰	0004644	Increased vertebrae number	0002946	Supernumerary vertebrae
8-2	Interrupted vertebral canal 脊柱管不連続	0004703	Abnormal vertebral column morphology	0000925	Abnormality of the vertebral column
8-3	Double vertebral canal 脊柱管二重	0004703	Abnormal vertebral column morphology	0000925	Abnormality of the vertebral column
8-4	Absent atlas 環椎欠損	0011576	Absent cervical atlas	0008440	C1-C2 vertebral abnormality
8-5	Fused atlas 環椎癒合	0010728	Fusion of atlas and occipital bones	0008440	C1-C2 vertebral abnormality
8-6	Misshapen atlas 環椎形態異常	0004607	Abnormal cervical atlas morphology	0008440	C1-C2 vertebral abnormality
8-7	Small atlas 環椎小型(化)	0004607	Abnormal cervical atlas morphology	0008440	C1-C2 vertebral abnormality
8-8	Fused cervical arch 頸椎弓癒合	0004620 / 0004613	Cervical vertebral fusion / Fusion of vertebral arches	0002949 / 0008438	Fused cervical vertebeae / Vertebral arch anomaly
8-9	Misshapen cervical arch 頸椎弓形態異常	0003048 / 0004599	Abnormal cervical vertebrae morphology / Abnormal vertebral arch morphology	0003319 / 0008438	Abnormality of the cervical spine / Vertebral arch anomaly
8-10	Split cervical vertebral arch 頸椎弓分離	0003048 / 0004599	Abnormal cervical vertebrae morphology / Abnormal vertebral arch morphology	0003319 / 0008438	Abnormality of the cervical spine / Vertebral arch anomaly
8-11	Thick cervical vertebral arch 頸椎弓肥厚(化)	0003048 / 0004599	Abnormal cervical vertebrae morphology / Abnormal vertebral arch morphology	0003319 / 0008438	Abnormality of the cervical spine / Vertebral arch anomaly
8-12	Thin cervical vertebral arch 頸椎弓菲薄(化)	0003048 / 0004599	Abnormal cervical vertebrae morphology / Abnormal vertebral arch morphology	0003319 / 0008438	Abnormality of the cervical spine / Vertebral arch anomaly
8-13	Isolated ossification site of the cervical vertebral arch 頸椎弓分離骨化部位	0005226	Abnormal vertebral arch development	0100569	Abnormal vertebral ossification
8-14	Absent cervical vertebral centrum 頸椎体欠損	0003048 / 0004668	Abnormal cervical vertebrae morphology / Absent vertebral body	0003319	Abnormality of the cervical spine

MP: Mouse phenotype
HP: Human phenotype
In some cases, MP and HP terms indicate a more general description for the Atlas term.

Table 2 Comparative List of This Atlas Findings, Mouse Phenotype, and Human Phenotype

Photo No.	Atlas Term	MP No.	MP Term	HP No.	HP Term
8-15	Fused cervical vertebral centrum 頸椎体癒合	0004620	Cervical vertebral fusion	0002949	Fused cervical vertebeae
		0004612	Fusion of vertebral bodies	0003305	Block vertebrae
8-16	Misshapen cervical vertebral centrum 頸椎体形態異常	0003048	Abnormal cervical vertebrae morphology	0003319	Abnormality of the cervical spine
		0000141	Abnormal vertebral body morphology	0003312	Abnormal form of the vertebral bodies
8-17	Split cervical vertebral centrum 頸椎体分離	0003048	Abnormal cervical vertebrae morphology	0003319	Abnormality of the cervical spine
		0000141	Abnormal vertebral body morphology	0003312	Abnormal form of the vertebral bodies
8-18	Dumbbell-shaped cervical vertebral centrum 頸椎体ダンベル状	0003048	Abnormal cervical vertebrae morphology	0003319	Abnormality of the cervical spine
		0000141	Abnormal vertebral body morphology	0003312	Abnormal form of the vertebral bodies
8-19	Absent cervical vertebra 頸椎欠損	0004646	Decreased cervical vertebrae number	0003319	Abnormality of the cervical spine
				0030305	Decreased number of vertebrae
9-1	Absent thoracic vertebral arch 胸椎弓欠損	0003047	Abnormal thoracic vertebrae morphology	0100711	Abnormal of the thoracic spine
		0004603	Absent vertebral arch	0008438	Vertebral arch anomaly
9-2	Fused thoracic vertebral arches 胸椎弓癒合	0004623	Thoracic vertebral fusion	0030039	Fused thoracic vertebrae
		0004613	Fusion of vertebral arches	0008438	Vertebral arch anomaly
9-3	Large thoracic vertebral arch 胸椎弓大型(化)	0003047	Abnormal thoracic vertebrae morphology	0100711	Abnormal of the thoracic spine
		0004599	Abnormal vertebral arch morphology	0008438	Vertebral arch anomaly
9-4	Misshapen thoracic vertebral arch 胸椎弓形態異常	0003047	Abnormal thoracic vertebrae morphology	0100711	Abnormal of the thoracic spine
		0004599	Abnormal vertebral arch morphology	0008438	Vertebral arch anomaly
9-5	Small thoracic vertebral arch 頸椎弓小型(化)	0003047	Abnormal thoracic vertebrae morphology	0100711	Abnormal of the thoracic spine
		0004599	Abnormal vertebral arch morphology	0008438	Vertebral arch anomaly
9-6	Isolated ossification site of the thoracic vertebral arch 胸椎弓分離骨化部位	0005226	Abnormal vertebral arch development	0100569	Abnormal vertebral ossification
9-7	Absent thoracic vertebral centrum 胸椎体欠損	0003047	Abnormal thoracic vertebrae morphology	0100711	Abnormal of the thoracic spine
		0004688	Absent vertebral body		
9-8	Fused thoracic vertebral centra 胸椎体癒合	0004623	Thoracic vertebral fusion	0030039	Fused thoracic vertebrae
		0004612	Fusion of vertebral bodies	0003305	Block vertebrae
9-9	Small thoracic vertebral centrum 胸椎体小型(化)	0003047	Abnormal thoracic vertebrae morphology	0100711	Abnormal of the thoracic spine
		0004670	Small vertebral body	0003312	Abnormal form of the vertebral bodies
9-10	Bipartite ossification of the thoracic vertebral centrum 胸椎体二分骨化	0005227	Abnormal vertebral body development	0100569	Abnormal vertebral ossification
9-11	Dumbbell ossification of thoracic vertebral centrum 胸椎体ダンベル状骨化	0005227	Abnormal vertebral body development	0100569	Abnormal vertebral ossification
9-12	Unossified thortacic vertebral centrum 胸椎体未骨化	0005227	Abnormal vertebral body development	0100569	Abnormal vertebral ossification

MP: Mouse phenotype
HP: Human phenotype
In some cases, MP and HP terms indicate a more general description for the Atlas term.

Table 2 Comparative List of This Atlas Findings, Mouse Phenotype, and Human Phenotype

Photo No.	Atlas Term	MP No.	MP Term	HP No.	HP Term
9-13	Absent thoracic vertebra 胸椎欠損	0004648	Decreased thoracic vertebrae number	0100711	Abnormal of the thoracic spine
				0030305	Decreased number of vertebrae
9-14	Thoracic hemivertebra 胸椎半椎	0008832	Hemivertebra	0008467	Thoracic hemivertebrae
10-1	Fused lumbar vertebral arches 腰椎弓癒合	0004621	Lumbar vertebral fusion	0008438	Vertebral arch anomaly
		0004613	Fusion of vertebral arches	0030040	Fused lumbar vertebrae
10-2	Misshapen lumbar vertebral arch 腰椎弓形態異常	0003049	Abnormal lumbar vertebrae morphology	0100712	Abnormality of the lumbar spine
		0004599	Abnormal vertebral arch morphology	0008438	Vertebral arch anomaly
10-3	Splayed lumbar vertebral arch 腰椎弓放散	0003049	Abnormal lumbar vertebrae morphology	0100712	Abnormality of the lumbar spine
		0004599	Abnormal vertebral arch morphology	0008438	Vertebral arch anomaly
10-4	Supernumerary site in lumbar vertebral arch 腰椎弓過剰部位	0003049	Abnormal lumbar vertebrae morphology	0100712	Abnormality of the lumbar spine
		0004599	Abnormal vertebral arch morphology	0008438	Vertebral arch anomaly
10-5	Increased ossification of the lumbar vertebral arch 腰椎弓骨化亢進	0005226	Abnormal vertebral arch development	0100569	Abnormal vertebral ossification
10-6	Fused lumbar vertebral centra 腰椎体癒合	0004621	Lumbar vertebral fusion	0030040	Fused lumbar vertebrae
		0004612	Fusion of vertebral body	0003305	Block vertebrae
10-7	Misaligned lumbar vertebral centra 腰椎体配列異常	0003049	Abnormal lumbar vertebrae morphology	0100712	Abnormality of the lumbar spine
		0000141	Abnormal vertebral body morphology	0003312	Abnormal form of the vertebral bodies
10-8	Bipartite ossification of lumbar vertebral centra 腰椎体二分骨化	0005227	Abnormal vertebral body development	0100569	Abnormal vertebral ossification
10-9	Absent lumbar vertebra 腰椎欠損	0004654	Absent lumbar vertebrae	0100712	Abnormality of the lumbar spine
		0004647	Decreased lumbar vertebrae number	0008465	Absent vertebrae
				0030305	Decreased number of vertebrae
10-10	Lumbar hemivertebra 腰椎半椎	0008832	Hemivertebra	0008439	Lumbar hemivertebrae
10-11	Supernumerary lumbar vertebrae 腰椎過剰	0004650	Increased lumbar vertebrae number	0002946	Supernumerary vertebrae
11-1	Fused sacral vertebral arches 仙椎弓癒合	0004622	Sacral vertebral fusion	0008438	Vertebral arch anomaly
		0004613	Fusion of vertebral arches	0003305	Block vertebrae
11-2	Misshapen sacral vertebral arch 仙椎弓形態異常	0003050	Abnormal sacral vertebrae morphology	0008438	Vertebral arch anomaly
		0004599	Abnormal vertebral arch morphology		
11-3	Sacral vertebral arch not fused 仙椎弓未癒合	0003050	Abnormal sacral vertebrae morphology	0008438	Vertebral arch anomaly
		0004599	Abnormal vertebral arch morphology		
11-4	Absent sacral vertebrae 仙椎欠損	0004656	Absent sacral vertebrae	0005107	Abnormality of the sacrum
				0008465	Absent vertebrae
11-5	Fused caudal vertebral centra 尾椎体癒合	0004619	Caudal vertebral fusion	0002948	Vertebral fision
		0004612	Fusion of vertebral body		

MP: Mouse phenotype
HP: Human phenotype
In some cases, MP and HP terms indicate a more general description for the Atlas term.

Table 2 Comparative List of This Atlas Findings, Mouse Phenotype, and Human Phenotype

Photo No.	Atlas Term	MP No.	MP Term	HP No.	HP Term
11-6	Misaligned caudal vertebral centrum 尾椎体配列異常	0000141	Abnormal vertebral body morphology	0003312	Abnormal form of the vertebral bodies
11-7	Incomplete ossification of caudal vertebral centra 尾椎体不完全骨化	0005225	Abnormal vertebrae development	0100569	Abnormal vertebral ossification
11-8	Unossified caudal vertebral centra 尾椎体未骨化	0005225	Abnormal vertebrae development	0100569	Abnormal vertebral ossification
11-9	Absent caudal vertebrae 尾椎欠損	0004653 0001539	Absent caudal vertebrae Decreased caudal vertebrae number	0008465 0030305	Absent vertebrae Decreased number of vertebrae
11-10	Caudal hemivertebra 尾椎半椎	0008833	Caudal hemivertebra	0002937	Hemivertebrae
11-11	Misaligned caudal vertebrae 尾椎配列異常	0002759	Abnormal caudal vertebrae morphology		
12-1	Malpositioned pelvic girdle (cranial, bilateral) 後肢帯両側(性)頭方位置異常				
12-2	Malpositioned caudal unilateral pelvic girdle 後肢帯片側(性)尾方位置異常				

MP: Mouse phenotype
HP: Human phenotype
In some cases, MP and HP terms indicate a more general description for the Atlas term.

Photographs of Normal Fetuses in Rats and Rabbits
正常写真（ラット、ウサギ）

Rats (Wistar Hannover)

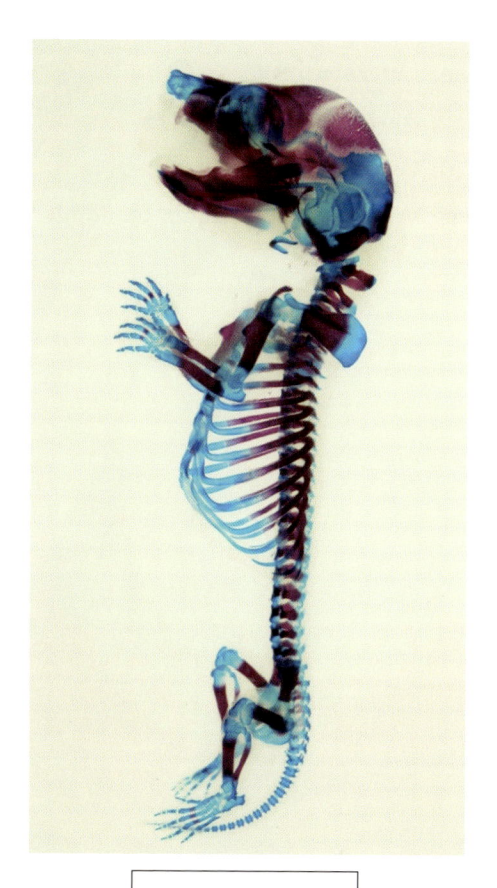

Lateral aspect

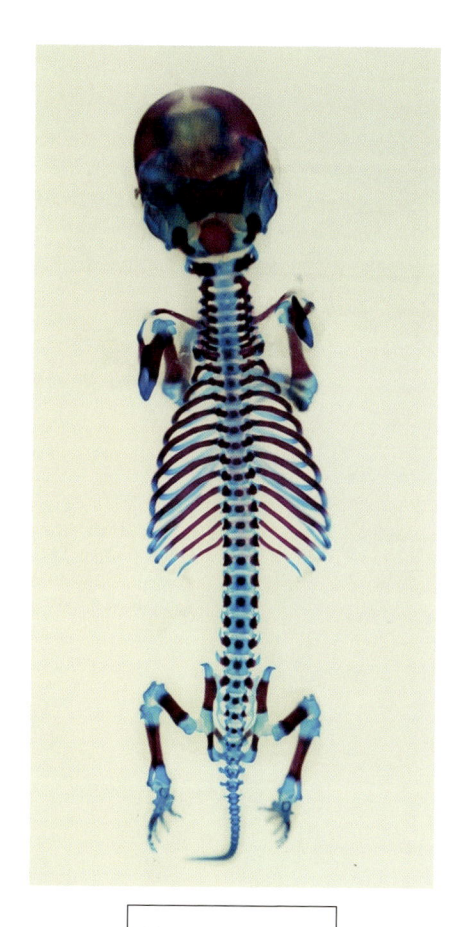

Dorsal aspect

Rats (Wistar Hannover)   Continued

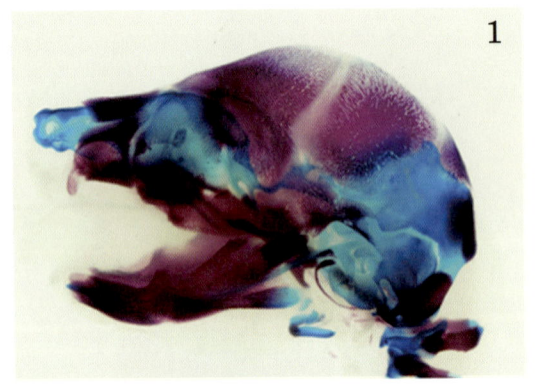

1. Head: Lateral aspect
2. Head: Dorsal aspect
3. Head: Ventral aspect with mandible
4. Head: Ventral aspect without mandible

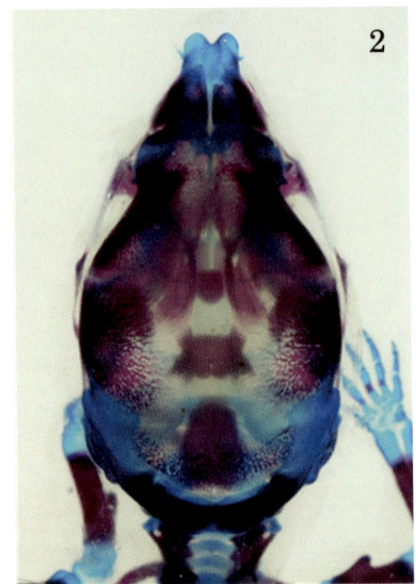

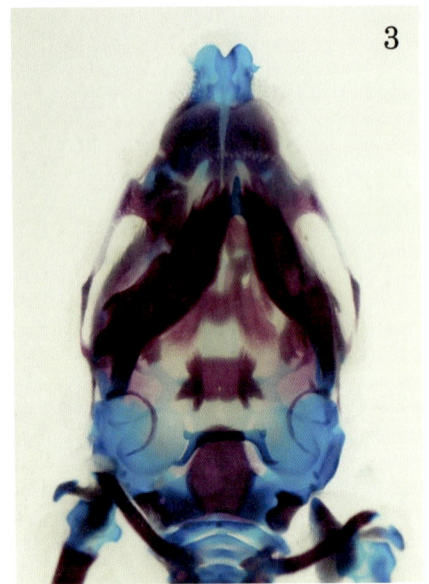

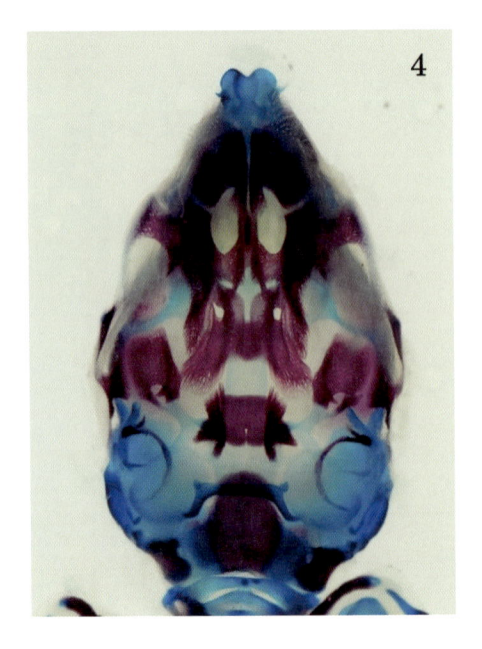

Rats (Wistar Hannover)   Continued

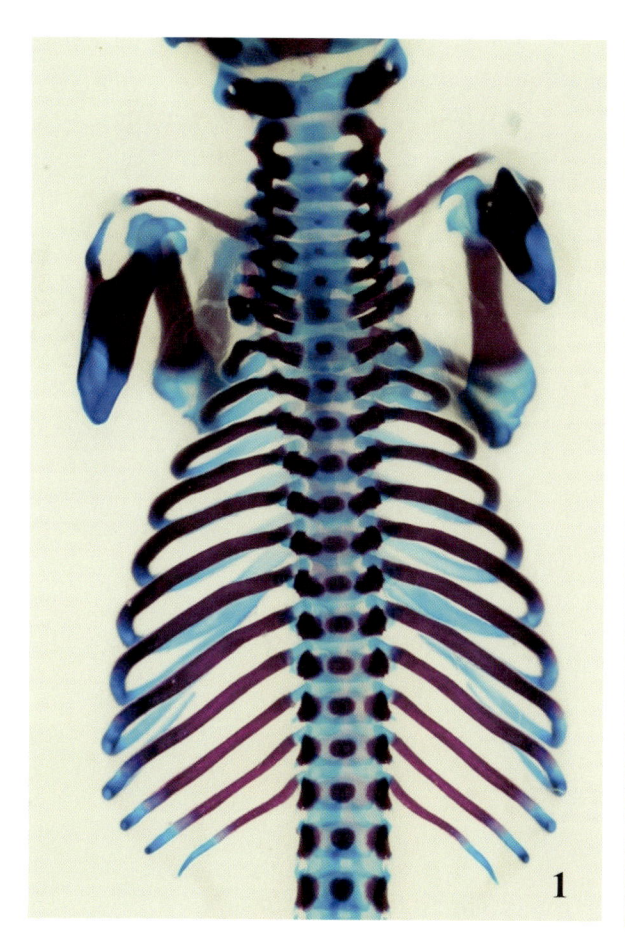

1. Cervical and thoracic vertebrae and ribs: Dorsal aspect
2. Lumbar and sacral vertebrae: Dorsal aspect
3. Caudal vertebra: Dorsal aspect

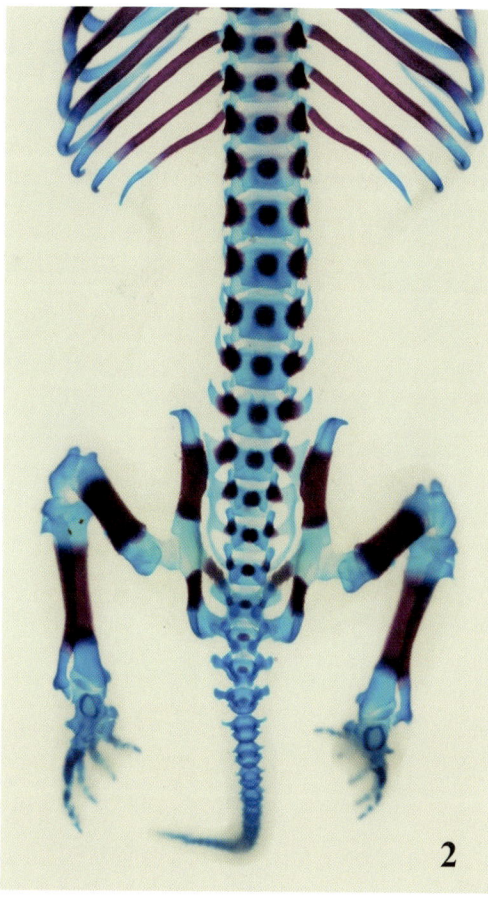

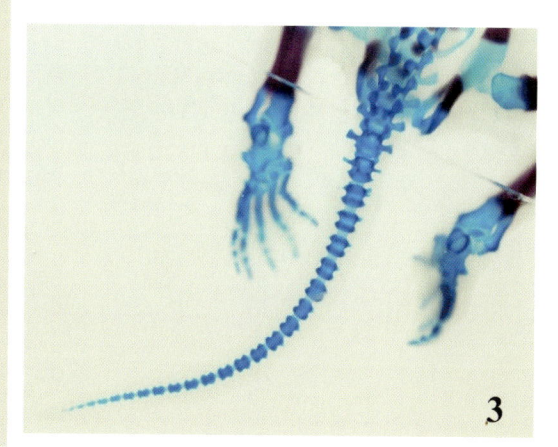

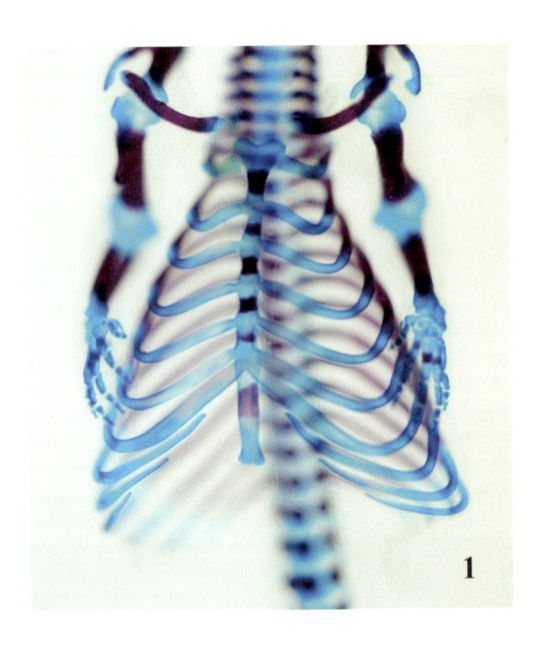

Rats (Wistar Hannover) Continued

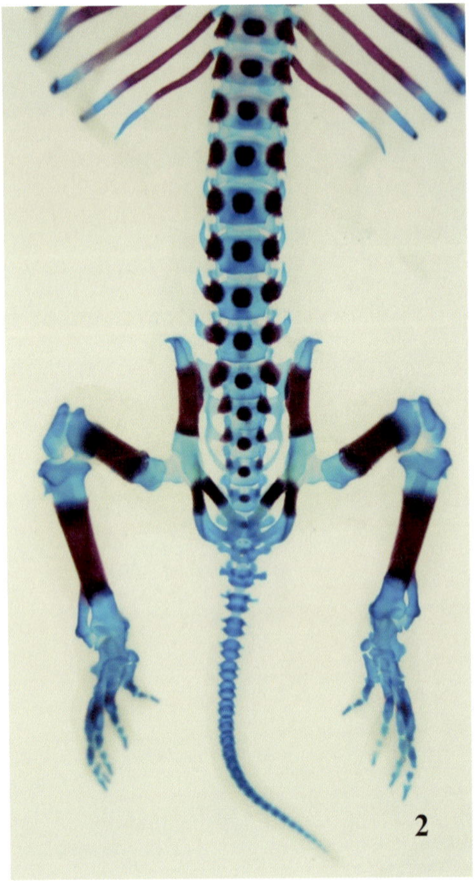

1. Sternum and Costal cartilage: Ventral aspect
2. Lumbar and sacral vertebrae and Pelvic girdle: Ventral aspect

Rats (Wistar Hannover) Continued

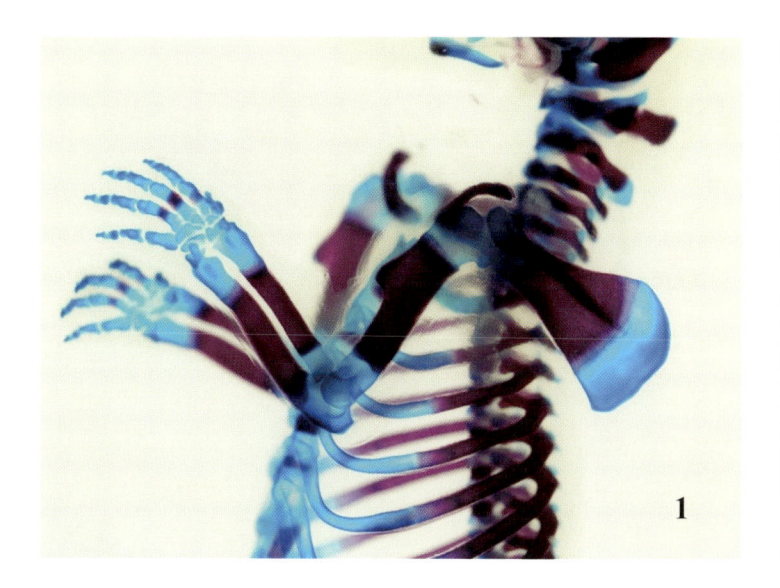

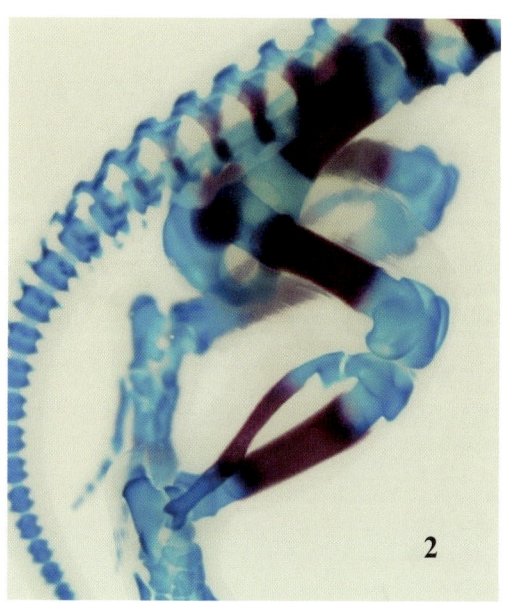

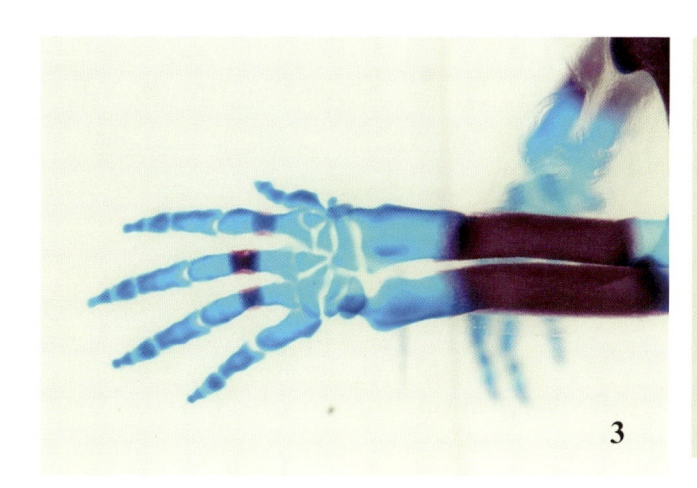

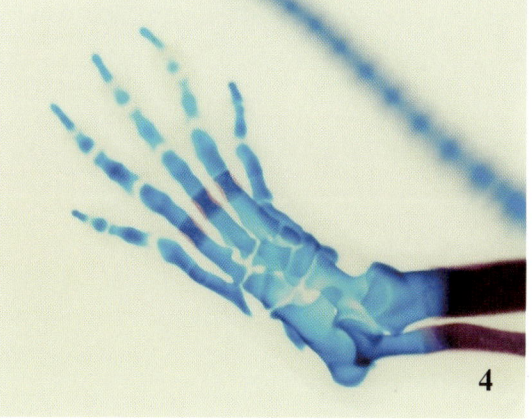

1. Forelimb: Lateral aspect
2. Hindlimb: Lateral aspect
3. Forepaw
4. Hindpaw

Rabbits (NZW)

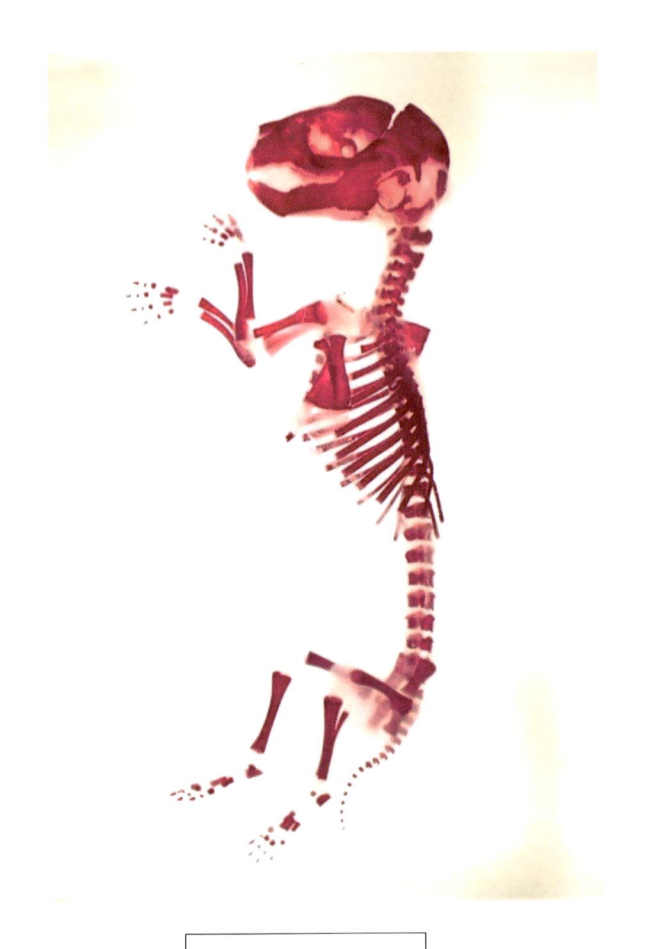

Lateral aspect

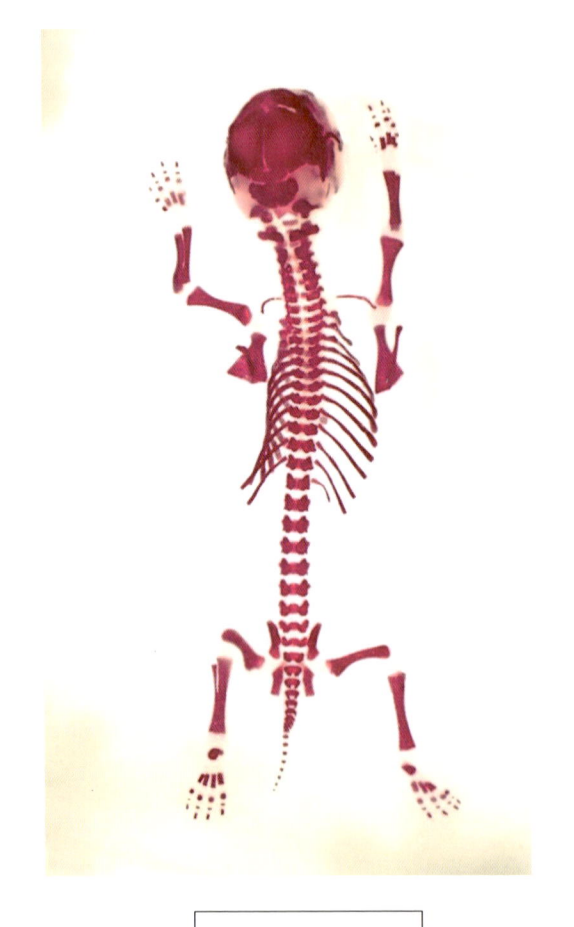

Dorsal aspect

Rabbits (NZW)

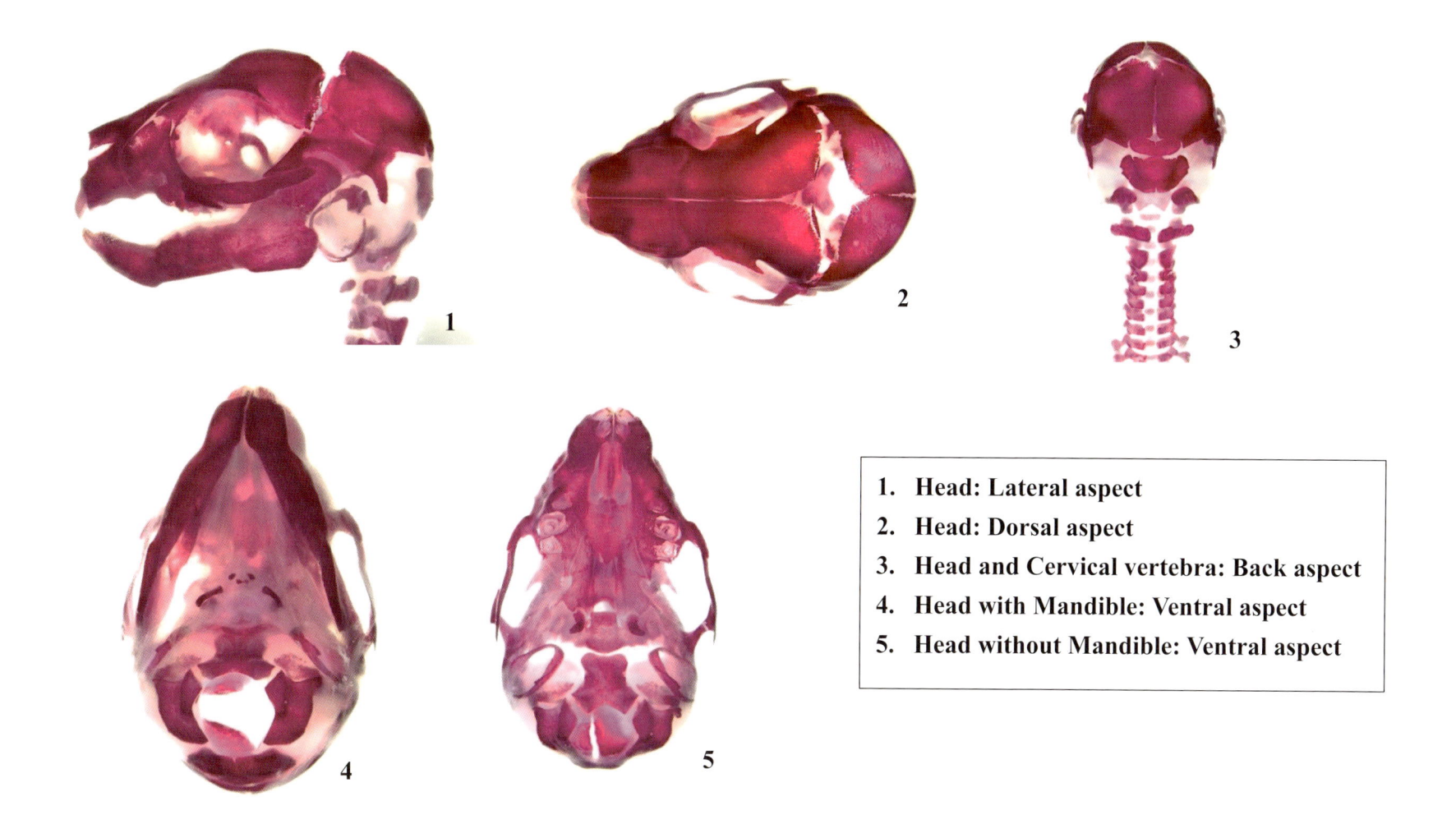

1. Head: Lateral aspect
2. Head: Dorsal aspect
3. Head and Cervical vertebra: Back aspect
4. Head with Mandible: Ventral aspect
5. Head without Mandible: Ventral aspect

Rabbits (NZW)   Continued

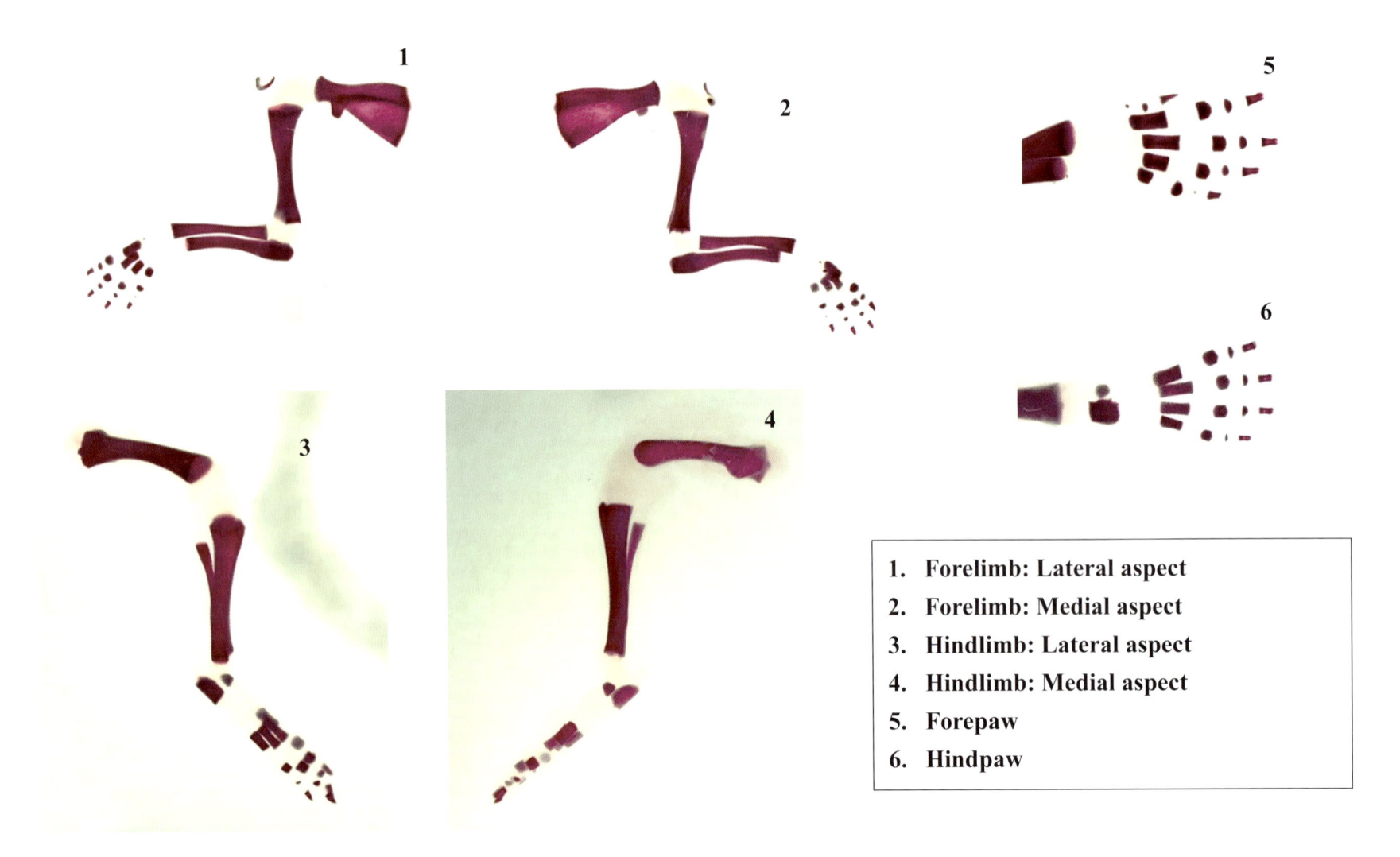

1. Forelimb: Lateral aspect
2. Forelimb: Medial aspect
3. Hindlimb: Lateral aspect
4. Hindlimb: Medial aspect
5. Forepaw
6. Hindpaw

Photographs of Skeletal Anomalies

1. Skull

1-1　Fused basioccipital bone　底後頭骨癒合　(10420)

Species	Mouse
Memo	Fused basioccipital and exoccipital bones: Basioccipital bone and exoccipital bones fused (thick arrow).
	底後頭骨外後頭骨癒合：底後頭骨と外後頭骨が癒合している（太矢印）。

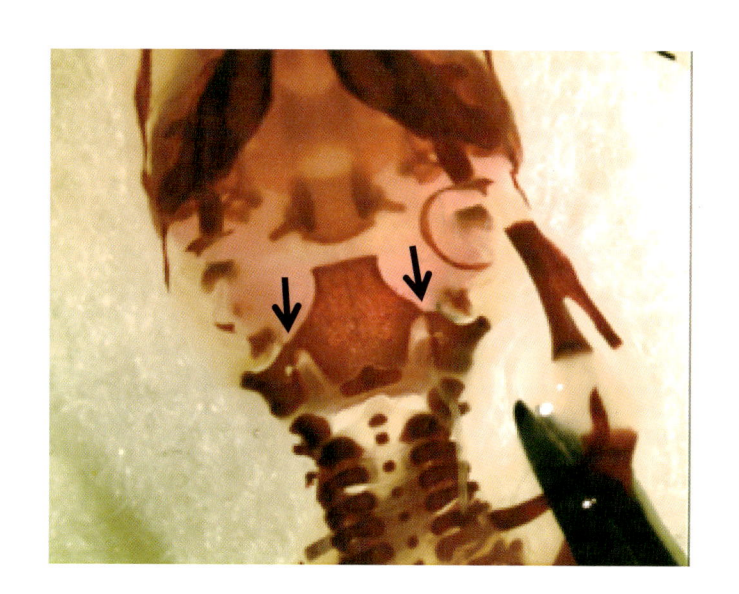

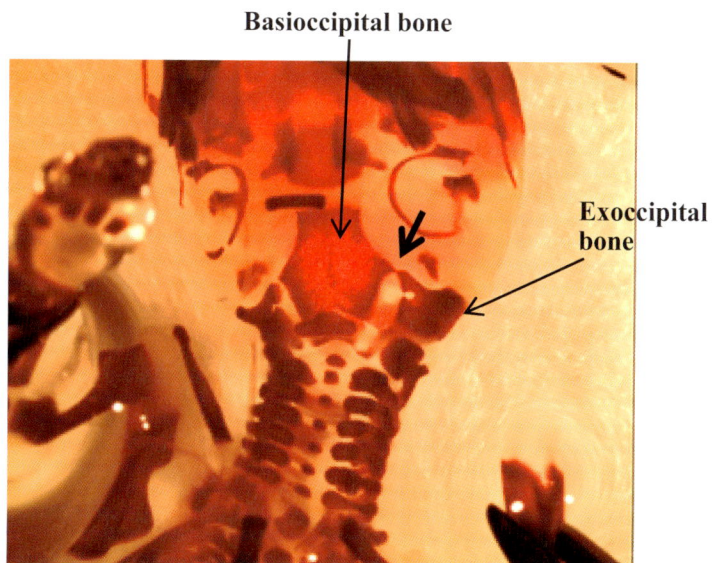

1-2 Misshapen basisphenoid bone　　底蝶形骨形態異常　(10429)

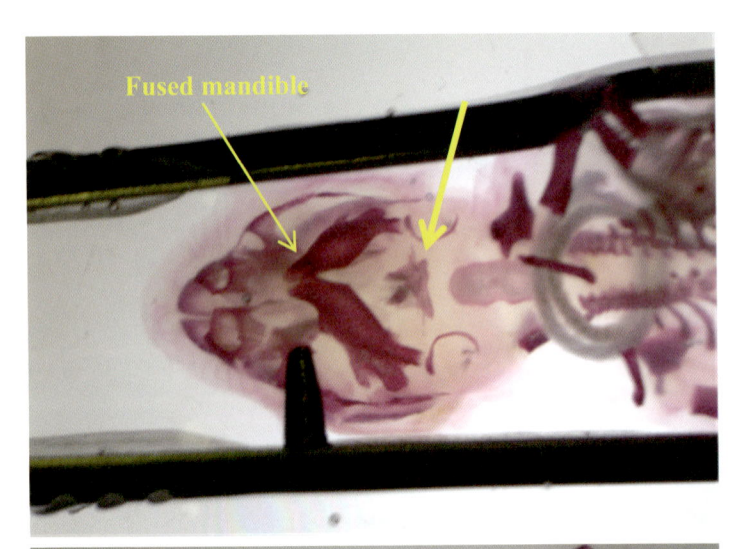

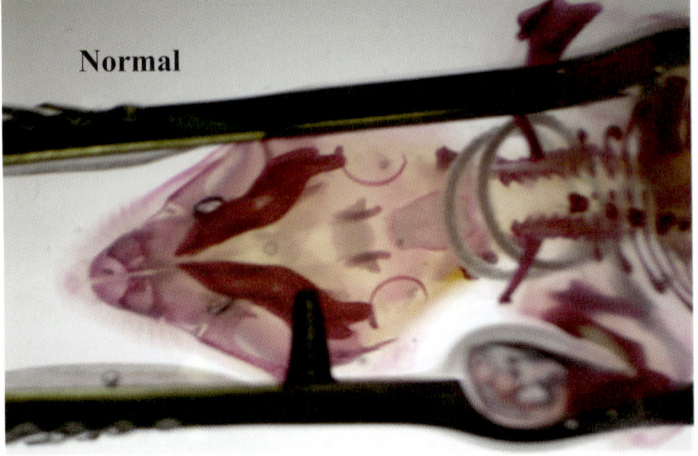

Fused mandible

Normal

Species	Rat, SD
Memo	Misshapen basisphenoid bone (thick arrow) with Fused mandible (10467, thin arrow): The shape of the basisphenoid bone is abnormal compared with that in a normal fetus (lower photograph).
	底蝶形骨形態異常（太矢印）：下顎骨癒合（10467、細矢印）を伴う。下写真は正常胎児。

1-3   Fused exoccipital bone   外後頭骨癒合   (10434)

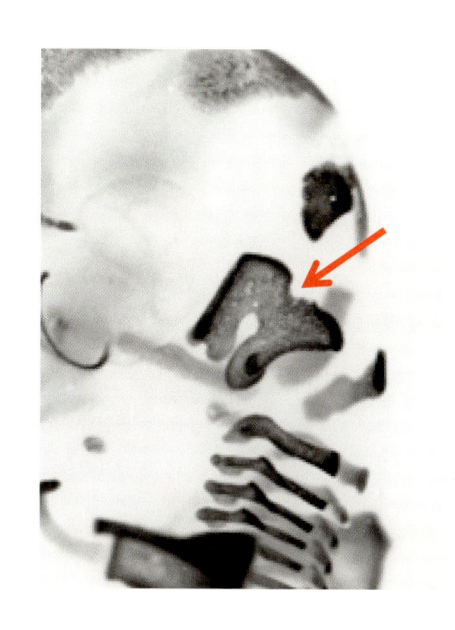

Species	Mouse
Memo	Fusion of exoccipital bone and atlas: Exoccipital bone fused with atlas (arrow).
	外後頭骨環椎癒合：外後頭骨と環椎が癒合している。（矢印）

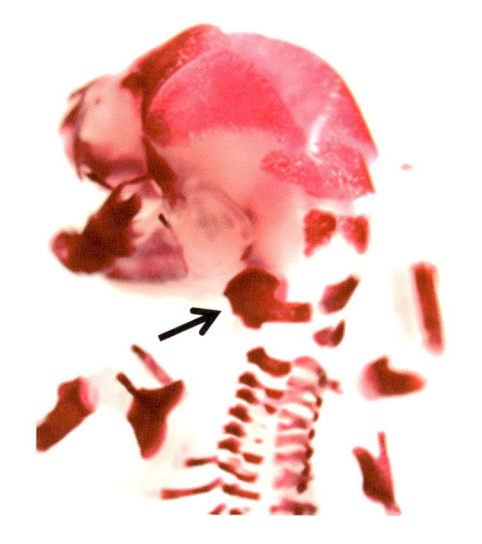

Species	Rat
Memo	Fusion of exoccipital bone and atlas: Exoccipital bone fused with atlas (arrow).
	外後頭骨環椎癒合：外後頭骨と環椎が癒合している。（矢印）

1-3 Continued

Species	Mouse
Memo	Fused exoccipital and basioccipital bones: Exoccipital and basioccipital bones fused (arrow).
	外後頭骨底後頭骨癒合：外後頭骨と底後頭骨が癒合している。（矢印）

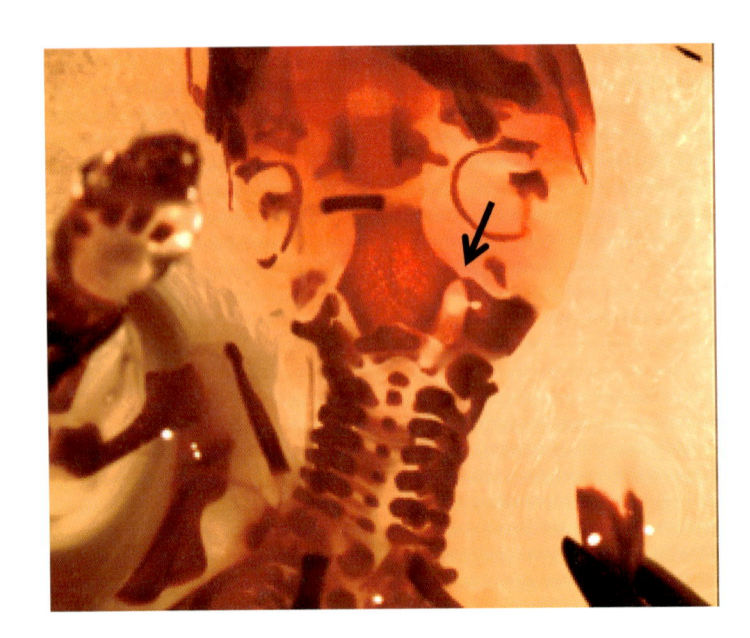

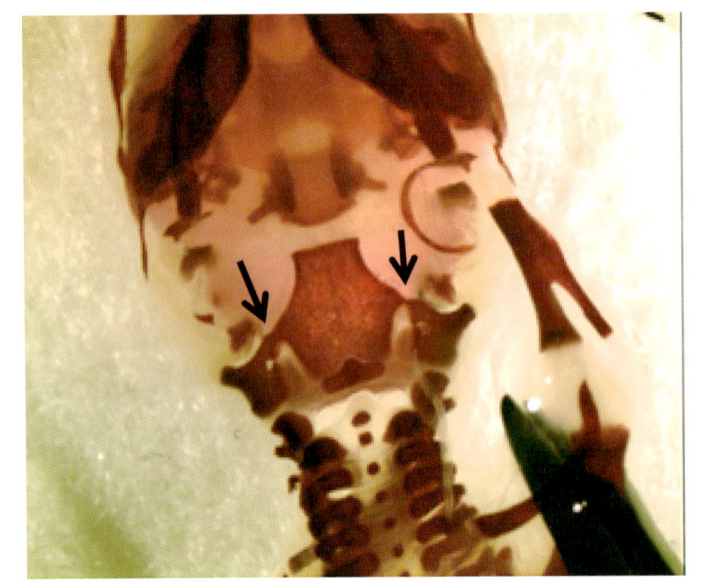

1-4 Fused frontal bone　　前頭骨癒合　(10441)

Species	Rabbit
Memo	Fused frontal bone: The right and left frontal bones fused (thick arrow, left and center fetuses). Split nasal bone (thin arrow) is also observed in the left fetus. Fused nasal bone (10479, long thin arrow) and hole in the parietal bone (10496, short thin arrow) are also observed in the center fetus. The right photograph shows normal features.
	前頭骨癒合：左右の前頭骨が癒合している（太矢印）。左胎児では鼻骨分離（New、細矢印）も見られる。中央胎児では鼻骨癒合（10479、長細矢印）及び頭頂骨孔（10496、短細矢印）も見られる。右は正常胎児

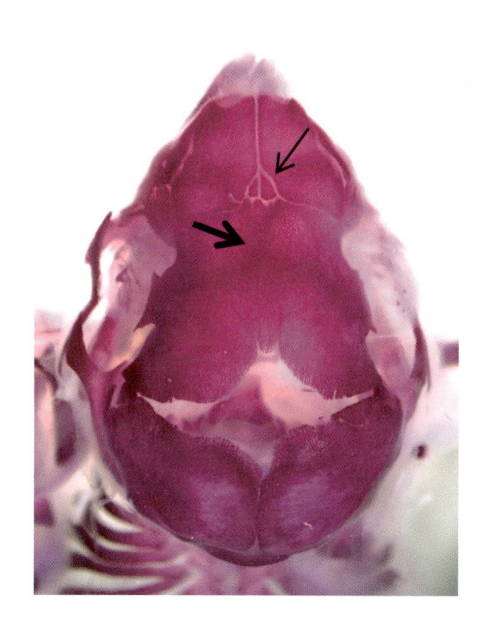

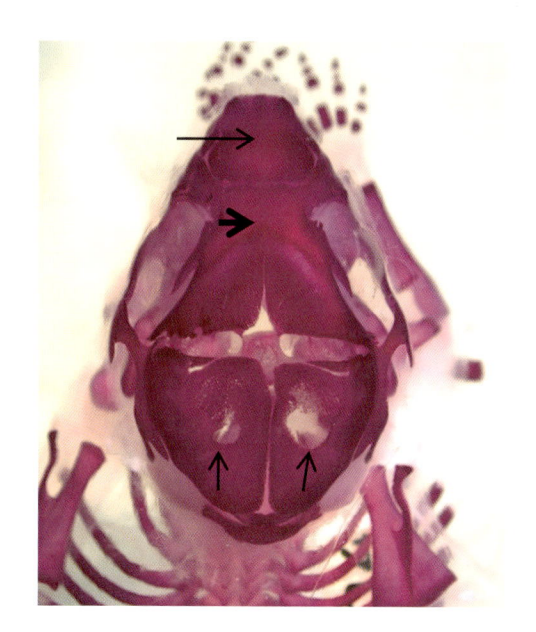

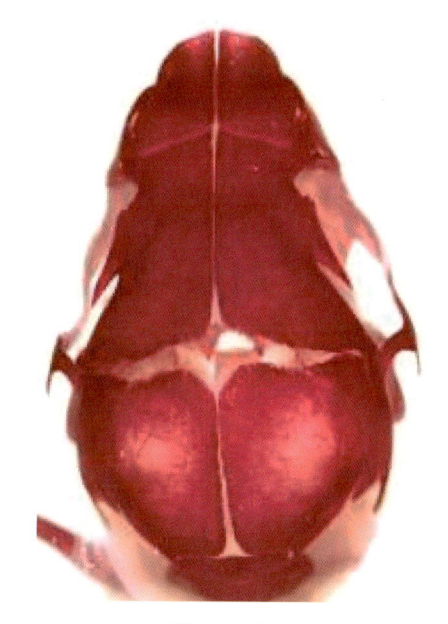

Normal

1-5 Misshapen frontal bone　　前頭骨形態異常　(10443)

Species	Rat
Memo	Misshapen frontal bone (thick arrow) with Misshapen parietal bone (10495), Small nasal bone (10483), Small premaxilla (10504), and Short mandible (New): This fetus may appear as "Domed head (10012)" in external examination. The left fetus shows normal features.
	前頭骨形態異常（太矢印）：本胎児は外表ではドーム状頭部（10012）であり、頭頂骨形態異常（10495）、鼻骨小型化（10483）、顎間骨小型化（10504）及び下顎骨短小（New）を伴う。左は正常胎児

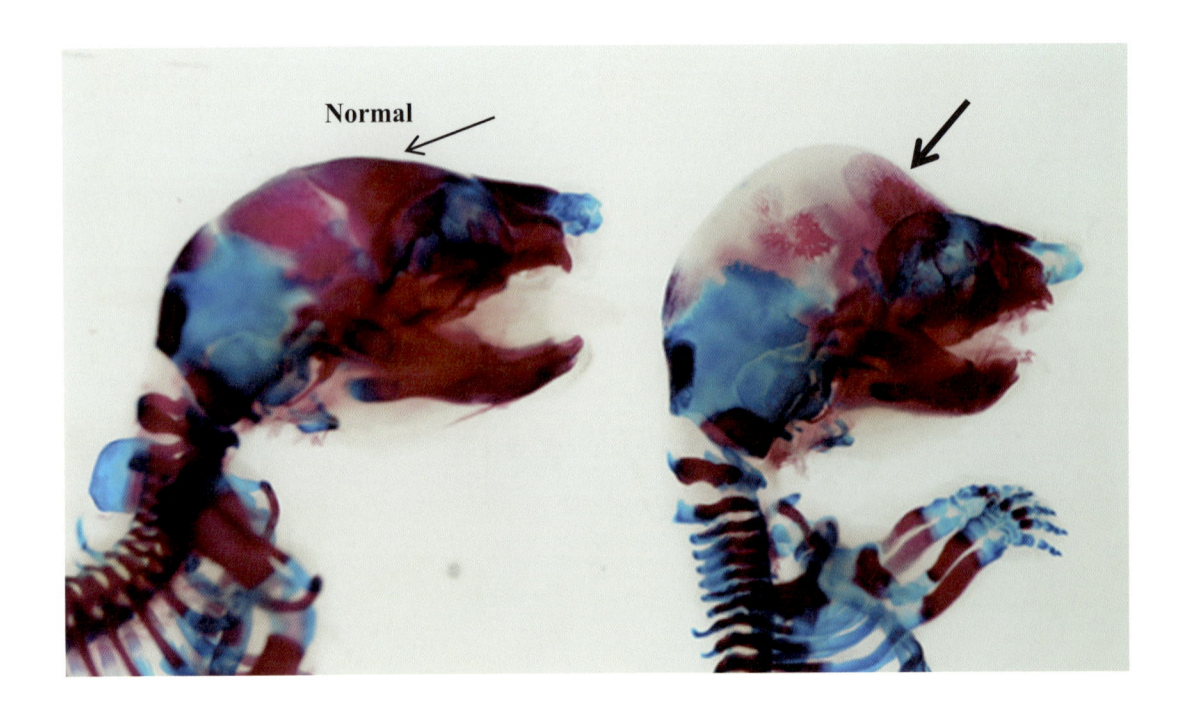

1-6　　Misshapen hyoid body　　舌骨体形態異常　　(10449)

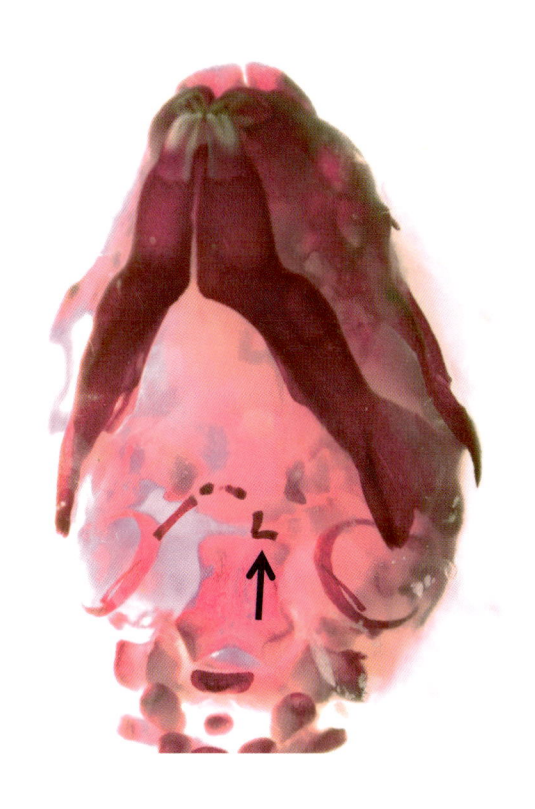

Species	Rabbit
Memo	Misshapen hyoid body: Hyoid body is abnormal shape (arrow).
	舌骨体形態異常：舌骨体が異常に屈曲している（矢印）。

1-7 Split hyoid body　　舌骨体分離　(New)

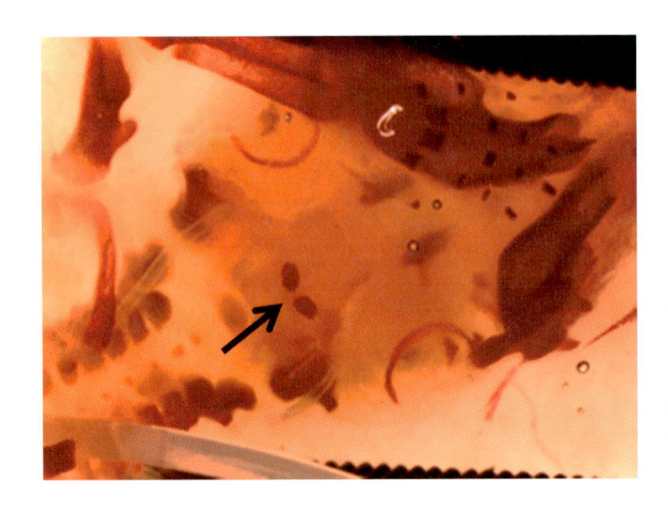

Species	Mouse: ICR
Memo	Split hyoid body: Hyoid body interrupted at the center (arrow). This may be considered as "Bipartite ossification of hyoid body (New)" because this fetus is only stained with alizarin red for the ossified area and its detail structure is unclear.
	舌骨体分離：舌骨体の中央部分が連続していない（矢印）。本胎児はアリザリンレッドによる単染色であり、舌骨体を詳細に観察できないことから、「舌骨体二分骨化（New）」の可能性もある。

1-8　Fused mandible　　下顎骨癒合　(10467)

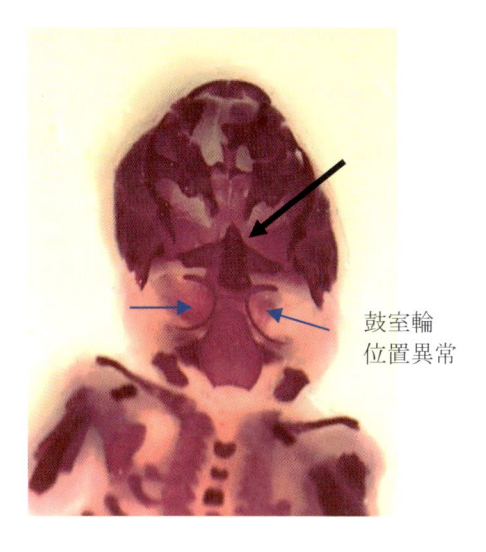

鼓室輪
位置異常

Species	Rat
Memo	Fused mandible (black arrow): This fetus also has Small mandible (10470) and Malpositioned tympanic annulus (New), so it may appear as "Otocephaly" in external observation.
	下顎骨癒合：下顎骨小型（10470）及び鼓室輪位置異常（New）を伴う。おそらく外表では耳頭症と考える。

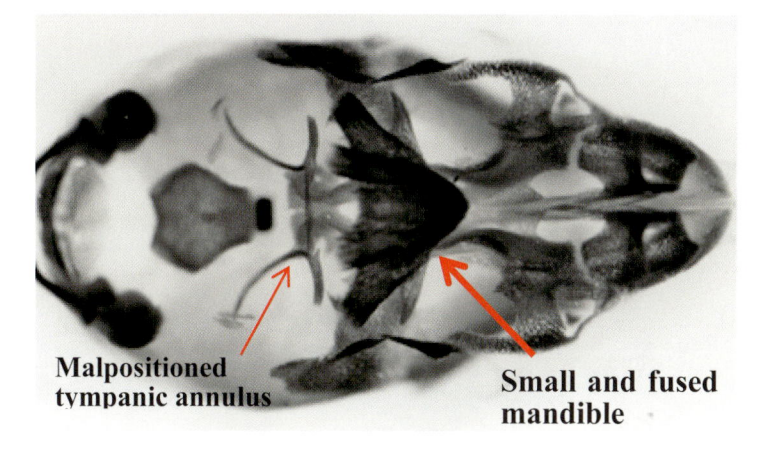

Malpositioned tympanic annulus

Small and fused mandible

Species	Rat
Memo	Fused mandible with Malpositioned tympanic annulus (New) and Small mandible (10470): This anomaly is usually observed in a fetus with "Otocephaly": Malpositioned auricle (10021) and Agnathia (Absent lower jaw, 10047).
	下顎癒合：鼓室輪位置異常（New）及び下顎骨小型（10470）も伴っている。外表で「耳頭症」＝耳介の位置異常（10021）及び下顎欠損（10047）が見られた胎児にこの所見が見られる。

1-8 Continued

Species	Rat, SD
Memo	Fused mandible (yellow thick arrow) with Misshapen basioccipital bone (10429): The lower photograph shows normal features.
	下顎骨癒合：底蝶形骨形態異常（10429）を伴う。下写真は正常。

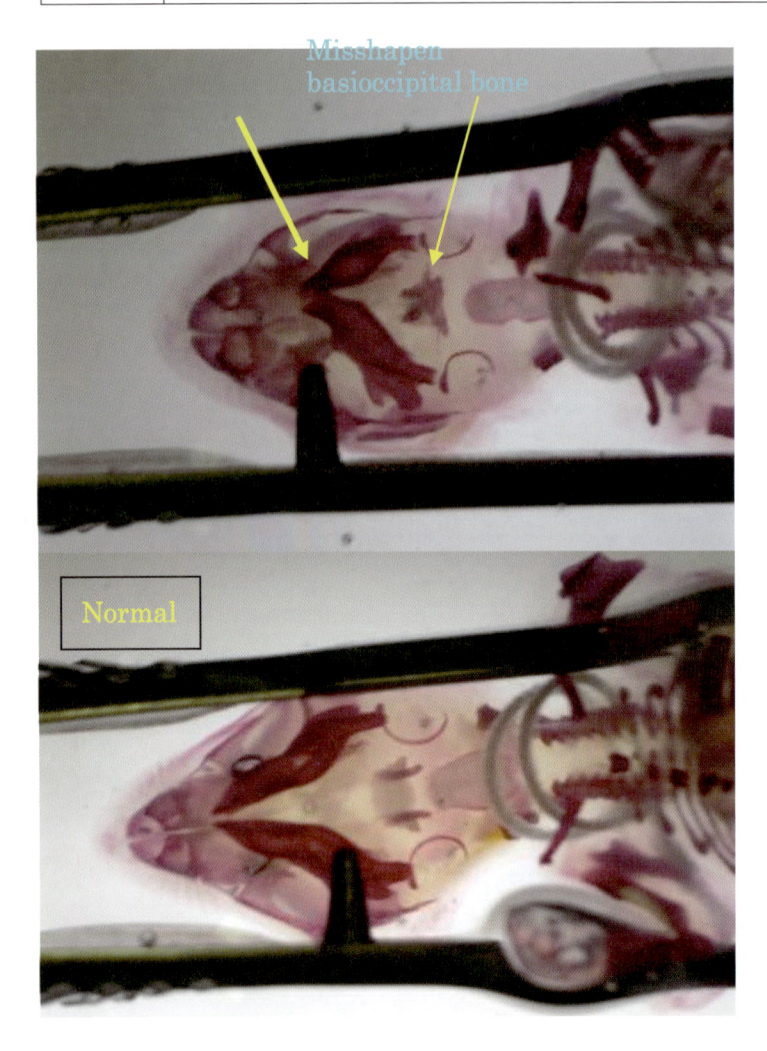

Species	Rat
Memo	Fused mandible (red arrow) with Small mandible (10470): This fetus may appear as "Otocephaly" in external observation.
	下顎骨癒合（赤矢印）：下顎骨小型（10470）を伴う。外表ではおそらく耳頭症（下顎欠損と耳の位置異常）

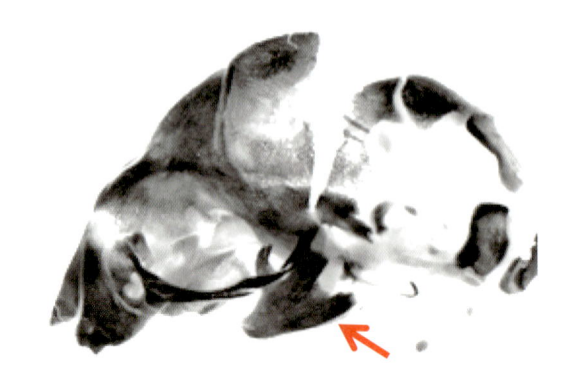

1-9　Misshapen mandible　　下顎骨形態異常　　(10469)

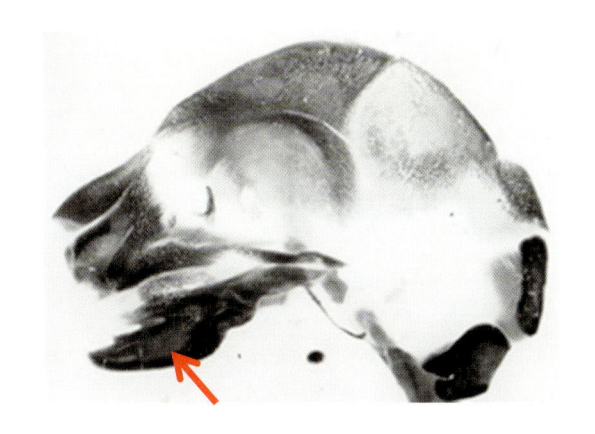

Species	Rat
Memo	Misshapen mandible (arrow) with Fused zygomatic arch (10541)
	下顎骨形態異常（矢印）：頬骨弓の癒合（10541）を伴う。

Species	Rat: Crl:CD(SD)
Memo	Misshapen mandible with Misshapen maxilla (10475) and Misshapen zygomatic arch (infraorbital foremen and zygomatic process: 10543): This mandible appears flatter than normal and has an abnormal shape of the condyloid process. The lower photograph shows normal features (arrow).
	下顎骨形態異常：下顎骨の全体が直線的であり、関節突起などの形状が異なる（矢印）。頬骨弓形態異常（10543）及び下顎骨形態異常（10469）を伴う。下写真は正常（矢印）

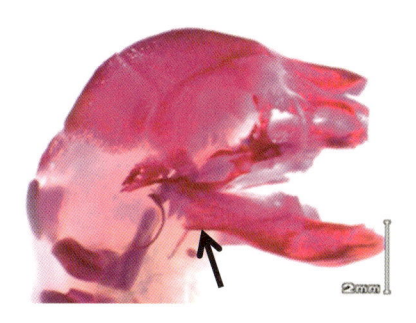

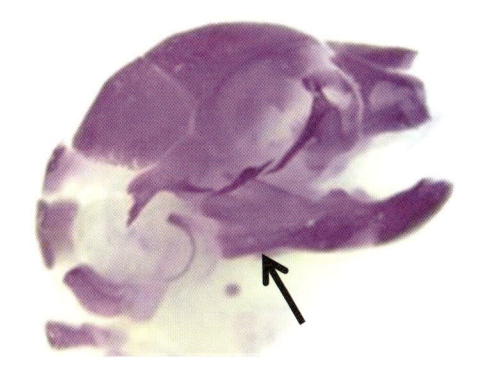

1-10   **Short mandible**   下顎骨短小（化）   **(New)**

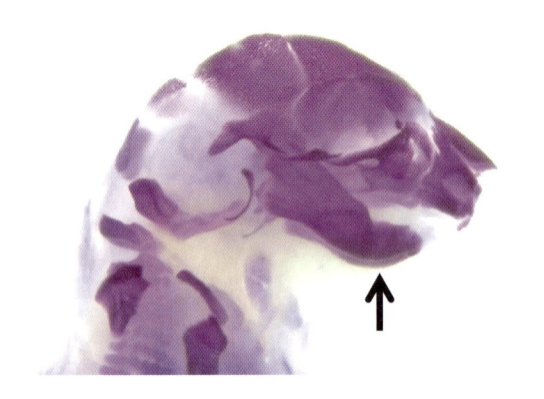

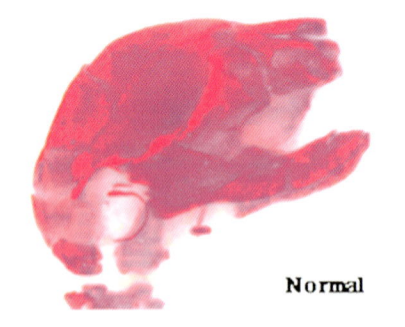

Species	Rat
Memo	Short mandible (arrow): This observation should be distinguished from Small mandible (10470). The lower photograph shows normal features.
	下顎骨短小（化）（矢印）：小型（10470）とは区分する。下写真は正常

1-10 Continued

Species	Rat
Memo	Short mandible (thick arrow) with Misshapen frontal bone (10443), Misshapen parietal bone (10495), Small nasal bone (10483), and Small premaxilla (10504): This fetus may appear as "Domed head (10012)" in external observation.
	下顎骨短小（化）（太矢印）：本胎児は外表ではドーム状頭部（10012）であり、前頭骨形態異常（10443）、頭頂骨形態異常（10495）、鼻骨小型（化）（10483）及び顎間骨小型（化）（10504）を伴う。

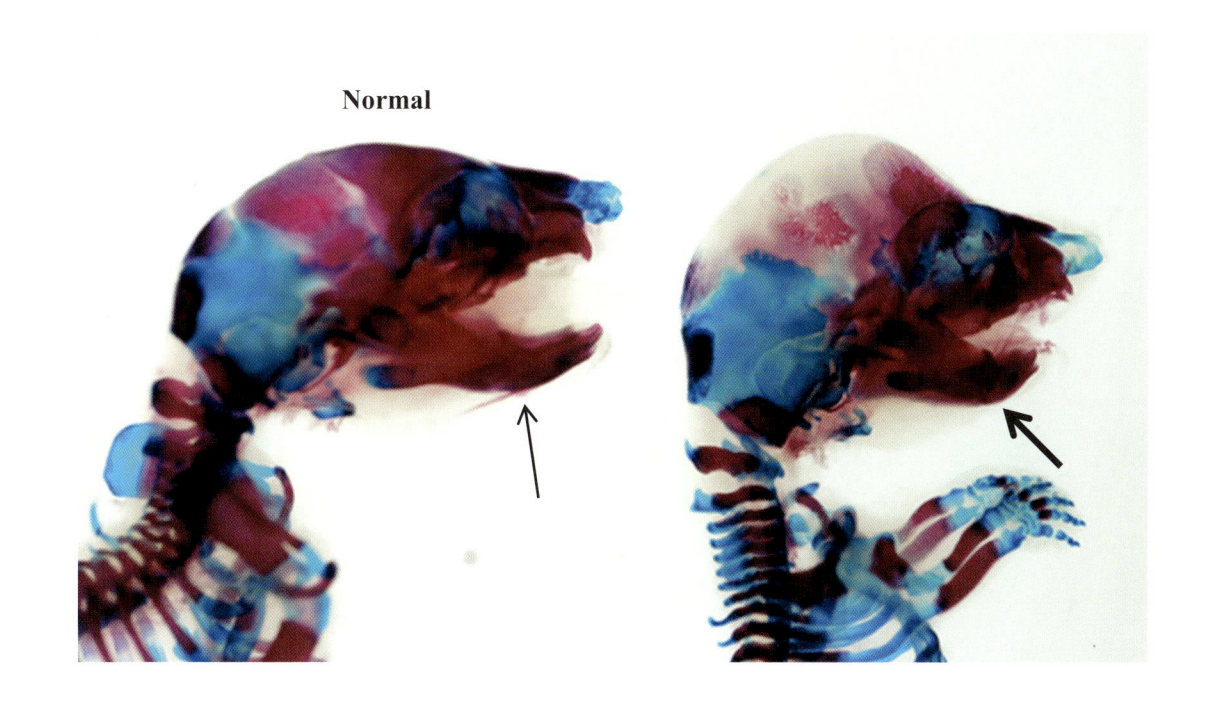

Normal

1-11 Small mandible   下顎骨小型（化）   (10470)

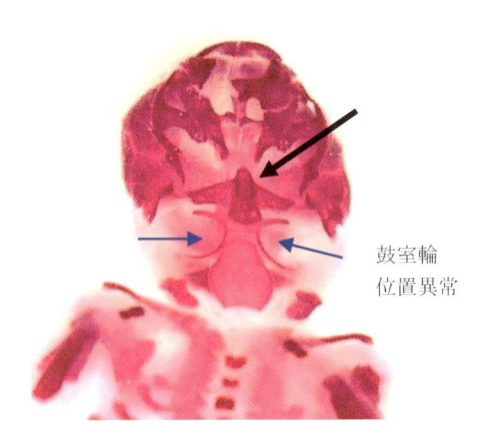

Species	Rat
Memo	Small mandible (arrow): This fetus also has Fused mandible (10467) and Malpositioned tympanic annulus (New), so it may appear as "Otocephaly" in external observation.
	下顎骨小型（化）：下顎骨癒合（10467）及び鼓室輪位置異常（New）を伴う。おそらく外表では耳頭症と考える。

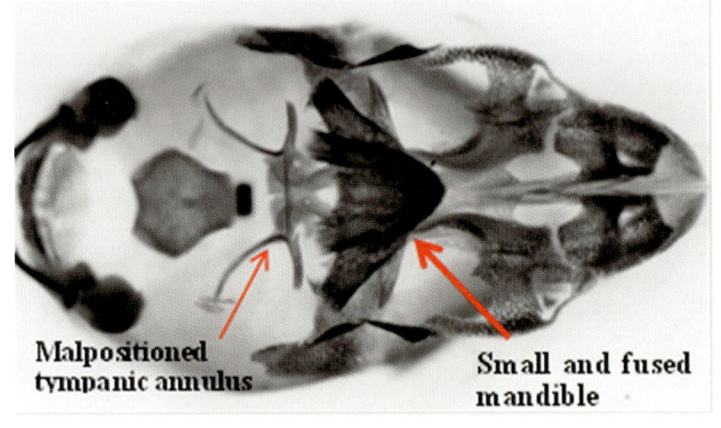

鼓室輪
位置異常

Species	Rat
Memo	Small mandible with Malpositioned tympanic annulus (New) and Fused mandible (10467): This anomaly is usually observed in a fetus with "Otocephaly": Malpositioned auricle (10021) and Agnathia (absent lower jaw, 10047).
	下顎骨小型（化）：鼓室輪位置異常（New）及び下顎骨癒合（10467）も伴っている。外表で「耳頭症」＝耳介の位置異常（10021）及び下顎欠損（10047）が見られた胎児にこの所見が見られる。

Malpositioned tympanic annulus

Small and fused mandible

1-12　　Misshapen maxilla　　　上顎骨形態異常　　(10475)

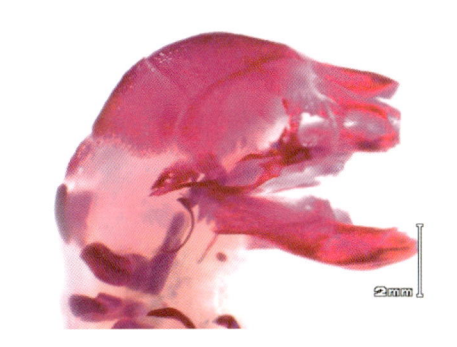

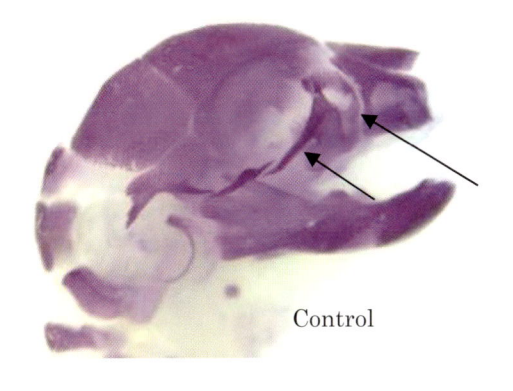

Control

Species	Rat: Crl:CD(SD)
Memo	Misshapen maxilla with Misshapen zygomatic arch (infraorbital foremen and zygomatic process: 10543) and Misshapen mandible (10469). The lower photograph shows normal features (arrow).
	上顎骨形態異常：上顎骨と頬骨のつながりが変化し、眼窩下孔及び頬骨突起の形が異なる（頬骨弓形態異常、10543）。下顎骨形態異常（10469）を伴う。下写真は正常（矢印）

1-12 Continued

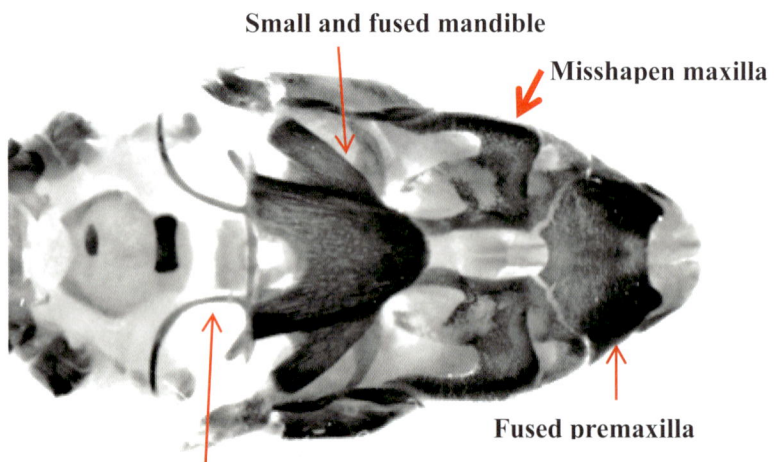

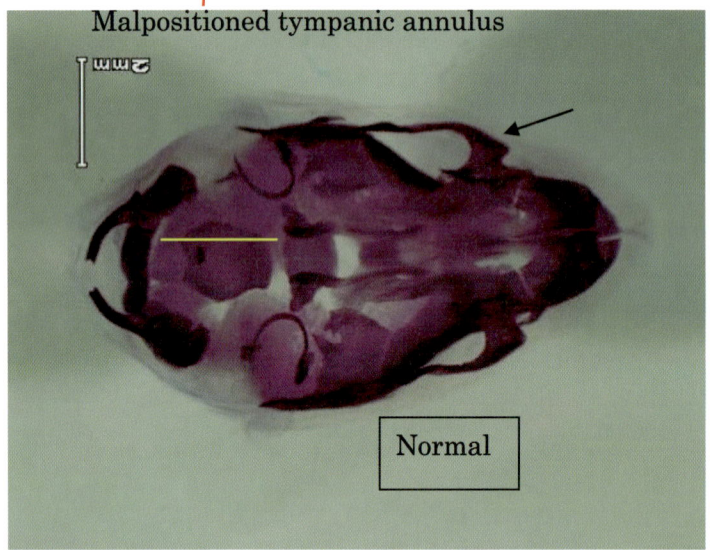

Small and fused mandible
Misshapen maxilla
Fused premaxilla
Malpositioned tympanic annulus

Normal

Species	Rat
Memo	Misshapen maxilla (red thick arrow) with Malpositioned tympanic annulus (New), Small (10470) and Fused (10467) mandible and Fused premaxilla (10500) The lower photograph shows normal features.
	上顎骨形態異常：鼓室輪位置異常（New）、下顎骨の小型（10470）及び癒合（10467）並びに顎間骨癒合（10500）も伴っている。

1-13 Small maxilla　　上顎骨小型（化）　**(10476)**

Species	Rabbit
Memo	Small maxilla with Small nasal bone (10483) and Small premaxilla (10504): The premaxilla (incisive bone) is abnormally shaped and the maxilla is slightly shorter than normal. The right photograph shows normal features.
	上顎骨小型（化）：顎間骨（切歯骨）側の形態異常があり、軽度に短縮している。鼻骨小型（化）（10483）及び顎間骨（切歯骨）小型（化）（10504）を伴う。

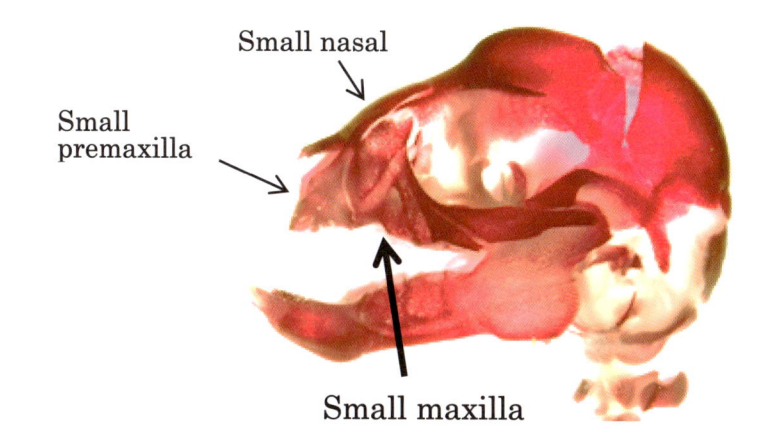

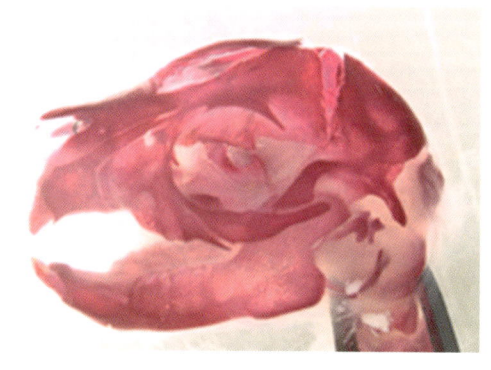

Small nasal
Small premaxilla
Small maxilla

Normal

1-14   Fused nasal bone   鼻骨癒合   (10479)

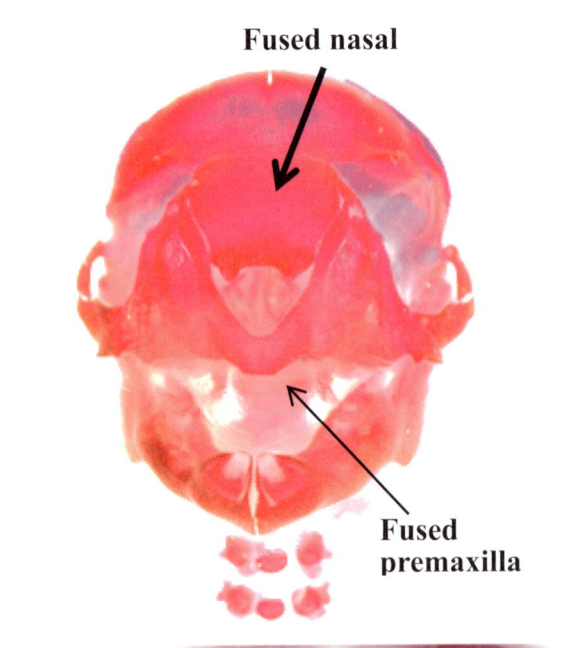

Fused nasal

Fused premaxilla

Species	Rabbit
Memo	Fused nasal bone with Fused premaxillae (10500): The right and left nasal bones fused.
	鼻骨癒合：左右が癒合している。顎間骨（切歯骨）癒合（10500）も伴う。

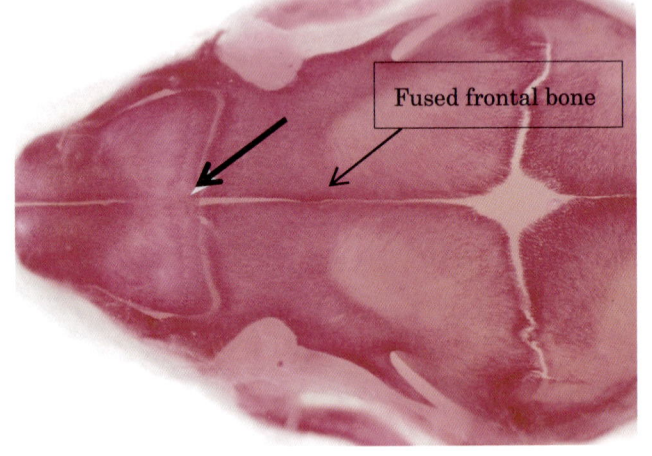

Fused frontal bone

Species	Rabbit
Memo	Fused nasal bone with Fused frontal bone (10441): The right and left nasal bones fused.
	鼻骨癒合：左右が癒合している。前頭骨癒合（10441）も伴う。

1-15 Misshapen nasal bones 鼻骨形態異常 (10481)

Species	Rat
Memo	Misshapen nasal bone: The nasal bones are small and fused, and the nasal cavity is considered to be single. This fetus has "Cyclopia (10027)" in the external examination. Cranio-facial bones are generally hypogenetic or grossly under-developed; the mandible is absent (10466); and the parietal and interparietal bones, maxilla, premaxilla and palatine, which form the skull and facial bones, are severely malformed. The external photograph of this fetus is shown on the right.
	鼻骨形態異常：鼻骨は矮小化及び癒合しており、単鼻腔と思われる。外表では単眼（10027）である。頭蓋・顔面骨には全体的に発生障害が認められる。特に下顎骨は欠損（10466）し、前頭・顔面を形成する前頭骨、頭頂骨、上顎骨、顎間骨（切歯骨）、口蓋骨は原型を留めていない。参考までに本胎児の外表写真を添付する。

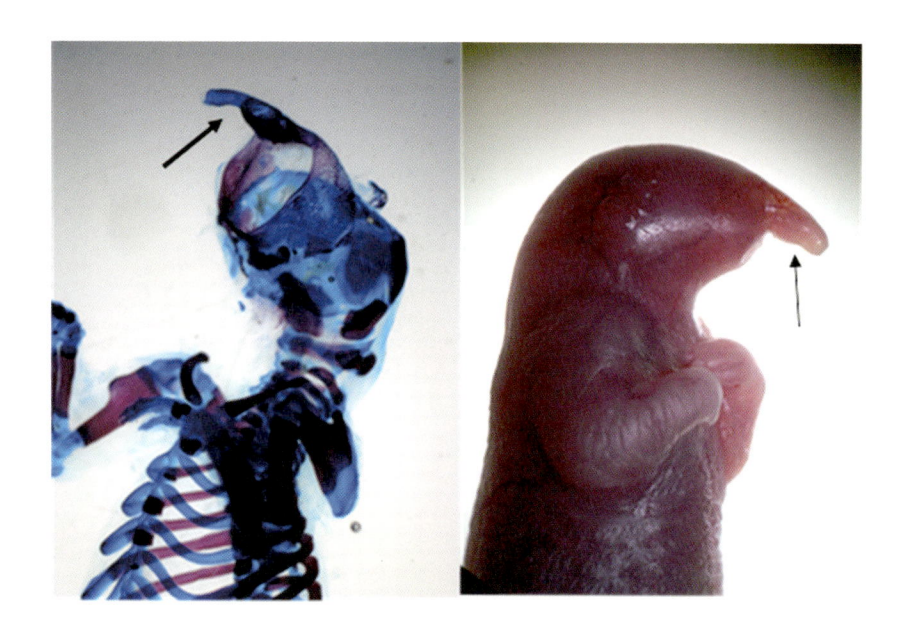

1-15 Continued

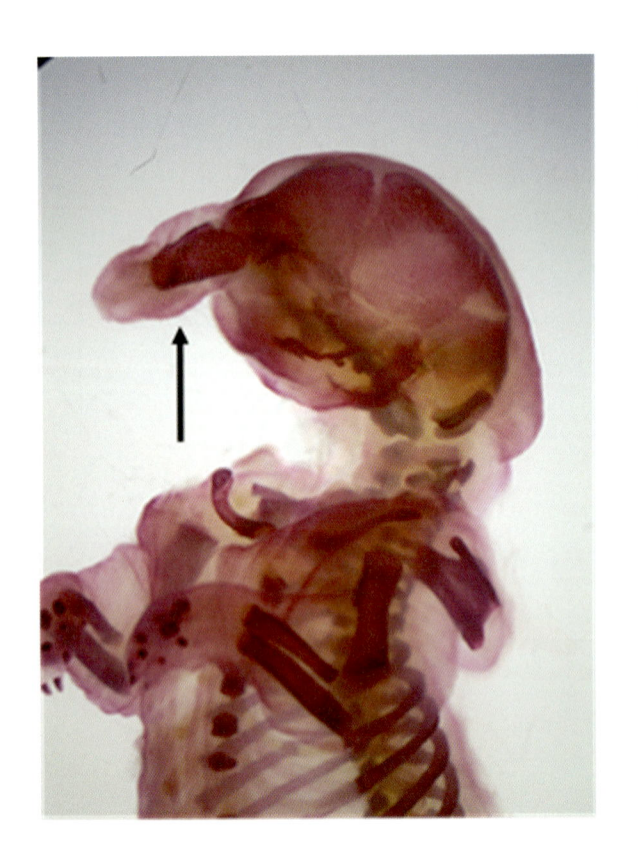

Species	Rat
Memo	Misshapen nasal bone: The nasal bones are small and fused, and the nasal cavity is considered to be single. This fetus has "Cyclopia (10027)" in the external examination. Facial bones are generally hypogenetic or grossly under-developed; the mandible is small (10470) and fused (10467), and the maxilla, premaxilla and palatine, which form the facial bones, are severely malformed.
	鼻骨形態異常：鼻骨は矮小化及び癒合しており、単鼻腔と思われる。外表では単眼（10027）である。顔面骨には全体的に発生障害が認められる。下顎骨は小型化（10470）、癒合（10467）し、口蓋骨、上顎骨及び顎間骨（切歯骨）は原型を留めていない。

1-16 Small nasal bone   鼻骨小型（化）   (10483)

Species	Rabbit
Memo	Small nasal bone with Small maxilla (10476) and Small premaxilla (10504)
	鼻骨小型（化）：上顎骨小型（化）（10476）及び顎間骨（切歯骨）小型（化）（10504）を伴う。

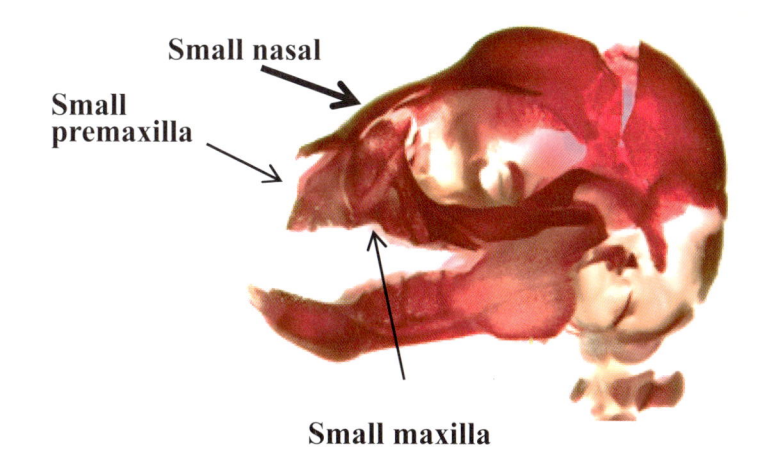

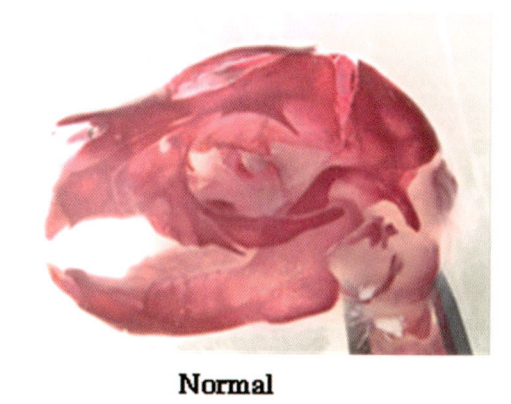

1-16 Continued

Species	Rat
Memo	Small nasal bone (thick arrow) with Misshapen frontal bone (10443), Misshapen parietal bone (10495), Small premaxilla (10504), and Short mandible (New): This fetus may appear as "Domed head (10012)" in the external examination.
	鼻骨小型（化）（太矢印）：本胎児は外表ではドーム状頭部（10012）であり、前頭骨形態異常（10443）、頭頂骨形態異常（10495）、顎間骨小型（化）（10504）及び下顎骨短小（化）（New）を伴う。

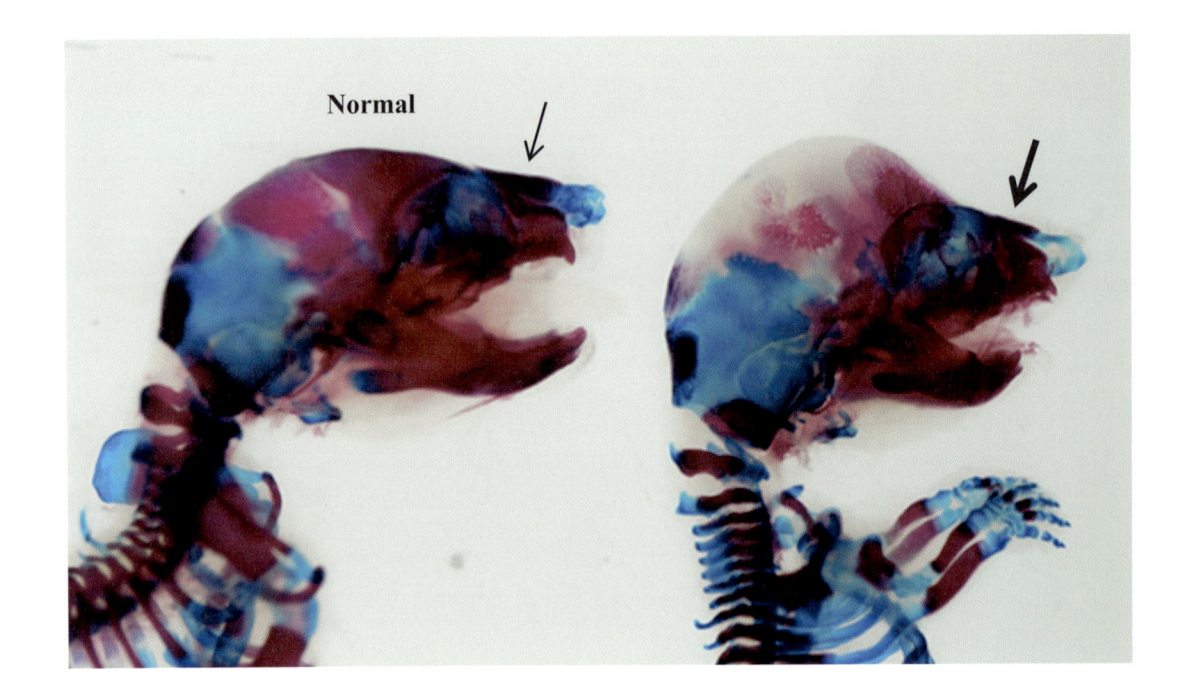

1-17 Hole in the parietal bone 　　頭頂骨孔　(10496)

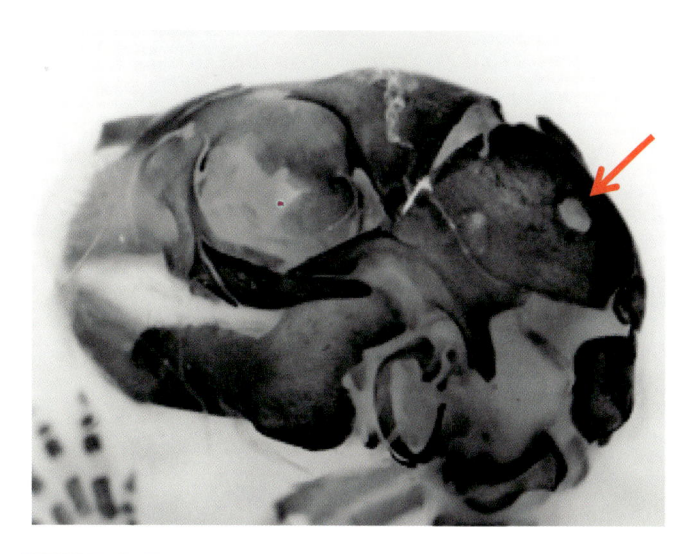

Species	Rabbit
Memo	Hole in the parietal bone (arrow)
	頭頂骨孔（矢印）

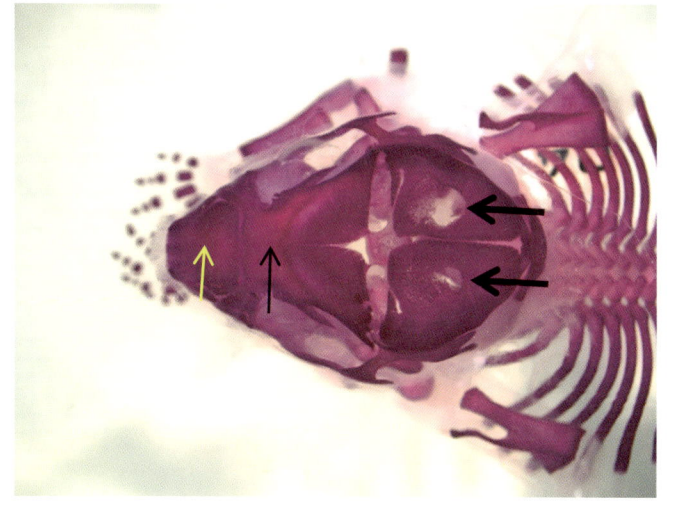

Species	Rabbit
Memo	Hole in the parietal bone (thick arrow) with Fused frontal bone (10441, black thin arrow) and Fused nasal bone (10479, yellow thin arrow)
	頭頂骨孔（太矢印）：前頭骨癒合（10441、細黒矢印）及び鼻骨癒合（10479、細黄矢印）を伴う。

1-18 Misshapen parietal bone   頭頂骨形態異常   (10495)

Species	Rat
Memo	Misshapen parietal bone (thick arrow) with Misshapen frontal bone (10443), Small nasal bone (10483), Small premaxilla (10504), and Short mandible (New): This fetus may appear as "Domed head (10012)" in external examination. The left fetus shows normal features.
	頭頂骨形態異常（太矢印）：本胎児は外表ではドーム状頭部（10012）であり、前頭骨形態異常（10443）、鼻骨小型化（10483）、顎間骨小型化（10504）及び下顎骨短小（New）を伴う。左は正常胎児。

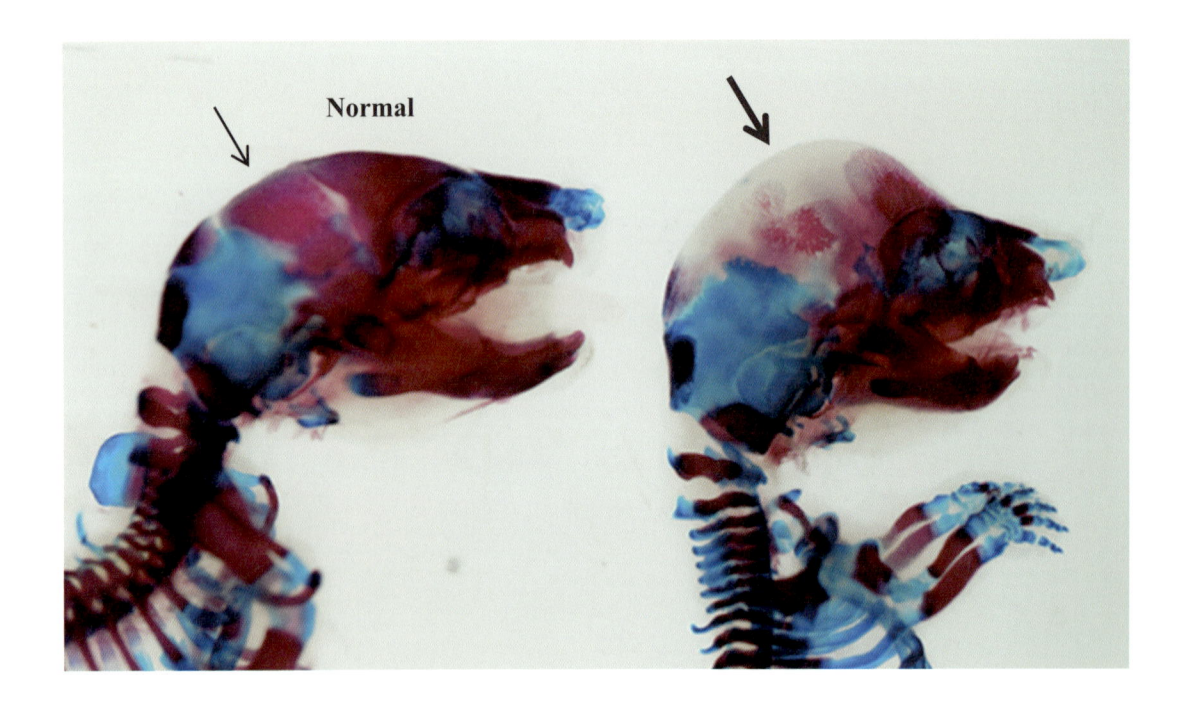

1-19　Split parietal bone　　頭頂骨分離　(New)

Species	Rabbit
Memo	Split parietal bone: A part of the parietal bone is isolated (arrow). The term, Split parietal bone, is recommended for the specimens below, although these may also be considered as "Supernumerary sutures in the skull (New)" or "Unossified line in the parietal bone (New)".
	頭頂骨分離：頭頂骨の一部が分離している（矢印）。頭蓋骨過剰縫合線（New）あるいは頭蓋骨線状未骨化（New）とも考えられるが、「頭頂骨分離」が推奨される。

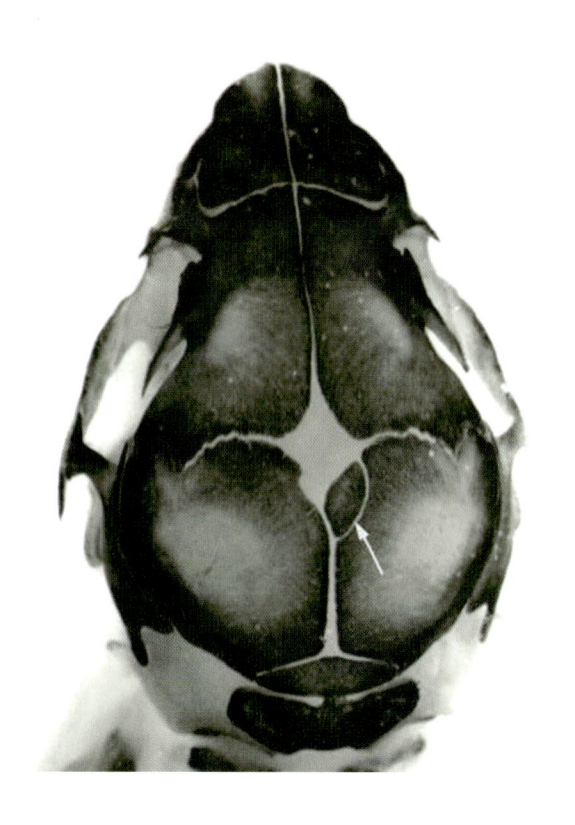

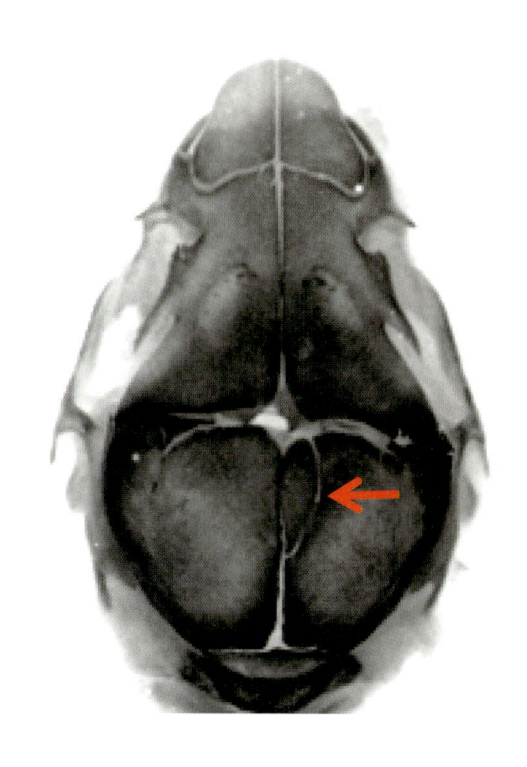

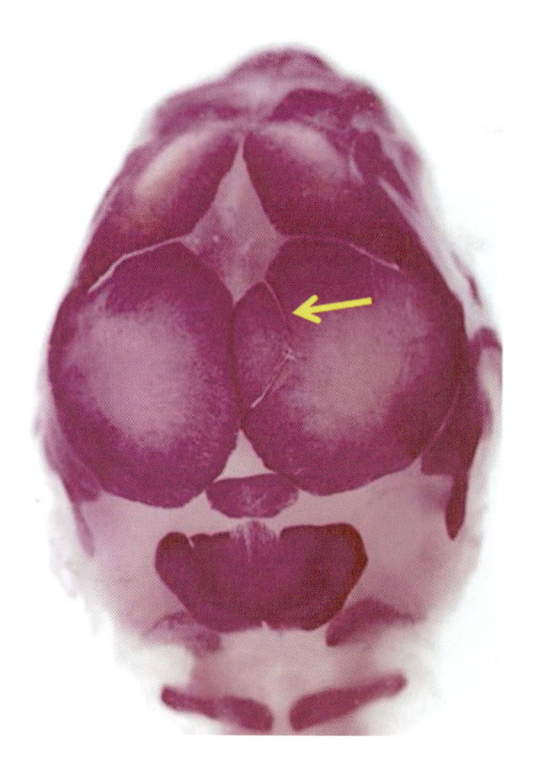

1-20   **Unossified area in the parietal bone**   頭頂骨未骨化領域   (New)

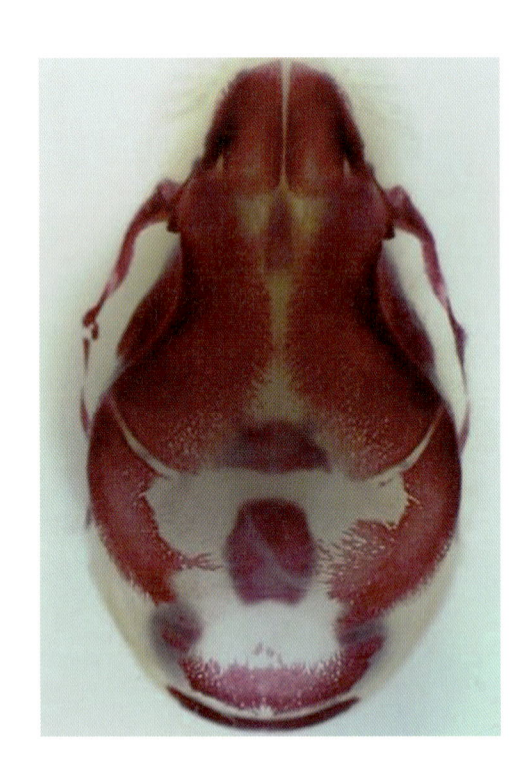

Species	Rat
Memo	Unossified area in the parietal bone: A part of the parietal bone dose not ossify.
	頭頂骨未骨化領域：頭頂骨の一部が骨化していない。

1-21　Fused premaxilla　　顎間骨（切歯骨）癒合　(10500)

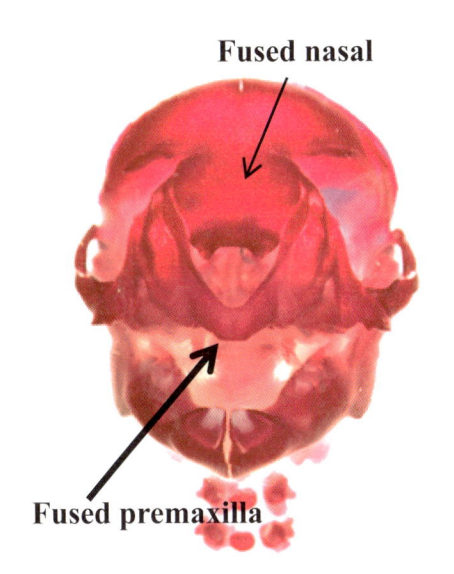

Species	Rabbit
Memo	Fused premaxilla with Fused nasal bone (10479): The right and left premaxillae fused.
	顎間骨（切歯骨）癒合：左右が癒合している。鼻骨癒合（10479）も伴う。

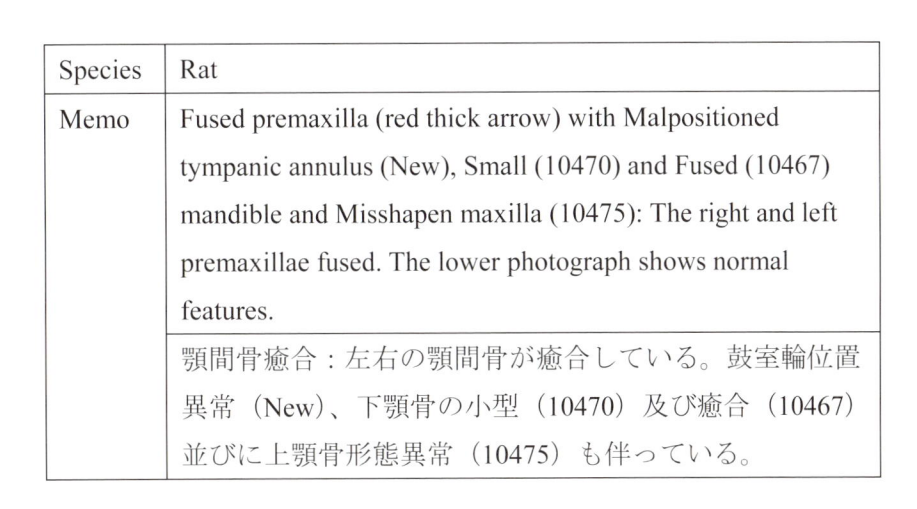

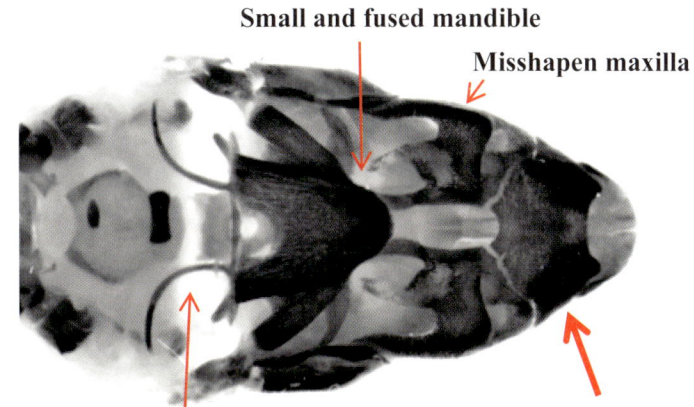

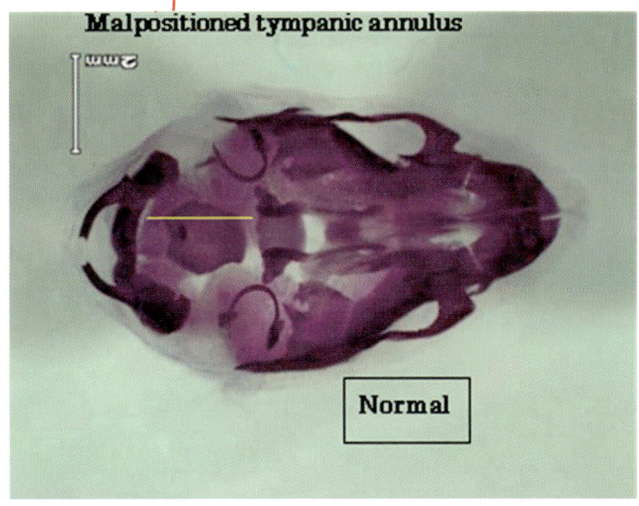

Species	Rat
Memo	Fused premaxilla (red thick arrow) with Malpositioned tympanic annulus (New), Small (10470) and Fused (10467) mandible and Misshapen maxilla (10475): The right and left premaxillae fused. The lower photograph shows normal features.
	顎間骨癒合：左右の顎間骨が癒合している。鼓室輪位置異常（New）、下顎骨の小型（10470）及び癒合（10467）並びに上顎骨形態異常（10475）も伴っている。

1-22 Malpositioned premaxilla 顎間骨（切歯骨）位置異常 (New)

Species	Rat、SD
Memo	Malpositioned premaxilla: The right and left premaxilla are misaligned at the frontal view, although the lateral view did not show any abnormality. The right photograph shows normal features.
	顎間骨（切歯骨）位置異常：左右顎間骨の位置が上下にずれている。側面からの観察では形態に異常はない。

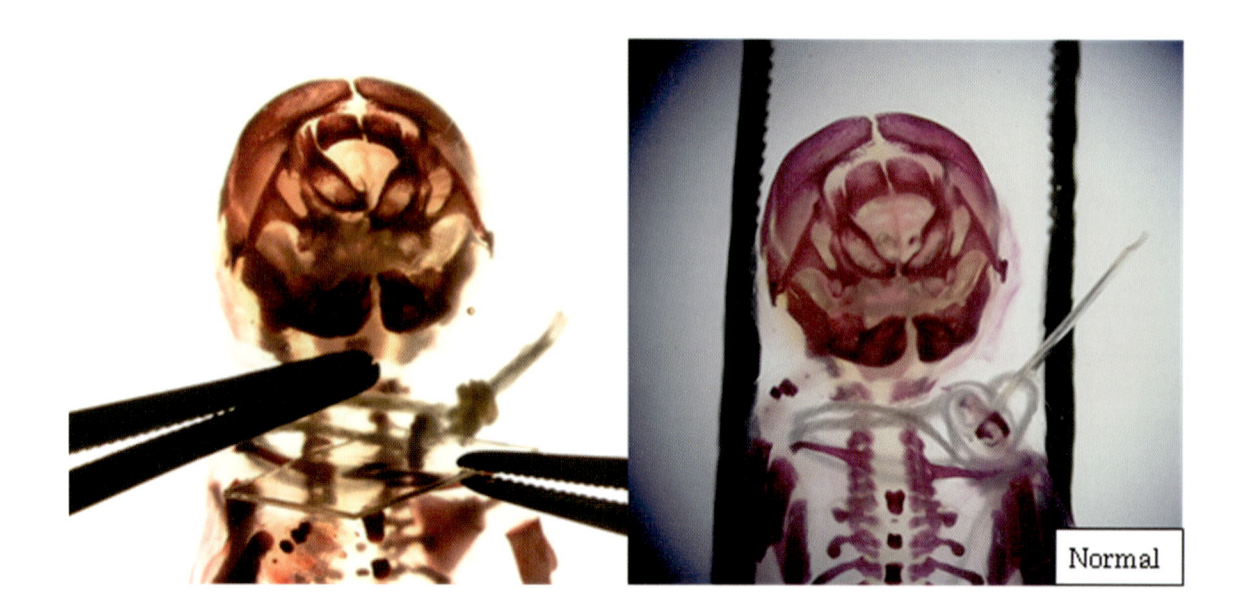

1-23　**Misshapen premaxilla**　顎間骨（切歯骨）形態異常　(10502)

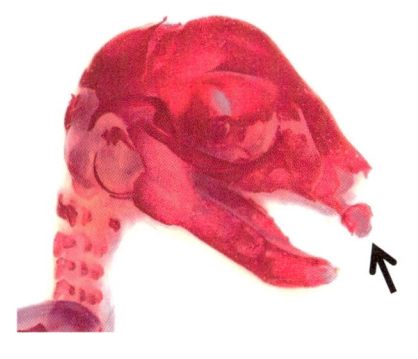

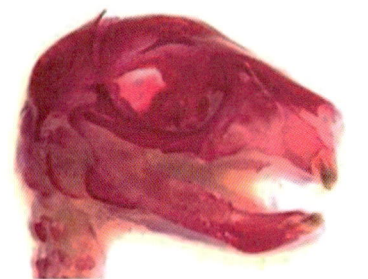

Species	Rabbit
Memo	Misshapen premaxilla (arrow): This bone may also be called incisive bone. The lower photograph shows normal features.
	顎間骨形態異常（切歯骨とも言う）、下写真は正常胎児

Normal

1-24 Small premaxilla　　顎間骨（切歯骨）小型（化）　**(10504)**

Species	Rabbit
Memo	Small premaxilla (thick arrow) with Small maxilla (10476) and Small nasal bone (10483): The right photograph shows normal features.
	顎間骨（切歯骨）小型（化）（太矢印）：上顎骨小型（化）（10476）及び鼻骨小型（化）（10483）を伴う。右写真は正常胎児

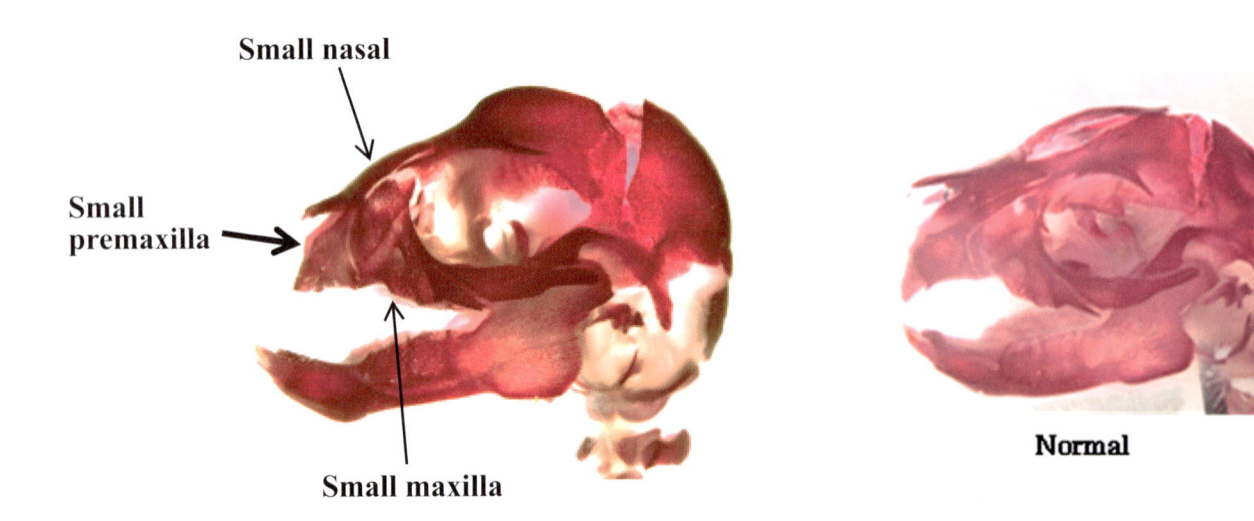

1-24 Continued

Species	Rat
Memo	Small premaxilla (thick arrow) with Misshapen frontal bone (10443), Misshapen parietal bone (10495), Small nasal bone (10483), and Short mandible (New): This fetus may appear as "Domed head (10012)" in the external examination.
	顎間骨（切歯骨）小型（化）（太矢印）：本胎児は外表ではドーム状頭部（10012）であり、前頭骨形態異常（10443）、頭頂骨形態異常（10495）、鼻骨小型（化）（10483）及び下顎骨短小（化）(New)を伴う。

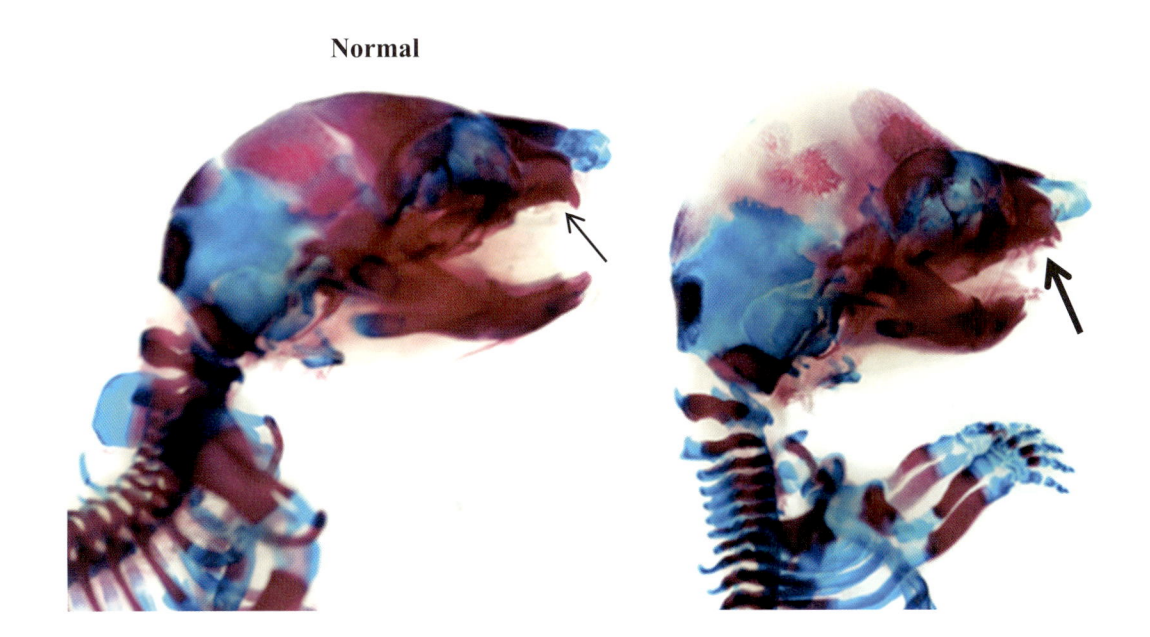

Normal

1-25　**Absent tympanic annulus**　　鼓室輪欠損　(10528)

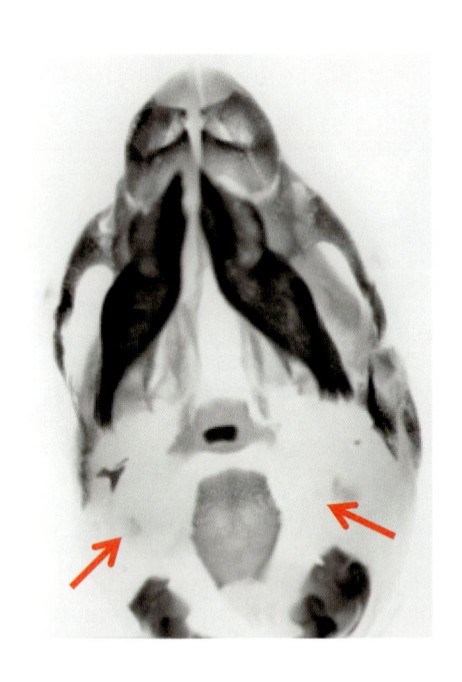

Species	Rat
Memo	Absent tympanic annulus (arrow): This should not be confused with "Unossified tympanic annulus (10533)".
	鼓室輪欠損（矢印）：鼓室輪の未骨化 (10533) の場合もあるので、観察に注意が必要。

1-26   Malpositioned tympanic annulus   鼓室輪位置異常   (New)

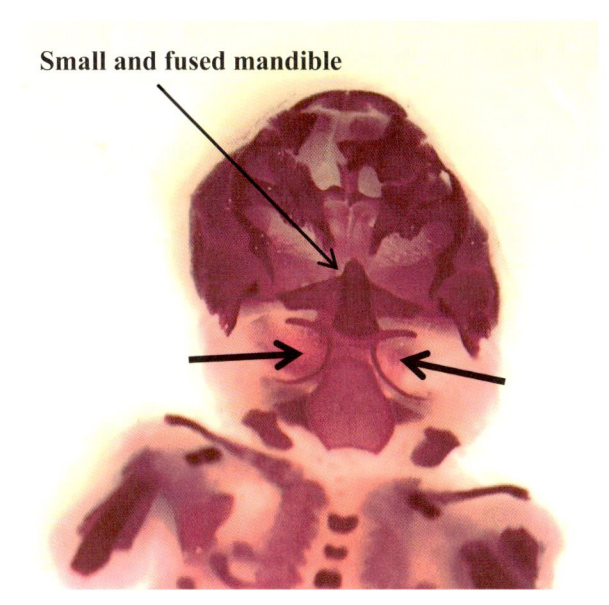

Small and fused mandible

Species	Rat
Memo	Malpositioned tympanic annulus: Both tympanic annuli moved to the center. This fetus had Small (10470) and Fused (10467) mandible, so it may appear as "Otocephaly" in external examination.
	鼓室輪位置異常：左右の鼓室輪が中央に寄っている。下顎骨の小型（10470）及び癒合（10467）を伴う。おそらく外表では耳頭症と考える。

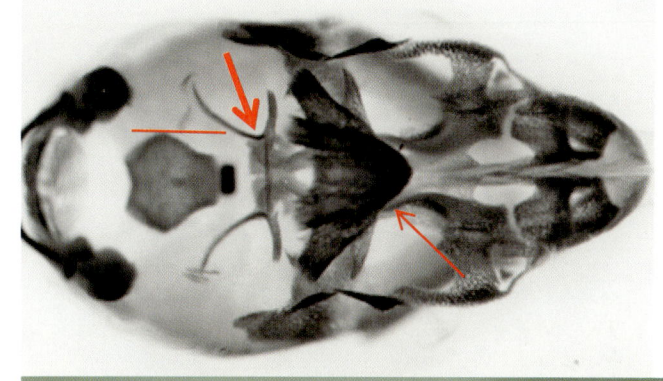

Species	Rat
Memo	Malpositioned tympanic annulus (thick arrow) with Small (10470) and Fused (10467) mandible (thin arrow): Tympanic annulus moves to the center. This anomaly is usually observed in a fetus with Malpositioned auricle (10021) (Otocephaly).
	鼓室輪位置異常：鼓室輪が中央に寄っている。外表で耳介の位置異常（10021）、特に「耳頭症」が見られた胎児にこの所見が見られる。下顎骨の小型（10470）及び癒合（10467）も伴っている。

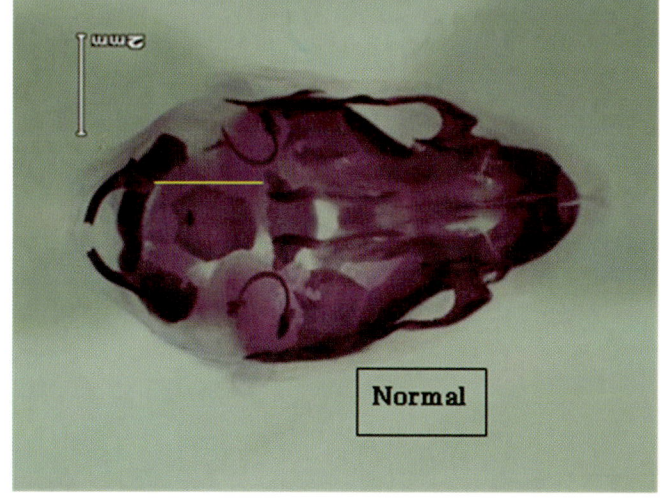

Normal

1-27   Fused zygomatic arch   頬骨弓癒合   (10541)

Species	Rat
Memo	Fused zygomatic arch (red arrow): The right photograph shows normal features.
	頬骨弓癒合（矢印）、右写真は正常胎児

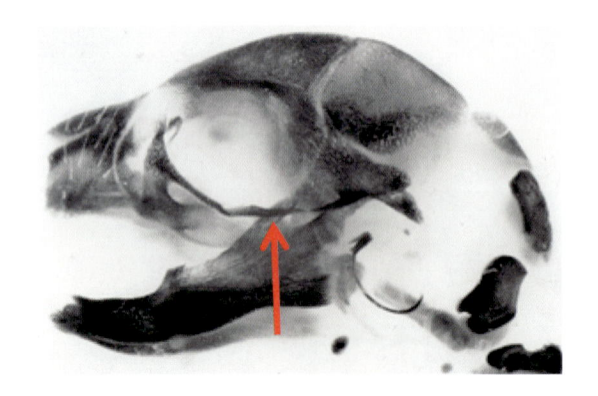

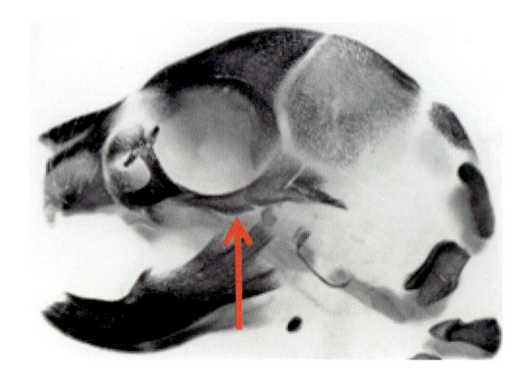

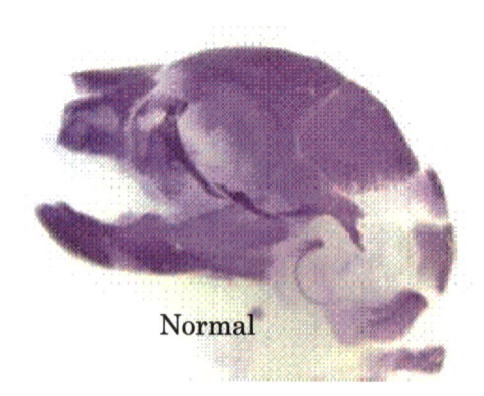

Normal

1-28　Misshapen zygomatic arch　　頬骨弓形態異常　(10543)

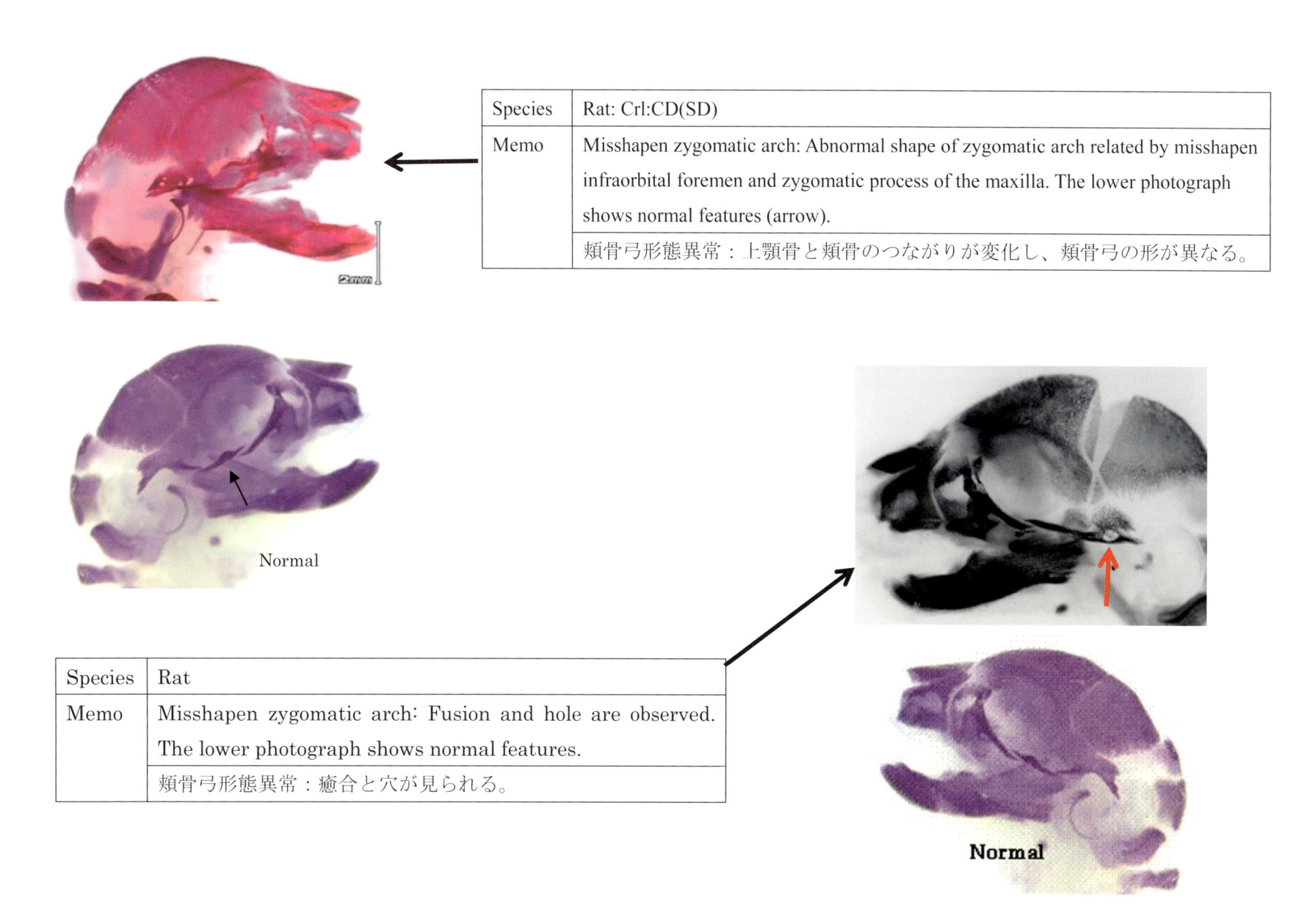

Species	Rat: Crl:CD(SD)
Memo	Misshapen zygomatic arch: Abnormal shape of zygomatic arch related by misshapen infraorbital foremen and zygomatic process of the maxilla. The lower photograph shows normal features (arrow).
	頬骨弓形態異常：上顎骨と頬骨のつながりが変化し、頬骨弓の形が異なる。

Species	Rat
Memo	Misshapen zygomatic arch: Fusion and hole are observed. The lower photograph shows normal features.
	頬骨弓形態異常：癒合と穴が見られる。

1-29　Large fontanelle　　泉門大型（化）　　(10405)

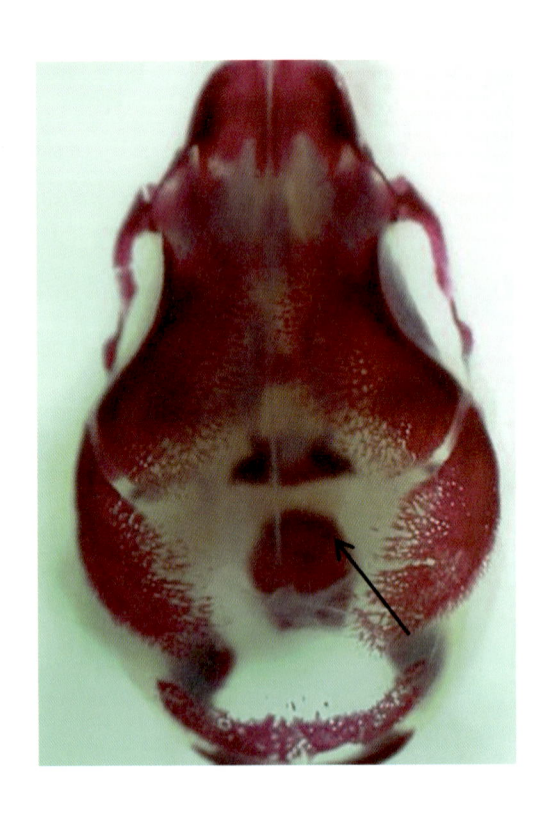

Species	Rat
Memo	Large fontanelle: Large unossified area in the skull. This finding is determined by a wide opening between the frontal and parietal bones (arrow) and a wide opening at the dome of the skull. Compare this with "Unossified area in the parietal bone (1-17)".
	頭蓋骨泉門大型（化）：前頭骨と頭頂骨の間が広く、また、頭部全体の形（幅が広い）から判断し、「泉門大型」とした。「頭頂骨未骨化領域（1-17）」と区分した。

1-30 Sutural bone   縫合骨   (New)

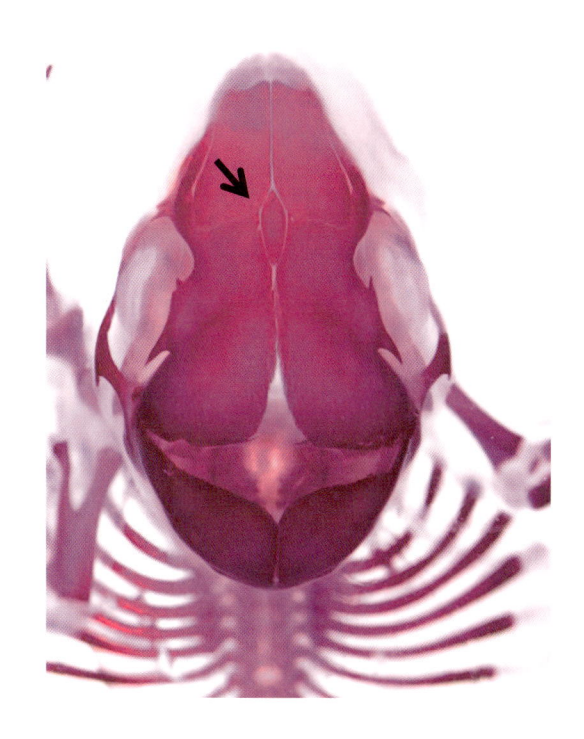

Species	Rabbit
Memo	Sutural bone, Isolated bone, or Supernumerary bone: Additional bone is observed in the area between the frontal and nasal bones (arrow).
	縫合骨、遊離骨、過剰骨：前頭骨と鼻骨の接合部に過剰な縫合骨がある（矢印）。

Photographs of Skeletal Anomalies

2. Clavicle and Scapula

2-1　Bent clavicle　　鎖骨弯曲　(10547)

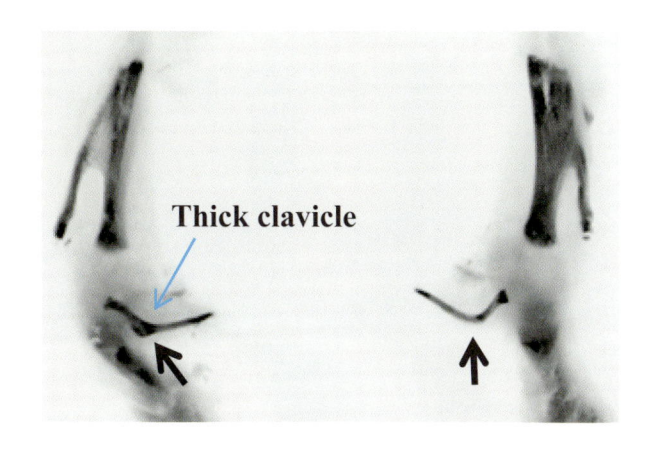

Species	Rabbit
Memo	Bent clavicle (arrow) with Thick clavicle (Partial, 10551)
	鎖骨弯曲（矢印）：鎖骨部分肥厚（10551）を伴う。

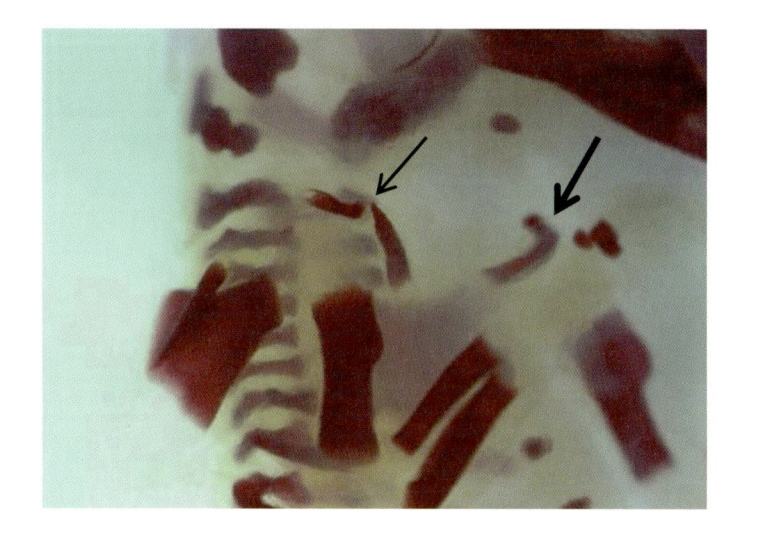

Species	Rat
Memo	Bent clavicle with Misshapen clavicle (10549): The left clavicle is bent (thick arrow), and the right clavicle splits at the center (thin arrow).
	鎖骨弯曲：左鎖骨が弯曲している（太矢印）。右鎖骨は分離している（細矢印、形態異常：10549）

2-2 Misshapen clavicle 鎖骨形態異常 (10549)

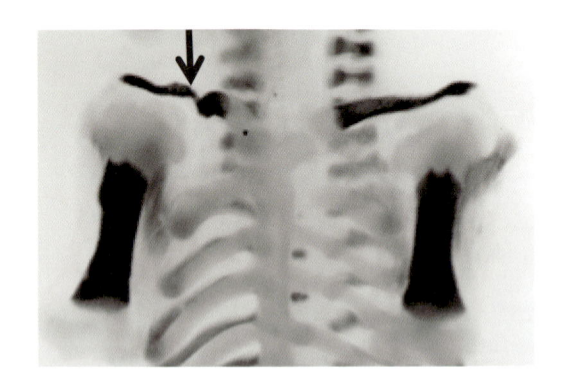

Species	Rat
Memo	Misshapen clavicle (arrow)
	鎖骨形態異常（矢印）

Species	Rat
Memo	Misshapen clavicle: with hole in the clavicle (arrow)
	鎖骨形態異常：鎖骨にホールあり（矢印）。

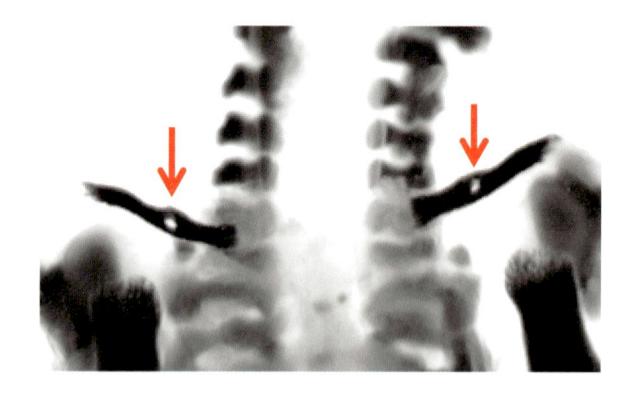

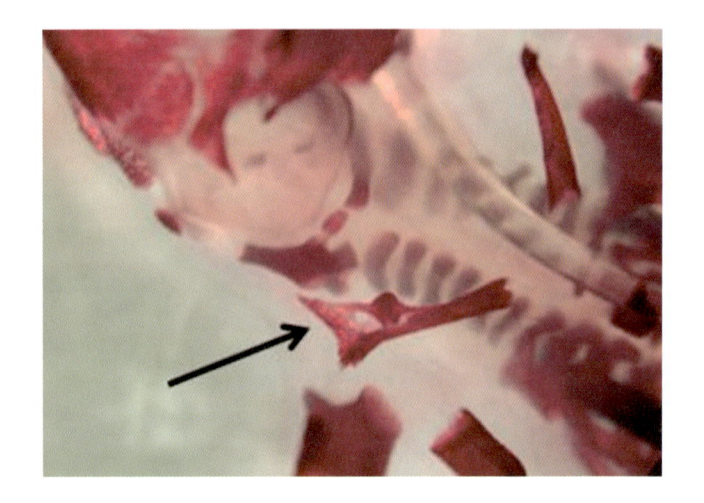

Species	Rat
Memo	Misshapen clavicle: Abnormally shaped clavicle which contains a hole (arrow).
	鎖骨形態異常：形が異常で、穴がある（矢印）。

2-3   **Thick clavicle**   鎖骨肥厚（化）   **(10551)**

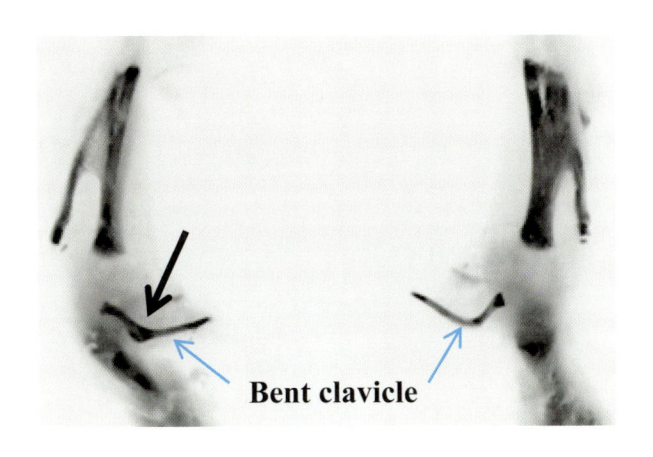

Species	Rabbit
Memo	Partially thick clavicle (black arrow) with Bent clavicle (blue arrow, 10547)
	鎖骨部分肥厚（化）：鎖骨弯曲（10547）を伴う。

2-4 Bent scapula　　肩甲骨弯曲　(10554)

Species	Rat
Memo	Bent scapula (thick arrow) and Bent humerus (10560)
	肩甲骨弯曲（太矢印）：上腕骨弯曲（10560）を伴う。

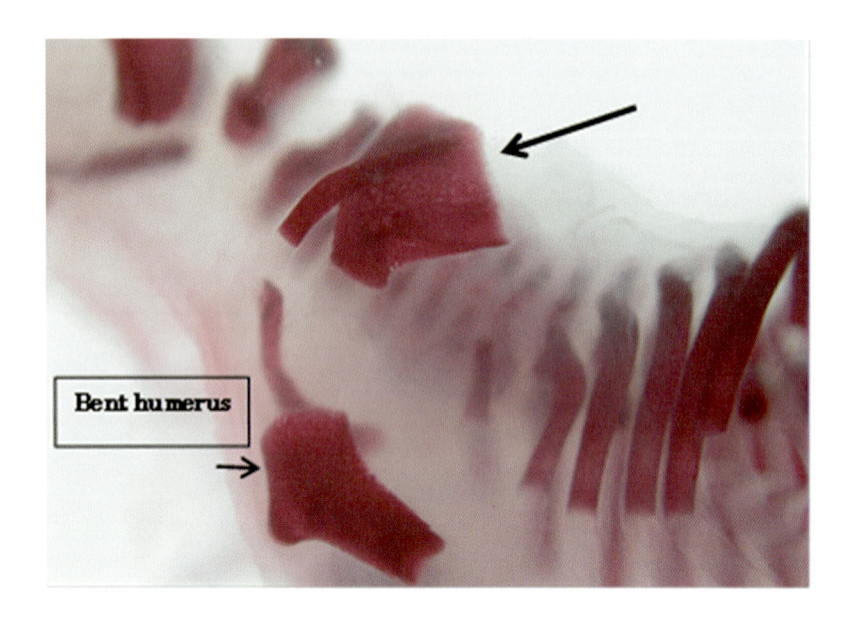

2-5 Misshapen scapula　　肩甲骨形態異常　(10556)

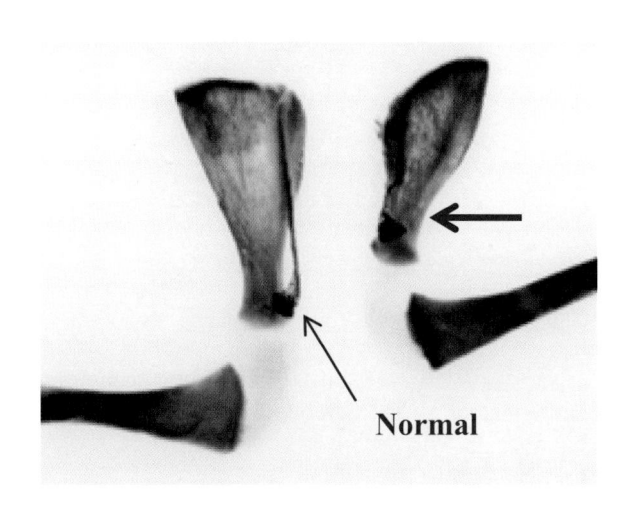

Species	Rabbit
Memo	Misshapen scapula (thick arrow): with abnormally shaped acromion process.
	肩甲骨形態異常：肩峰突起の形態異常（太矢印）

2-6　**Small scapula**　　肩甲骨小型（化）　　**(New)**

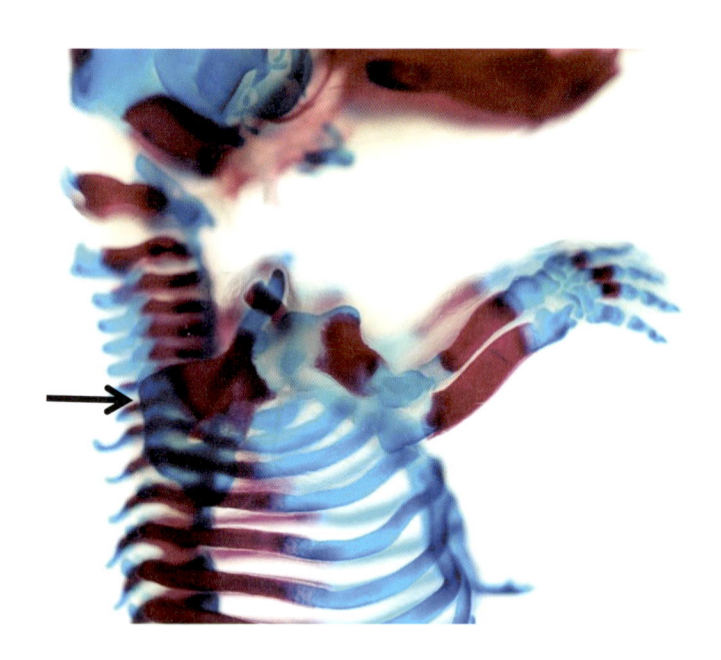

Species	Rat
Memo	Small scapula (thick arrow) with Short humerus (10565), Short radius (10574) and Short ulna (10583)
	肩甲骨小型（化）（太矢印）：上腕骨短小（化）（10565）、橈骨短小（化）（10574）及び尺骨短小（化）（10583）を伴う。

Photographs of Skeletal Anomalies

3. Forelimb

3-1 Misshapen humerus 上腕骨形態異常 (10564)

Species	Rat
Memo	Misshapen humerus (red arrow) with Short femur (10806), Short tibia (10824) and Short fibula (10815): The deltoid tuberosity is absent in this fetus. The right photograph shows normal features.
	上腕骨形態異常（赤矢印）：三角筋粗面の欠損。大腿骨の短小（10806）、脛骨の短小（10824）、腓骨の短小（10815）を伴う。右写真は正常胎児。

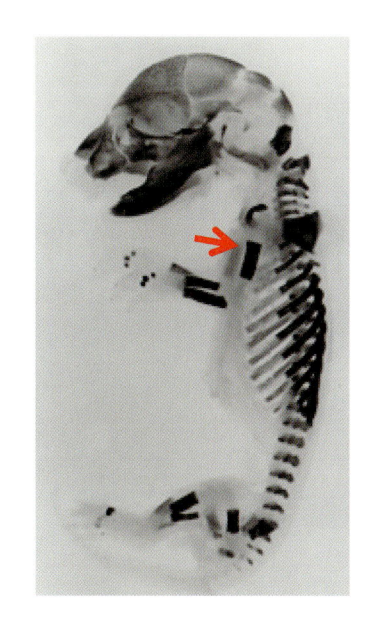

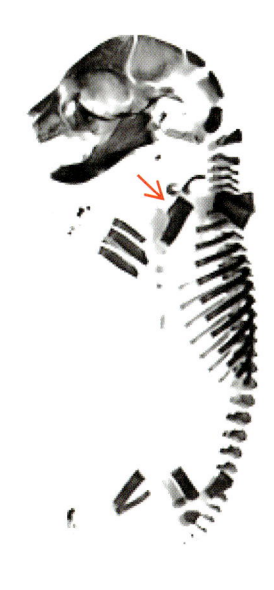

Normal

3-1 Continued

Species	Rat
Memo	Misshapen humerus (red arrow) with Absent forepaw phalanx (10602): The deltoid tuberosity is absent in this fetus.
	上腕骨形態異常（赤矢印）：三角筋粗面の欠損。指節骨欠損（10602）を伴う。

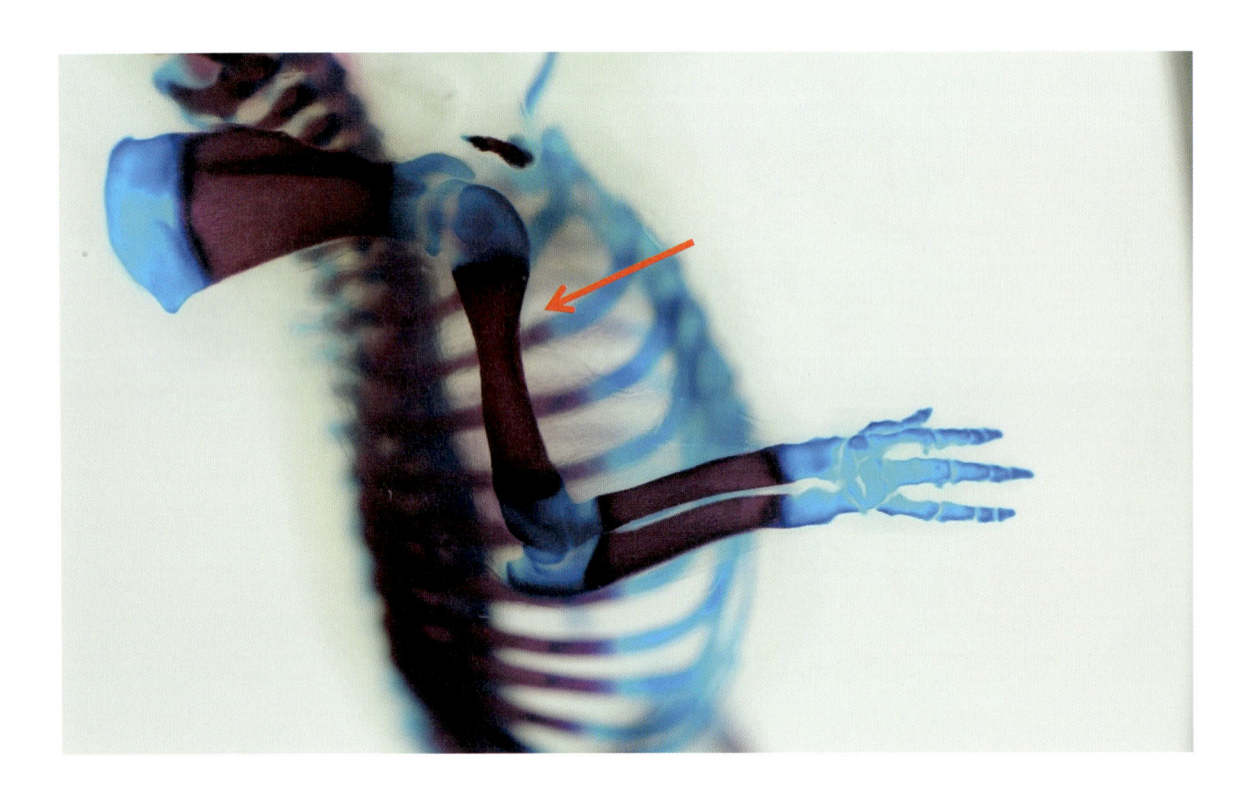

3-2 Short humerus　　上腕骨短小（化）　　**(10565)**

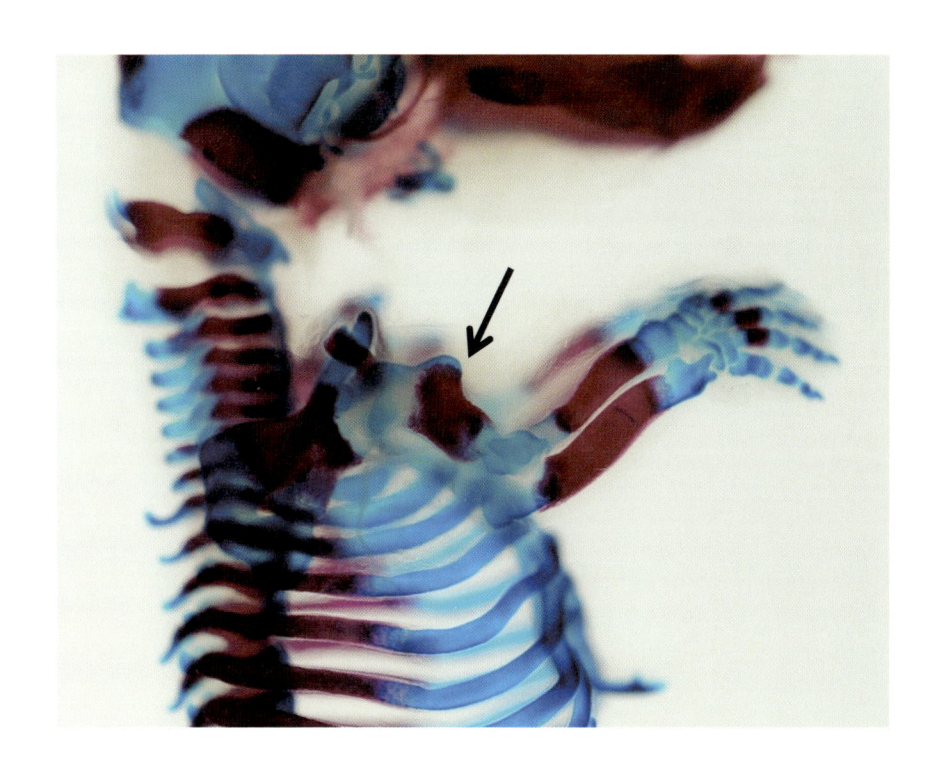

Species	Rat
Memo	Short humerus (arrow) with Small scapula (New), Short radius (10574) and Short ulna (10583): The humerus is short and shaped abnormally
	上腕骨短小（化）（矢印）：肩甲骨小型（化）（New）、橈骨短小（化）（10574）及び尺骨短小（化）（10583）を伴う。

3-3 Absent radius   橈骨欠損   (10568)

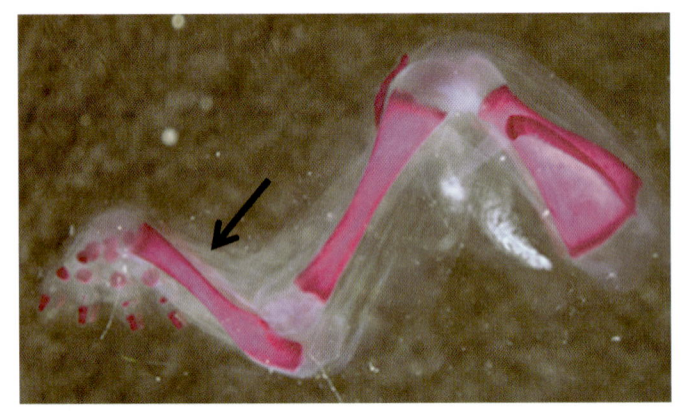

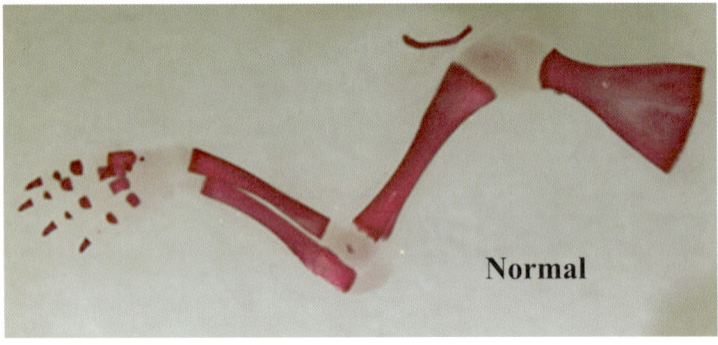

Species	Rabbit
Memo	Absent radius (thick arrow). The lower photograph shows normal features.
	橈骨欠損（太矢印）、下写真は正常胎児

Normal

3-4 Bent radius   橈骨弯曲 (10569)

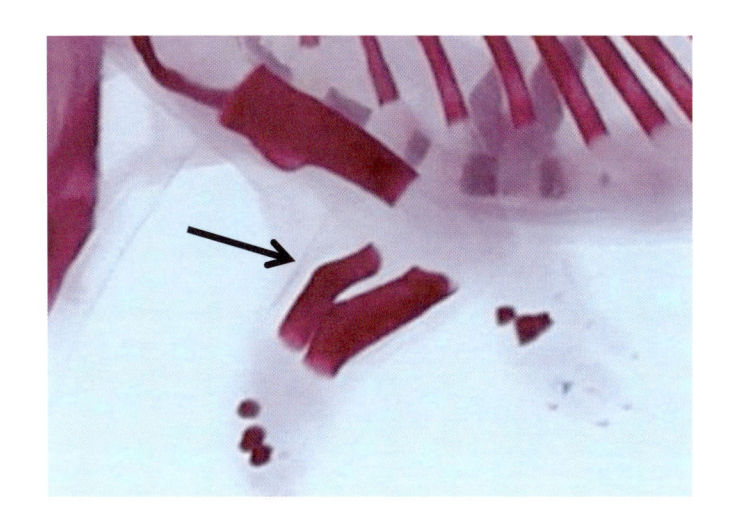

Species	Rat
Memo	Bent radius (arrow) with Bent ulna (10578)
	橈骨弯曲（矢印）：尺骨弯曲（10578）を伴う。

3-5 Misshapen radius 橈骨形態異常 (10573)

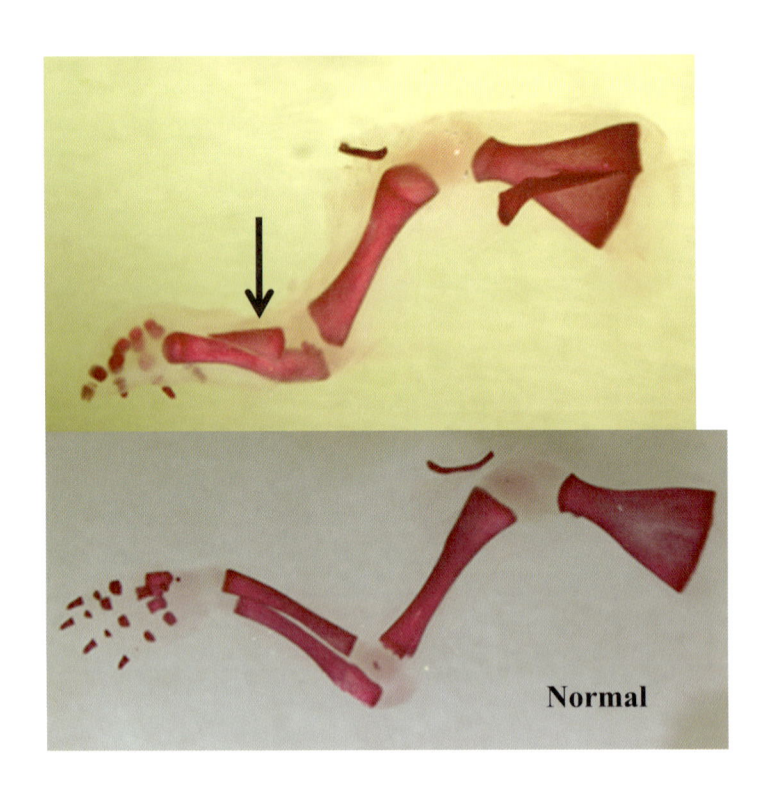

Species	Rabbit
Memo	Misshapen radius (thick arrow): The radius is short and cone-shaped. The lower photograph shows normal features.
	橈骨形態異常（太矢印）：短く、三角状になっている。下写真は正常胎児。

3-6 Short radius 橈骨短小（化） (10574)

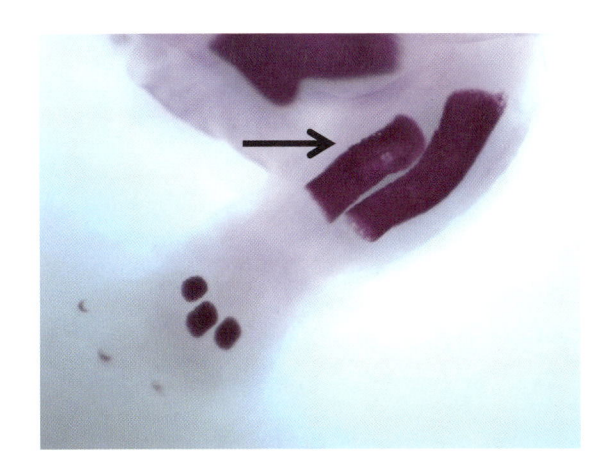

Species	Rat: Crl:CD(SD)
Memo	Short radius (arrow) and Bent ulna (10578)
	橈骨短小（化）（矢印）：尺骨弯曲（10578）を伴う。

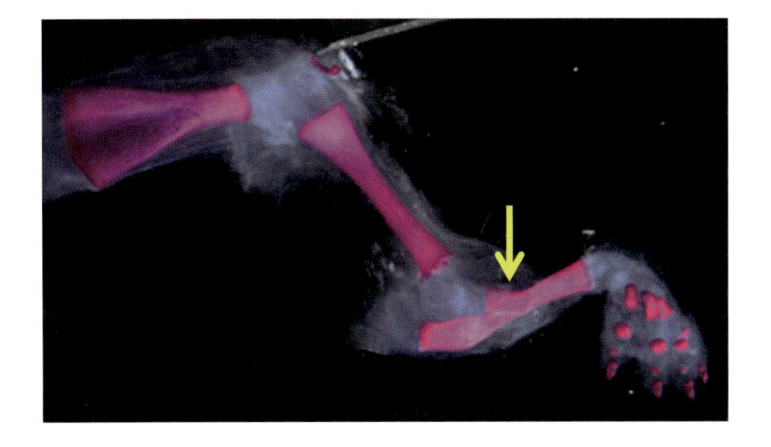

Species	Rabbit
Memo	Short radius (yellow arrow): This fetus shows Flexed paw (10087) and Oligodactyly (10081) in external observation.
	橈骨短小（化）（黄矢印）：外表では過屈曲手（10087）及び欠指（10080）を伴う。

3-7　Absent ulna　尺骨欠損　(10577)

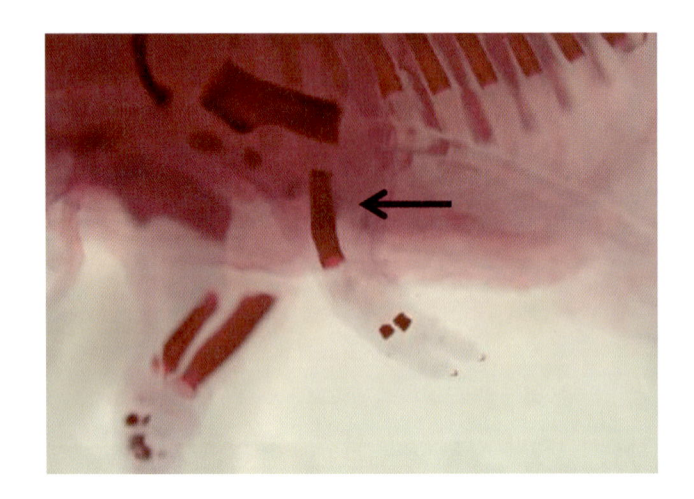

Species	Rat
Memo	Absent ulna (arrow) with Absent forepaw phalanx (10602)
	尺骨欠損（矢印）：指節骨欠損 (10602) を伴う。

3-8　Bent ulna　　尺骨弯曲　(10578)

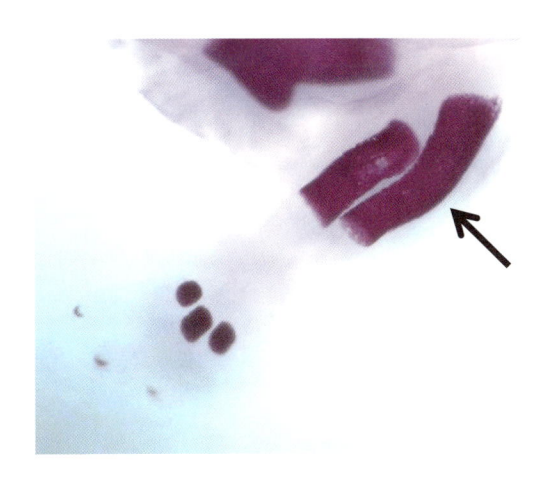

Species	Rat: Crl:CD(SD)
Memo	Bent ulna (arrow) and Short radius(10574)
	尺骨弯曲（矢印）：橈骨短小（10574）を伴う。

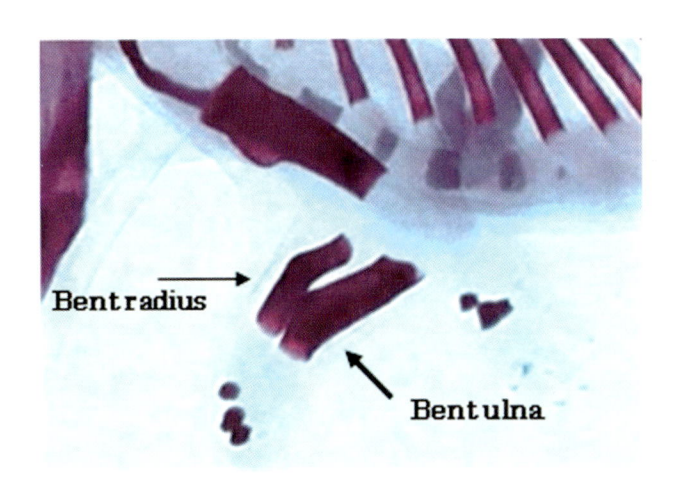

Species	Rat
Memo	Bent ulna (thick arrow) and Bent radius (10569)
	尺骨弯曲（太矢印）：橈骨弯曲（10569）を伴う。

Photographs of Skeletal Anomalies

4. Hindlimb

4-1　Bent femur　　大腿骨弯曲　(10801)

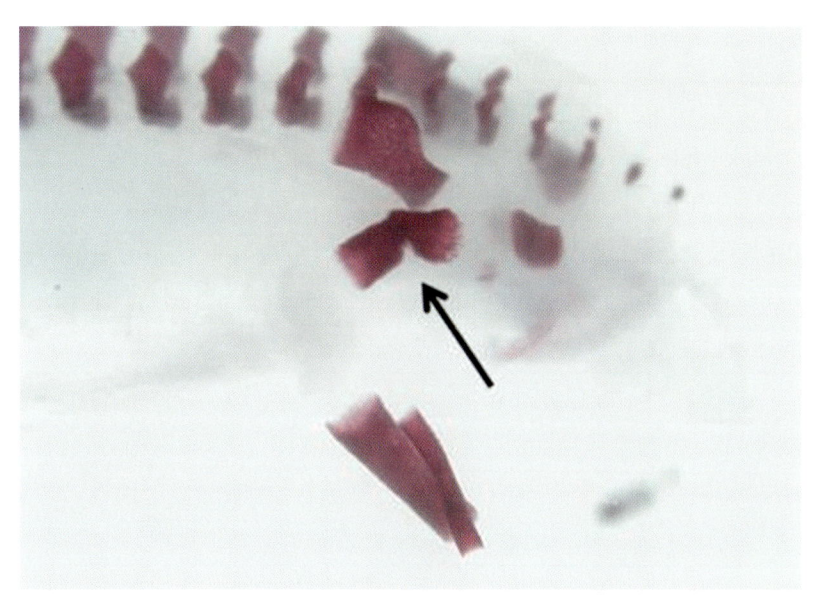

Species	Rat
Memo	Bent femur (arrow)
	大腿骨弯曲（矢印）

4-2　Misshapen femur　　大腿骨形態異常　(10805)

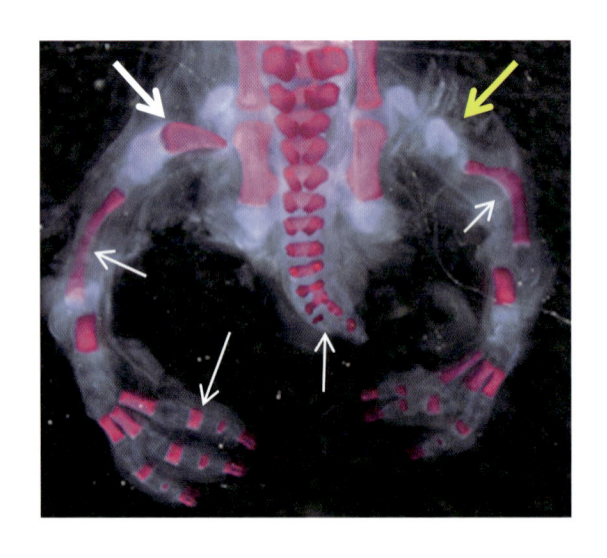

Species	Rabbit, Kbl:JW
Memo	Misshapen femur (thick white arrow) with Absent tibia (10818), Bent fibula (10810), Absent hindpaw phalanx (10860), Absent caudal vertebrae (10769), and Fused caudal vertebral arches (10753): Short and abnormally shaped right femur (thick white arrow) and small and unossified (10808) left femur (thick yellow arrow) are observed. This fetus may appear as "Phocomelia (10074)" in external examination.
	大腿骨形態異常（太矢印）：右大腿骨は短く、変形（白太矢印）、左大腿骨は小さく、未骨化（黄太矢印）である（10808）。脛骨欠損（10818）、腓骨弯曲（10810）、趾節骨欠損（10860）及び尾椎欠損（10769）、尾椎弓癒合（10753）を伴う。本胎児では外表異常としてフォコメリアが観察されている。

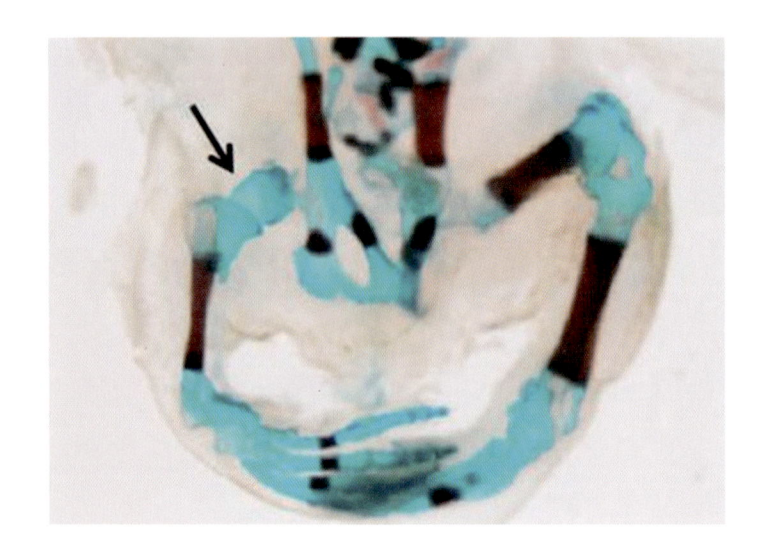

Species	Rat
Memo	Misshapen femur (arrow) with Absent tibia (10818) and Absent caudal vertebrae (10769): Unossified femur (10808) is confirmed in this double-stained specimen (arrow).
	大腿骨形態異常（矢印）：脛骨欠損（10818）及び尾椎欠損（10769）を伴う。未骨化の大腿骨（10808）が確認できる（矢印）二重染色標本

4-3 Short femur   大腿骨短小（化）   (10806)

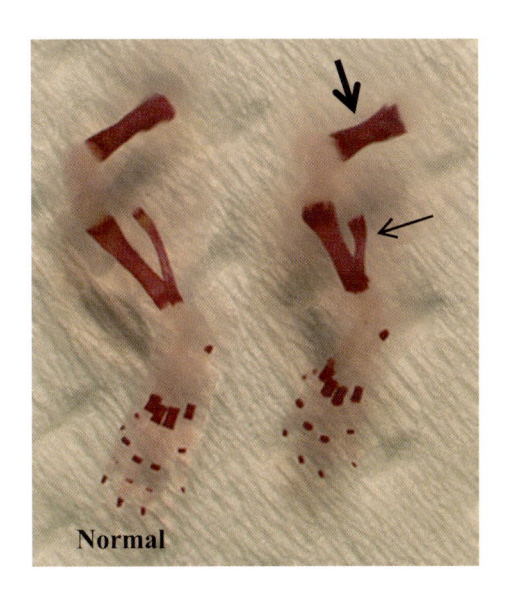

Species	Mouse
Memo	Short femur (thick arrow) with Short fibula (10815). The left specimen in the photograph shows normal features.
	大腿骨短小（化）（太矢印）：腓骨短小（化）（10815）を伴う。写真左は正常胎児。

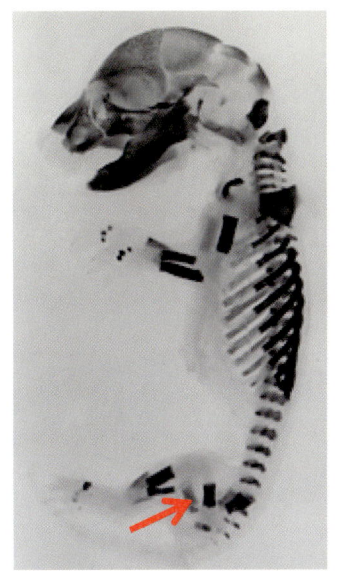

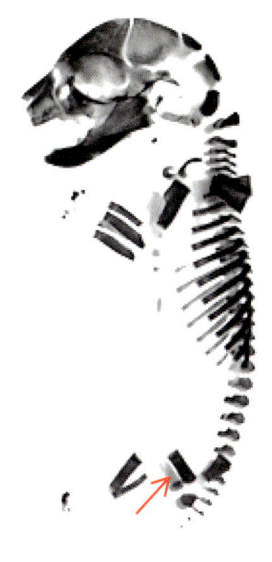

Species	Rat
Memo	Short femur (red arrow) with Misshapen humerus (10564), Short tibia (10824) and Short fibula (10815). The right photograph shows normal features.
	大腿骨の短小（化）（赤矢印）：上腕骨形態異常（10564）、脛骨の短小（化）（10824）、腓骨（10815）の短小（化）を伴う。右写真は正常胎児。

4-4　Bent fibula　　腓骨弯曲　(10810)

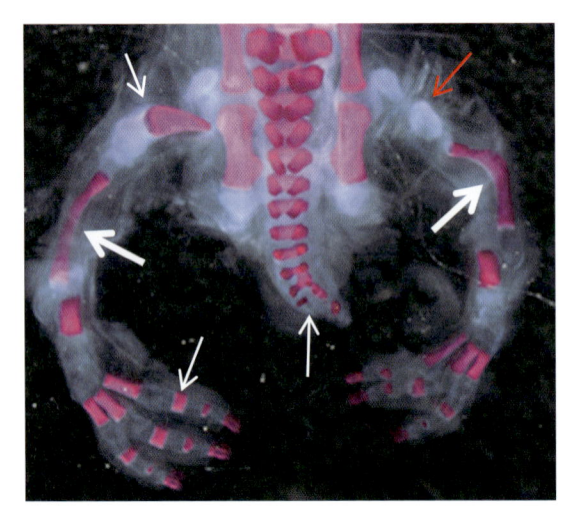

Species	Rabbit, Kbl:JW
Memo	Bent fibula (thick arrow) with Misshapen femur (10805), Unossified femur (red thin arrow, 10808), Absent tibia (10818), Absent caudal vertebrae (10769), and Fused caudal arches (10753).
	腓骨弯曲（太矢印）：大腿骨形態異常（10805）、大腿骨未骨化（赤細矢印、10808）、脛骨欠損（10818）、趾節骨欠損（10860）、尾椎欠損（10769）及び尾椎弓癒合（10753）を伴う。

4-5　Short fibula　腓骨短小（化）　(10815)

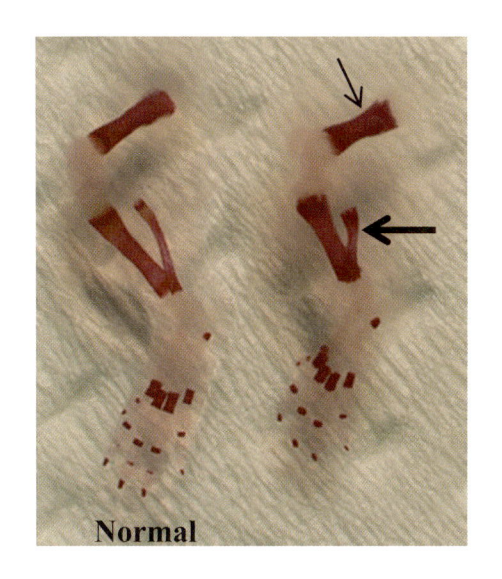

Species	Mouse
Memo	Short fibula (thick arrow) with Short femur (10806). The left specimen in the photograph shows normal features.
	腓骨短小（化）（太矢印）：大腿骨短小（化）（10806）を伴う。写真左は正常胎児

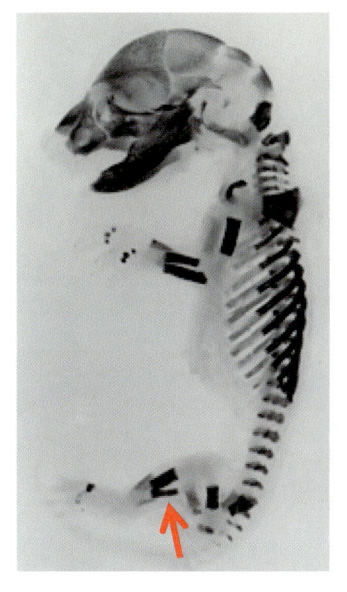

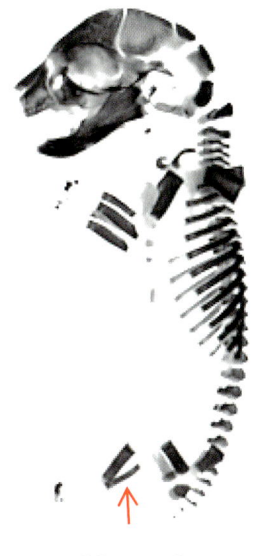

Species	Rat
Memo	Short fibula (red arrow) with Misshapen humerus (10564), Short tibia (10824) and Short femur (10806): The fetus in the right photograph shows normal features.
	腓骨短小（化）（赤矢印）：上腕骨形態異常（10564）、大腿骨の短小（化）（10806）、脛骨の短小（化）（10824）を伴う。

4-6　Absent tibia　　脛骨欠損　(10818)

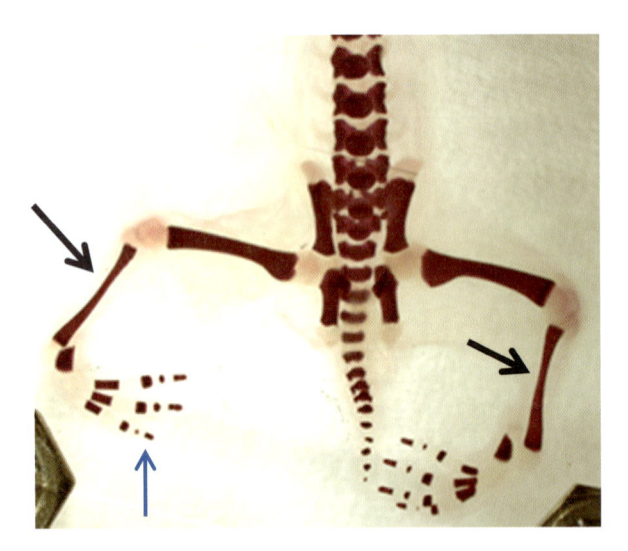

Species	Rabbit: Kbl:JW
Memo	Absent tibia (black arrow) in both limbs with Absent hindpaw phalanx (blue arrow, 10860)
	脛骨欠損（黒矢印）：両側の脛骨が欠損。趾節骨欠損（青矢印、10860）を伴う。

4-7 Misshapen tibia   脛骨形態異常   (10823)

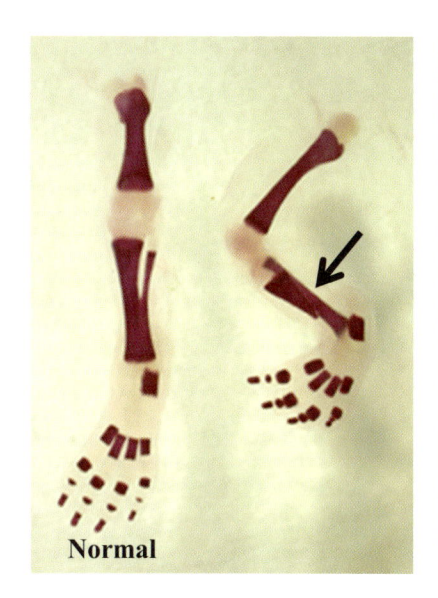

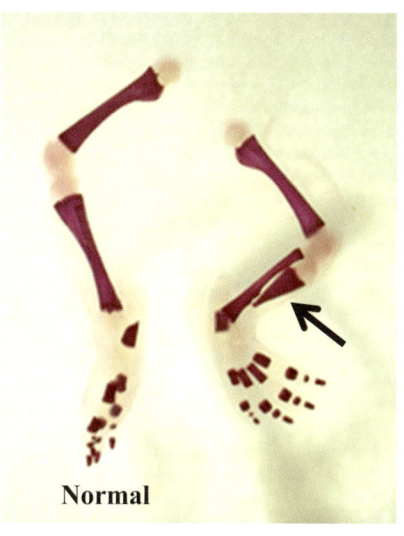

Species	Rabbit: Kbl:JW
Memo	Misshaped tibia (arrow): Tibia was short and abnormally shaped. The left specimens in both photographs show normal features.
	脛骨形態異常（矢印）：脛骨が短く三角状。写真左は正常胎児

4-8　Short tibia　脛骨短小（化）　(10824)

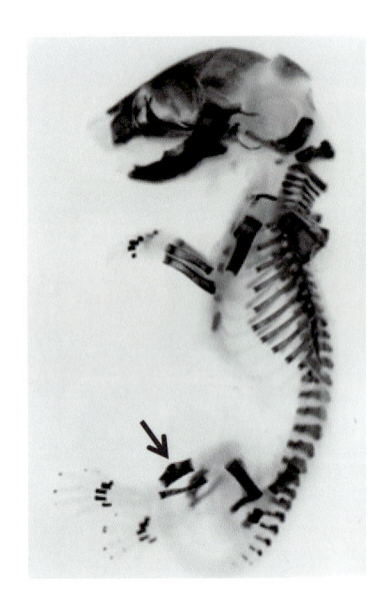

Species	Mouse
Memo	Short tibia (arrow) with Thick tibia (arrow, 10825).
	脛骨短小（化）（矢印）：脛骨部分肥厚（化）（矢印、10825）を伴う。

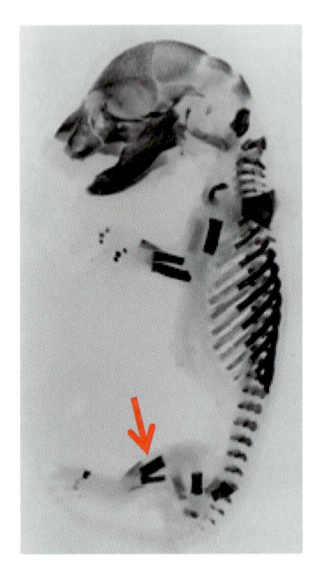

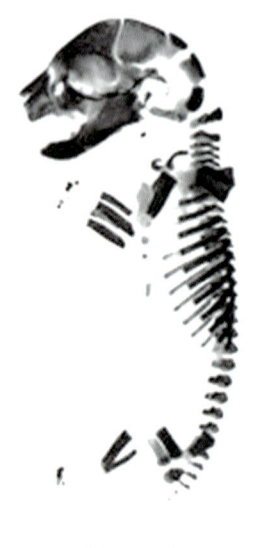

Species	Rat
Memo	Short tibia (red arrow) with Misshapen humerus (10564), Short fibula (10815) and Short femur (10806). The right photograph shows normal features.
	脛骨短小（化）（赤矢印）：上腕骨形態異常（10564）、大腿骨の短小（化）（10806）、腓骨の短小（化）（10815）を伴う。右写真は正常胎児。

Normal

4-9   **Thick tibia**   脛骨肥厚（化）   **(10825)**

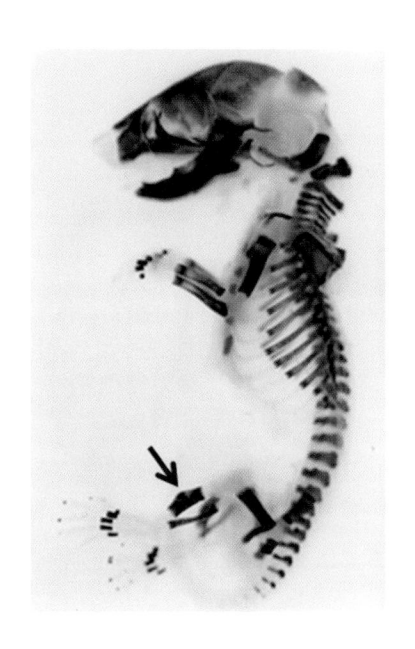

Species	Mouse
Memo	Thick tibia (arrow) with Short tibia (10824).
	脛骨部分肥厚（化）（矢印）：脛骨短小（化）（10824）を伴う。

Photographs of Skeletal Anomalies

5. Phalanx of fore- and hind-paw

5-1 Absent forepaw phalanx 指節骨欠損 (10602)

Species	Rabbit
Memo	Absent 1st forepaw phalanx (in circle): Pre-axial oligodactyly in the external examination.
	指節骨欠損（円中）：軸前性、外表観察では第一指の欠指

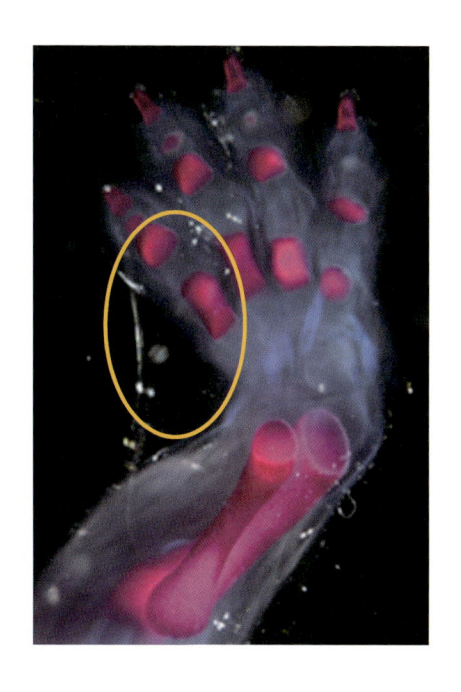

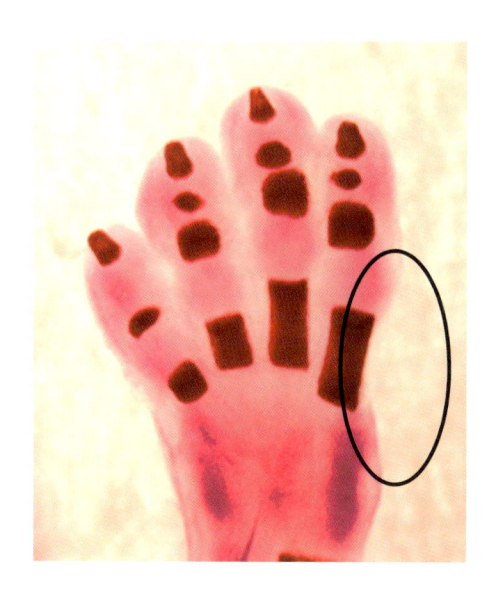

5-1 Continued

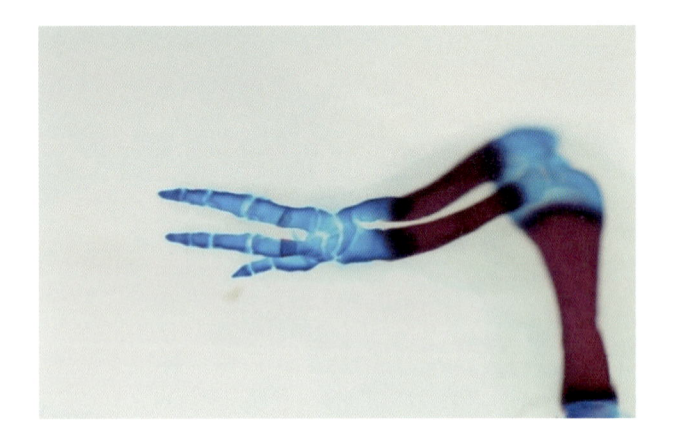

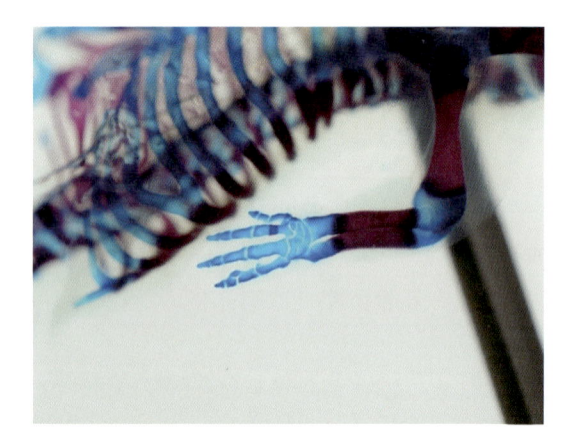

Species	Rat
Memo	Absent forepaw phalanx
	指節骨欠損

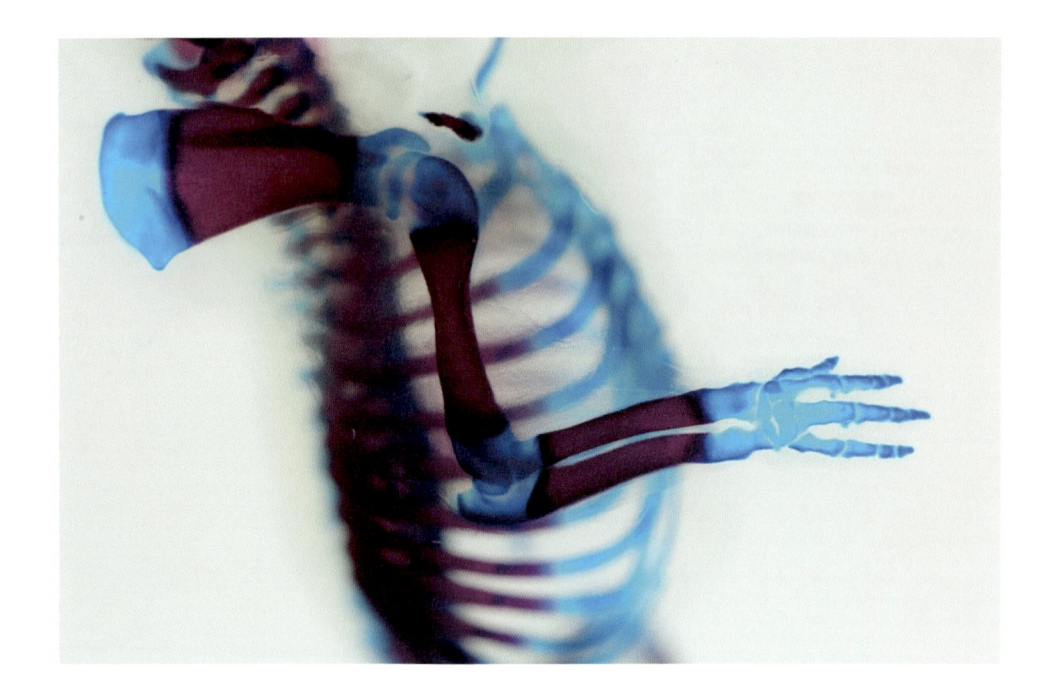

Species	Rat
Memo	Absent forepaw phalanx with Misshapen humerus (10564, see 3-1, Absent deltoid tuberosity)
	指節骨欠損：上腕骨形態異常（10564、三角筋粗面の欠損）を伴う。

5-2　Fused forepaw phalanx　　指節骨癒合　(10603)

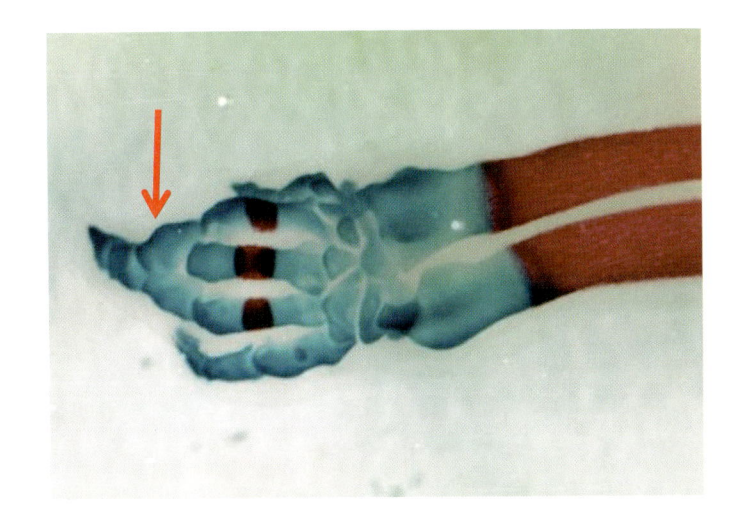

Species	Rat
Memo	Fused forepaw phalanx (red arrow): The 2nd, 3rd and 4th digits fused.
	指節骨癒合（赤矢印）：第 2-4 指が癒合している。

5-3 Supernumerary forepaw phalanx 指節骨過剰 (10608)

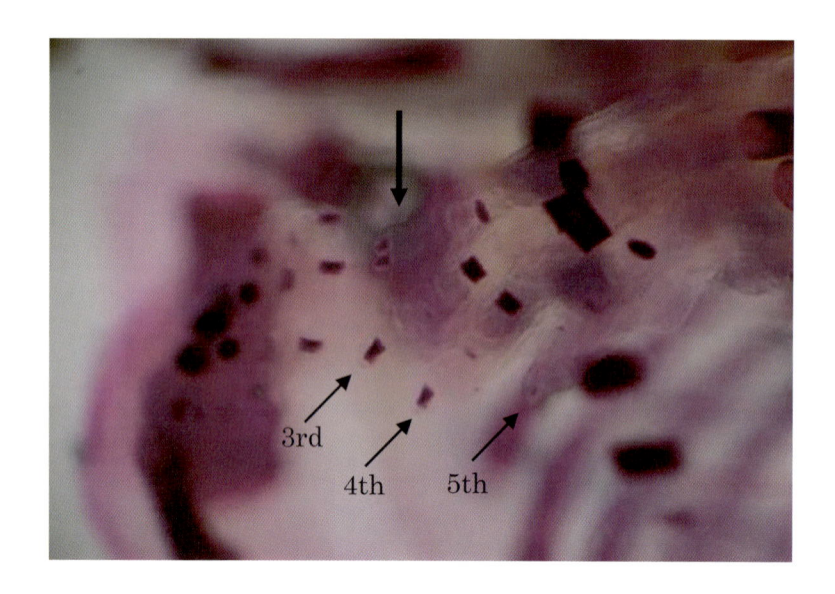

Species	Mouse, ICR
Memo	Supernumerary forepaw phalanx: The 2nd phalanx is duplicated (thick arrow).
	指節骨過剰：第2指指節骨の一部が重複（太矢印）。

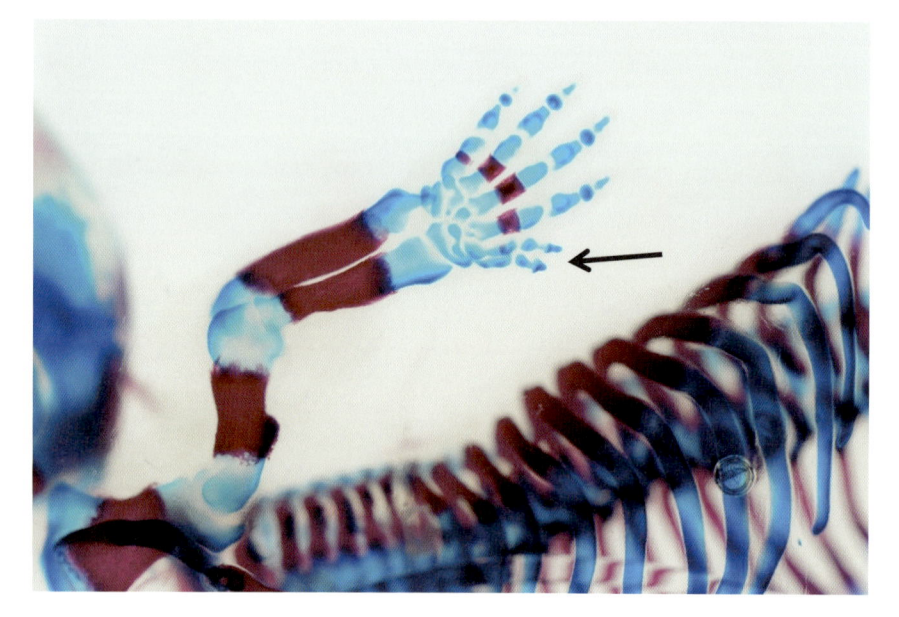

Species	Rat
Memo	Supernumerary forepaw phalanx (pre-axial): The 1st phalanx is duplication (arrow). This fetus may appear as "Polydactyly (10088)" in external observation.
	指節骨過剰：軸前性の過剰（矢印）。外表では多指（10088）。

5-4 Absent hindpaw phalanx   趾節骨欠損   (10860)

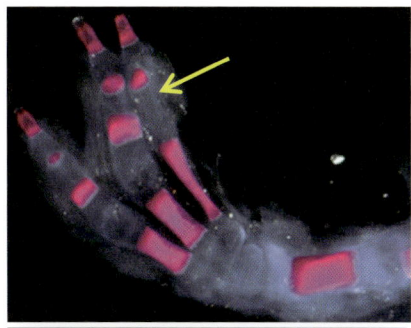

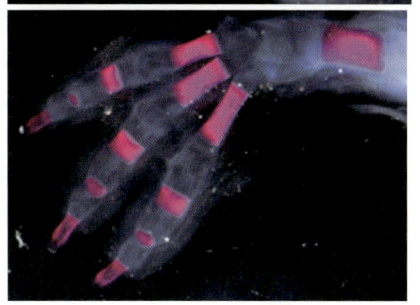

Species	Rabbit: Kbl:JW
Memo	Absent hindpaw phalanx: The number of phalanges is 3. In the upper specimen, Absent phalanx proximalis (yellow arrow) and Misshapen metatarsal bone (long, 10856) are also observed. This fetus has Oligodactyly (10080) and Syndactyly (10091, cutaneous) in external observation.
	趾節骨欠損：趾が 3 本。上写真では、基節骨の欠損（矢印）中足骨の形態異常（長い、10856）を伴う。外表では欠趾（10080）及び趾癒合（10091、皮膚性）もみられる。

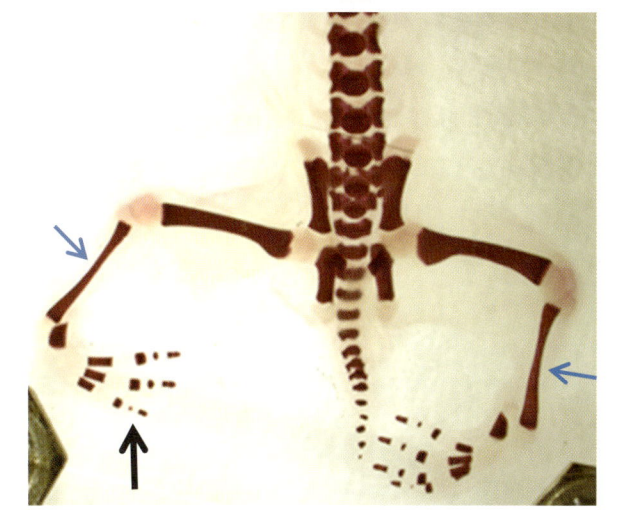

Species	Rabbit: Kbl:JW
Memo	Absent hindpaw phalanx (black arrow) with Absent tibia (blue arrow) in both limbs (10818): This fetus has Oligodactyly (10080) in external observation.
	趾節骨欠損（黒矢印）：両側の脛骨が欠損している（青矢印、10818）。外表では欠趾（10080）である。

5-4 Continued

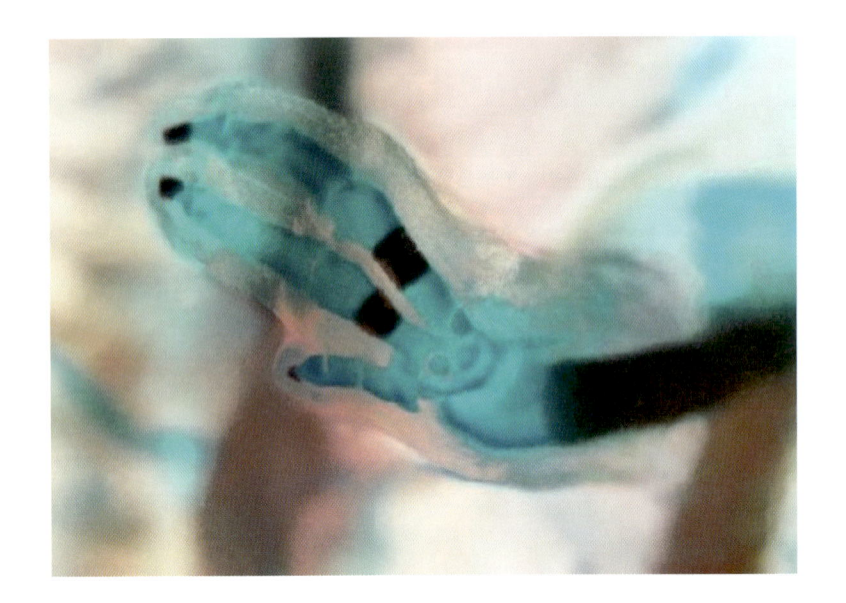

Species	Rat
Memo	Absent hindpaw phalanx
	趾節骨欠損

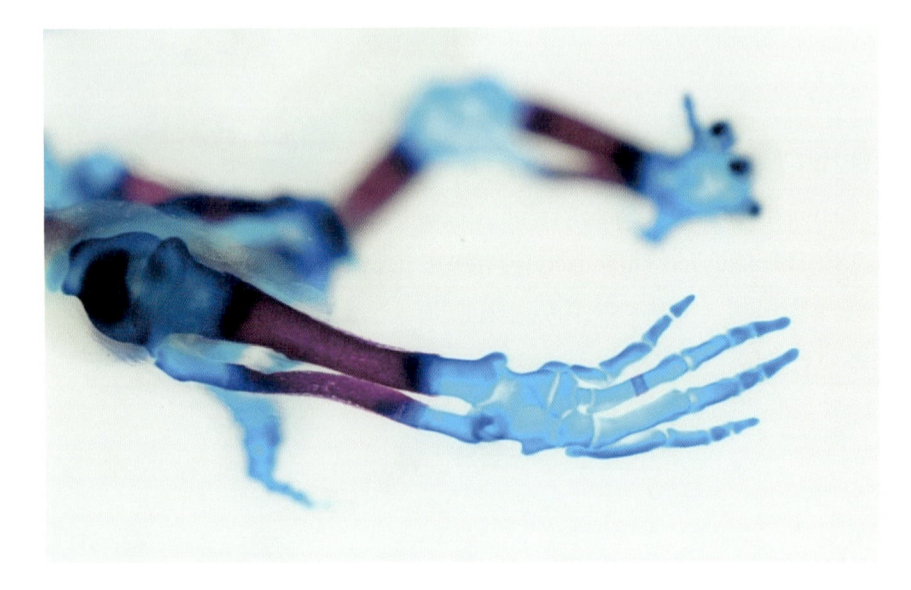

Species	Rat
Memo	Absent hindpaw phalanx with Unossified hindpaw phalanx (10868)
	趾節骨欠損：趾節骨未骨化（10868）を伴う。

5-5　Supernumerary hindpaw phalanx　　趾節骨過剰　(10866)

Species	Rat
Memo	Supernumerary hindpaw phalanx (pre-axial): The 1st phalanx is duplicated (arrow). This fetus has "Polydactyly (10088)" in external observation.
	趾節骨過剰：軸前性の過剰（矢印）。外表では多趾（10088）。

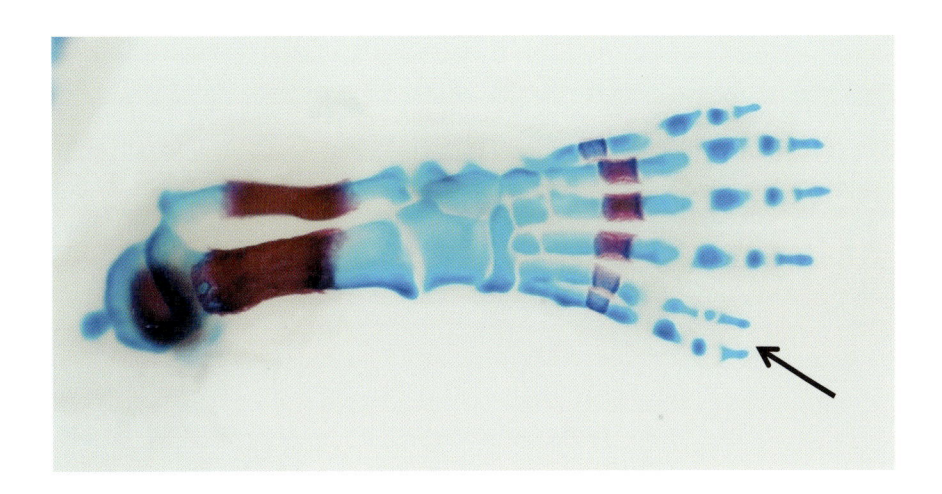

Photographs of Skeletal Anomalies

6. Sternebra

6-1 Fused sternebrae   胸骨分節癒合   (10614)

Species	Rabbit
Memo	Fused sternebrae
	胸骨分節癒合

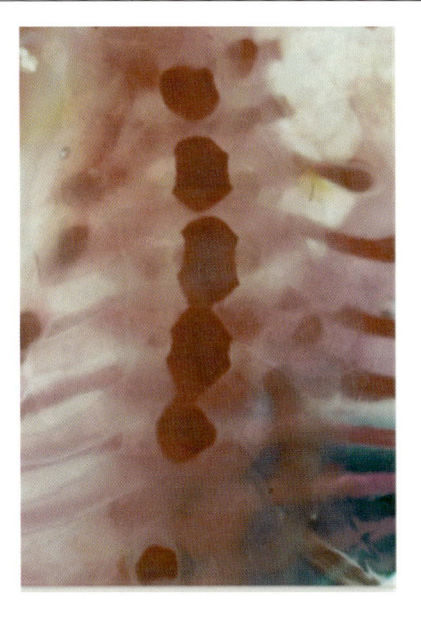

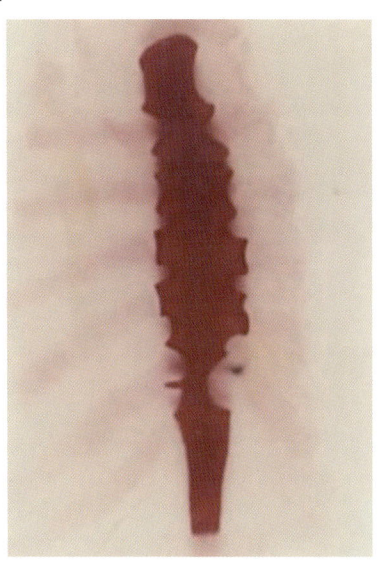

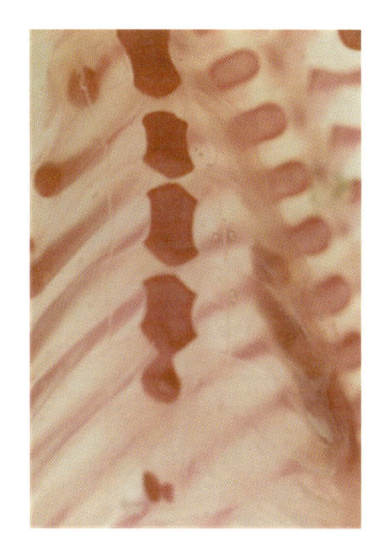

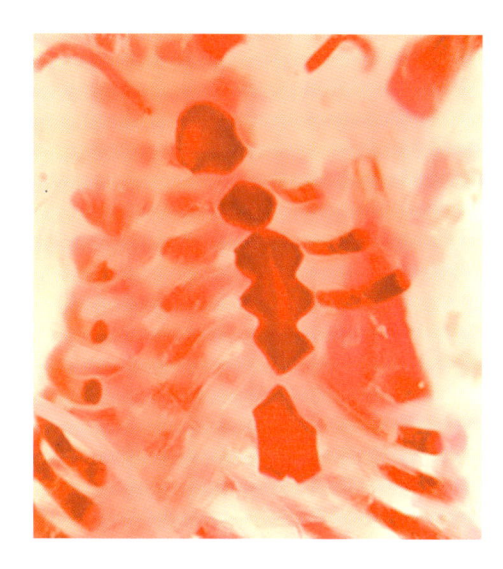

Species	Rabbit
Memo	Fused sternebrae (peduncular) (arrow)
	胸骨分節（糸状）癒合（矢印）

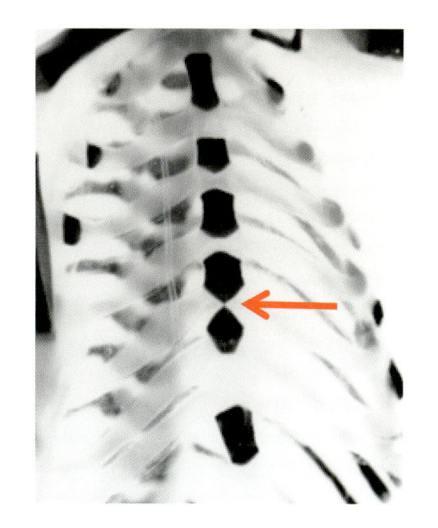

6-2　**Misaligned sternebrae**　　胸骨分節配列異常　　(10617)

Species	Mouse, Rat, Rabbit
Memo	Misaligned sternebrae
	胸骨分節配列異常

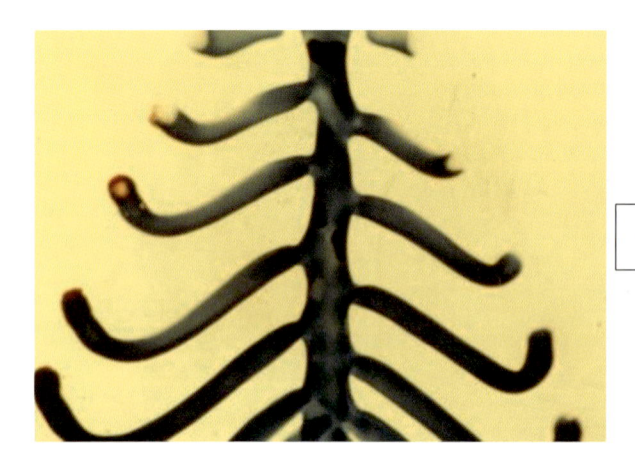

Rat

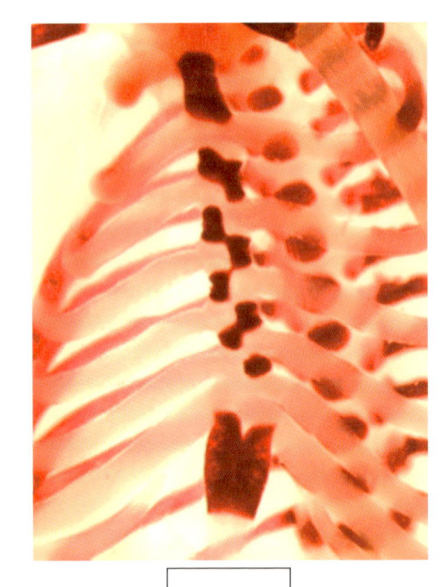

Mouse

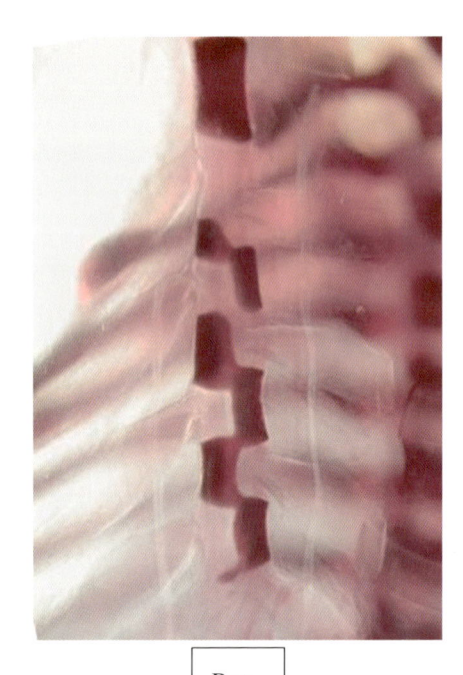

Rat

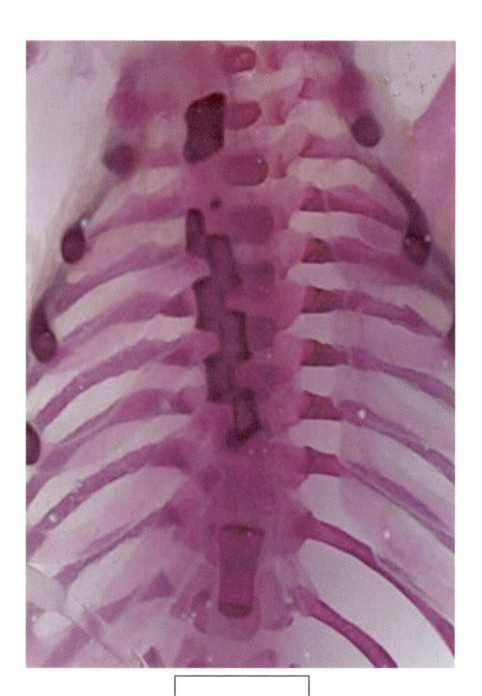

Rabbit

6-3　Misshapen sternebrae　　胸骨分節形態異常　(10618)

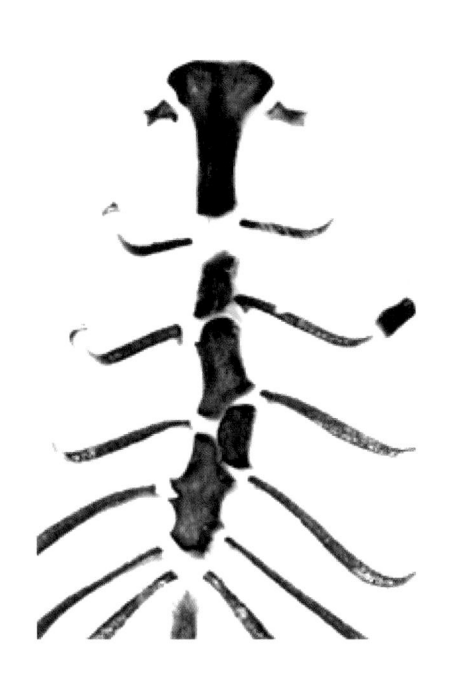

Species	Rat (Weanling)
Memo	Misshapen sternebrae: This may be considered to be "Hemisternebra (New)".
	胸骨分節形態異常：半胸骨分節（New）でも良い。

6-4　Split sternebra　　胸骨分節分離　(New)

Species	Rat
Memo	Split sternebra: This should be distinguished from Split sternum (10619) observed in fetus that has Ectopia cordis (10108) or Thoracogastroschisis (10121) in external observation.
	胸骨分節分離：外表異常として「心臓逸所（10108）」や「胸腹壁裂（10121）」を持つ「胸骨分離（10619）」とは区分する。

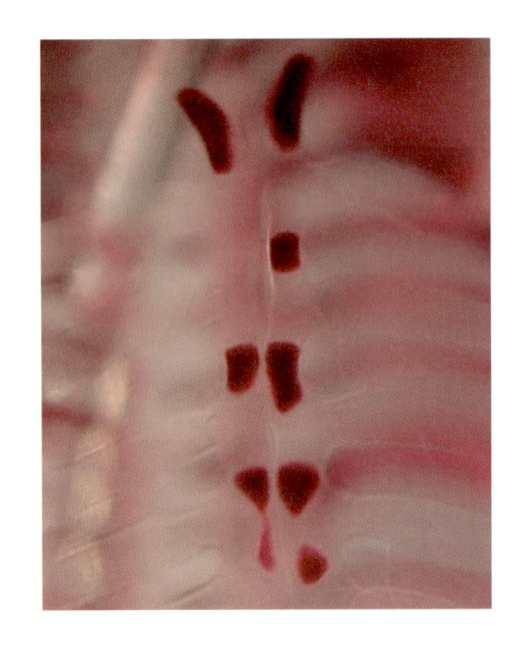

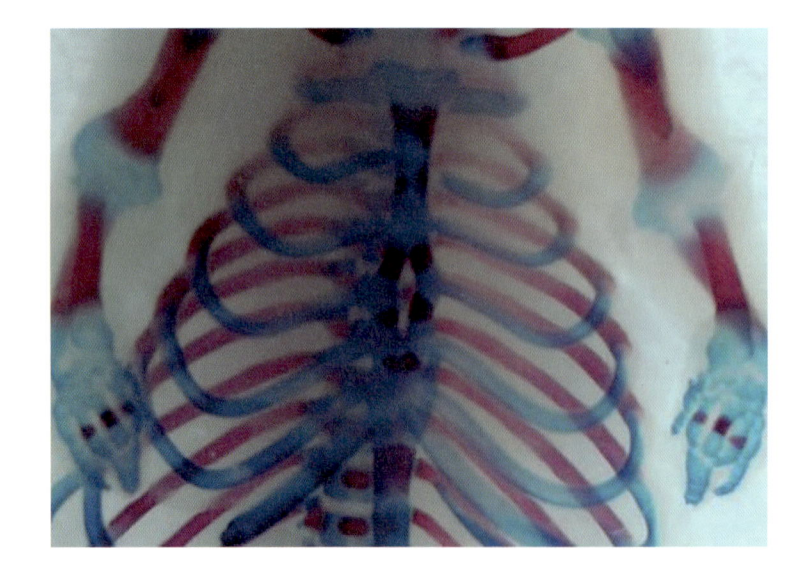

6-5 Asymmetric ossification of sternebra   胸骨分節非対称骨化   (New)

Species	Rat
Memo	Asymmetric ossification of sternebra: Alizarin red stain uptake is greater in one hemicenter than the other (arrow). Both costal cartilages are almost symmetrical.
	胸骨分節非対称骨化：一方の胸骨分節の骨化（アリザリンレッドの染色性）が強い（矢印）。肋軟骨はほぼ左右対称である。

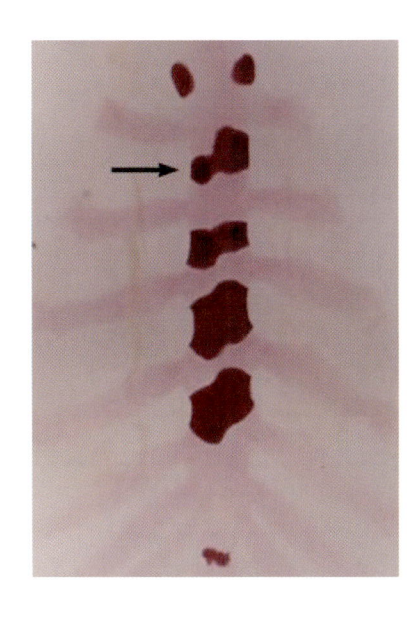

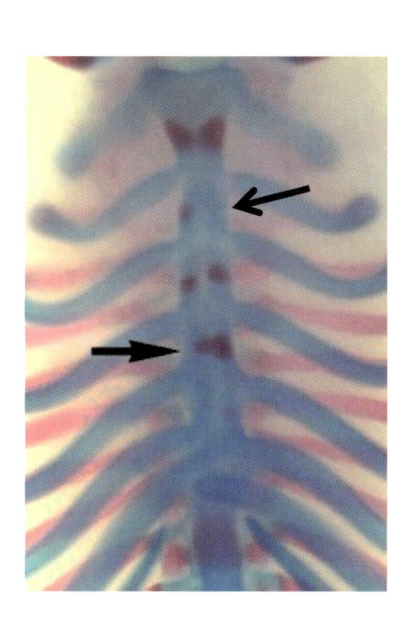

6-6 Bipartite ossification of sternebra 胸骨分節二分骨化 (10612)

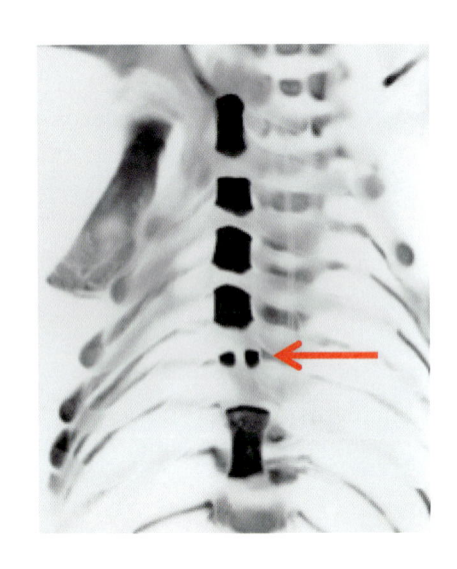

Species	Rabbit
Memo	Bipartite ossification of sternebra (arrow): Two ossification sites are observed in one sternebra.
	胸骨分節二分骨化：一つの胸骨内に二つに分離した骨化部位がみられる。

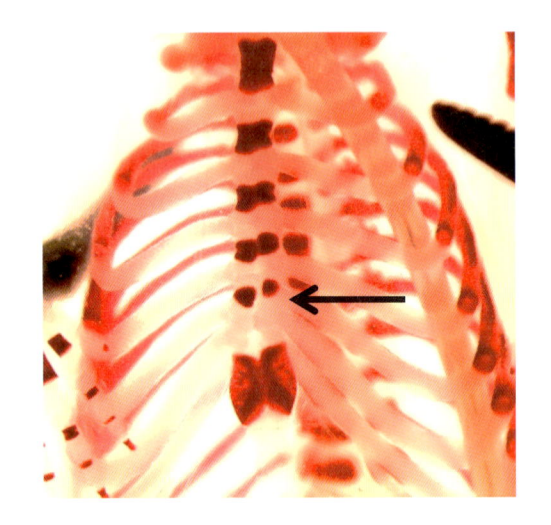

Species	Mouse
Memo	Bipartite ossification of sternebra (arrow): Two ossification sites are observed in one sternebra.
	胸骨分節二分骨化：一つの胸骨内に二つに分離した骨化部位がみられる。

6-7 Unilateral ossification of sternebra　　胸骨分節片側性骨化　(New)

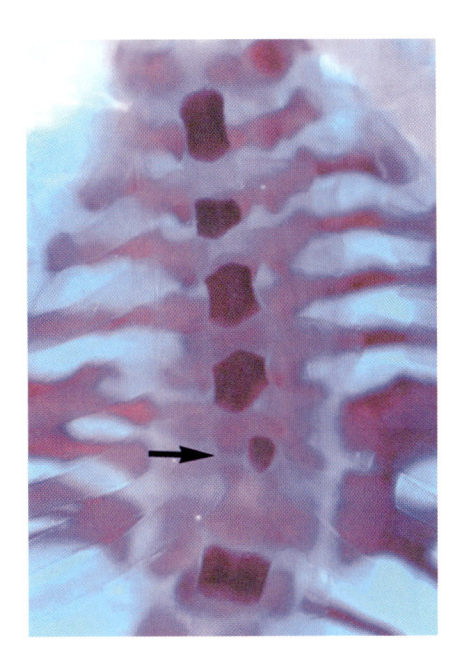

Species	Rat
Memo	Unilateral ossification of sternebra
	胸骨分節片側性骨化

6-8　Split xiphoid cartilage　　剣状軟骨分離　(New)

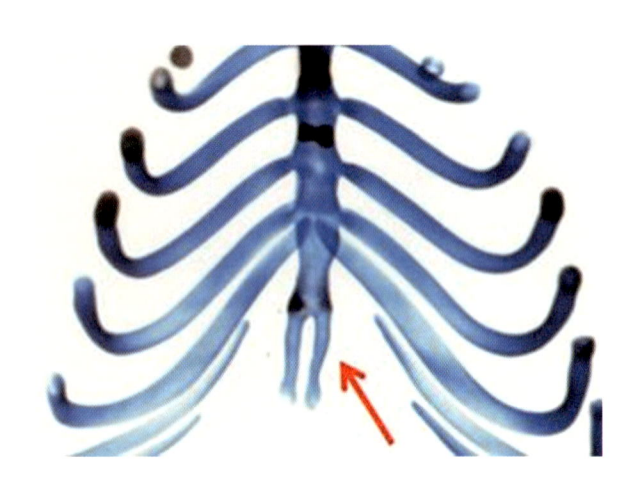

Species	Rat
Memo	Split xiphoid cartilage (arrow)
	剣状軟骨分離（矢印）

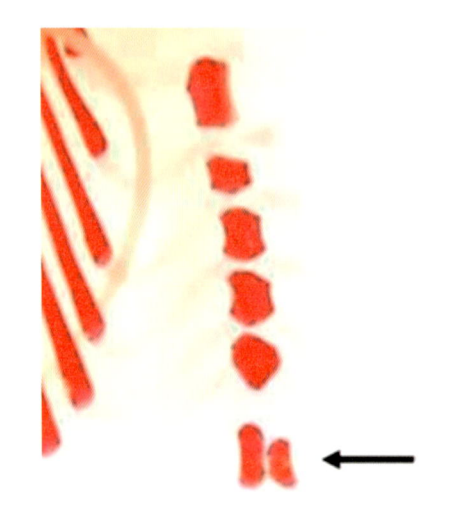

Species	Rabbit
Memo	Split xiphoid cartilage (arrow)
	剣状軟骨分離（矢印）：単染色の場合、軟骨部分を良く確認する。

6-9　Misshapen sternum　　胸骨形態異常　(New)

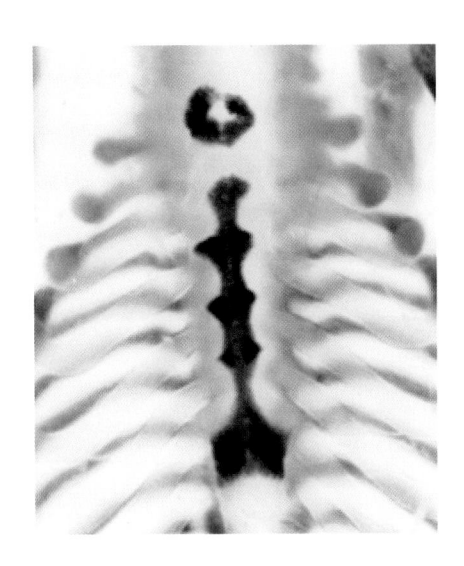

Species	Rabbit
Memo	Misshapen sternum with Fused sternebrae (10614)
	胸骨形態異常：胸骨分節癒合（10614）を伴う。

6-10　**Split sternum**　　胸骨分離　　(10619)

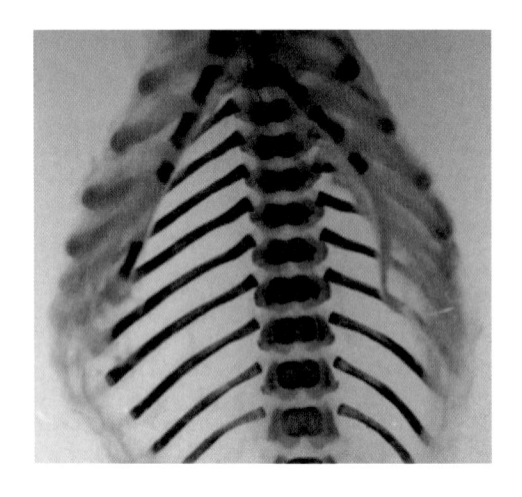

Species	Rabbit
Memo	Split sternum or Sternoschisis: This fetus has Thoracogastroschisis (10121) in external observation.
	胸骨分離、胸骨裂：外表観察では胸腹壁裂（10121）の個体

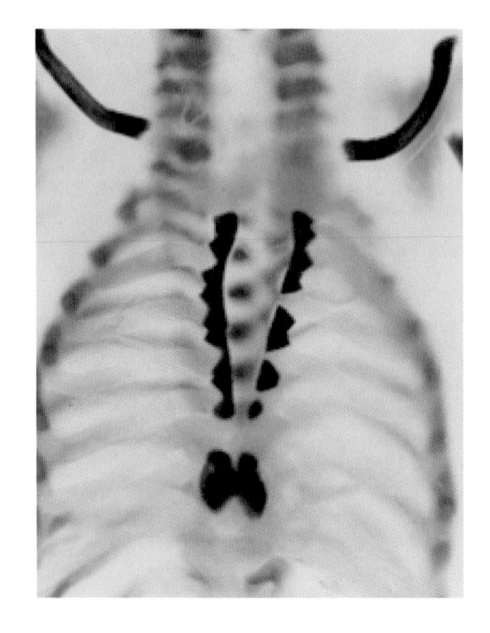

Species	Rat
Memo	Split sternum or Sternoschisis
	胸骨分離、胸骨裂

6-10 Continued

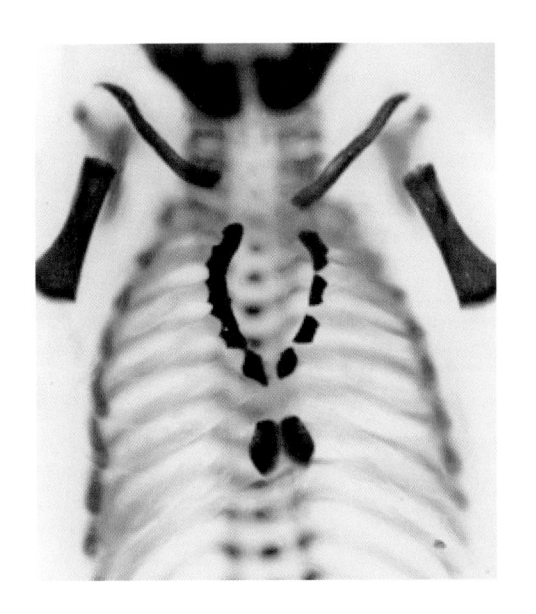

Species	Rat
Memo	Split sternum or Sternoschisis: This fetus has Ectopia cordis (10108) in external observation.
	胸骨分離、胸骨裂：外表観察では心臓逸所（10108）

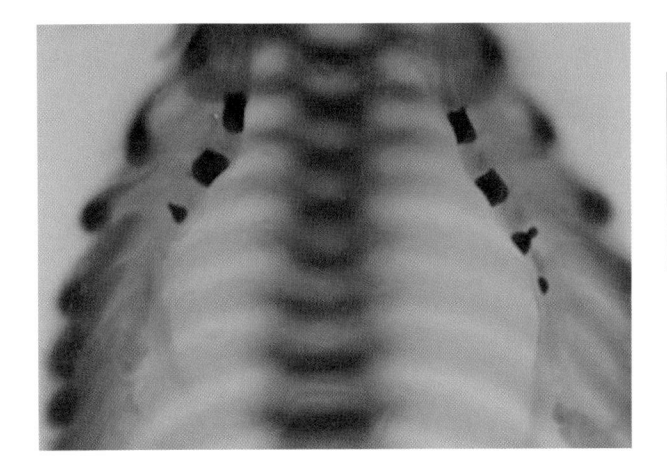

Species	Rabbit
Memo	Split sternum or Sternoschisis: This fetus has Thoracogastroschisis (10121) in external observation.
	胸骨分離、胸骨裂：外表観察では胸腹壁裂（10121）の個体

6-11　**Supernumerary ossification site of sternum**　　胸骨過剰骨化部位　**(New)**

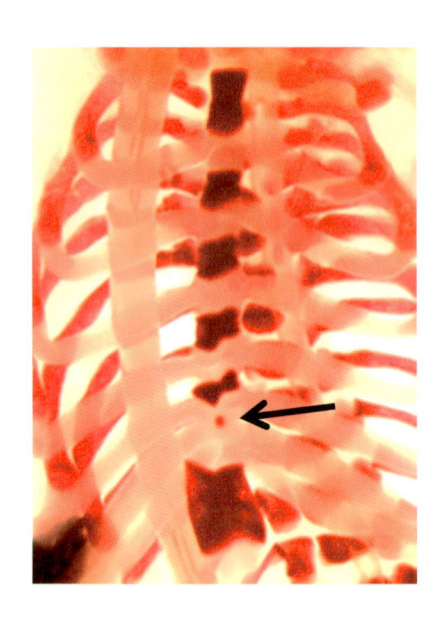

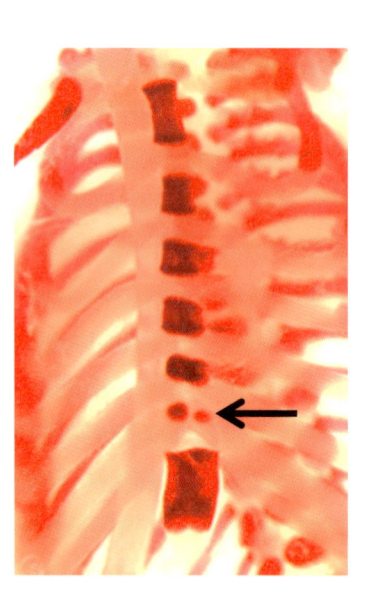

Species	Mouse
Memo	Supernumerary ossification site of sternum (arrow)
	胸骨過剰骨化部位（矢印）

Photographs of Skeletal Anomalies

7. Rib

7-1 Absent rib　　肋骨欠損　(10621)

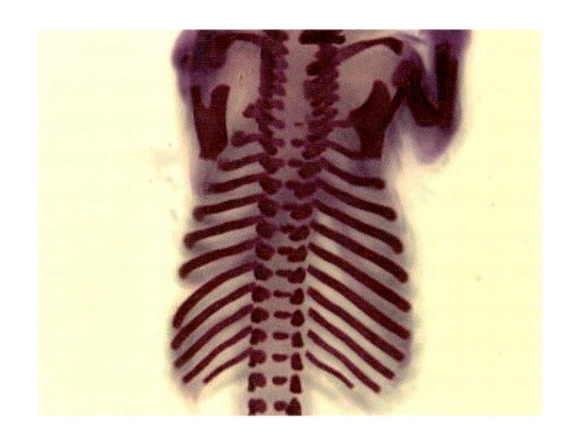

Species	Rat
Memo	Absent rib with Absent thoracic vertebrae (10694): This may be considered as "Reduced number of ribs" because the number of ribs and thoracic vertebrae are reduced bilaterally to 12 pairs, and their shapes are normal.
	肋骨欠損：胸椎の欠損（10694）も伴う。本所見は、左右とも 12 対に減少しており、また、それらの形態に異常性は認められないことから、「肋骨数の減少」でも良い。

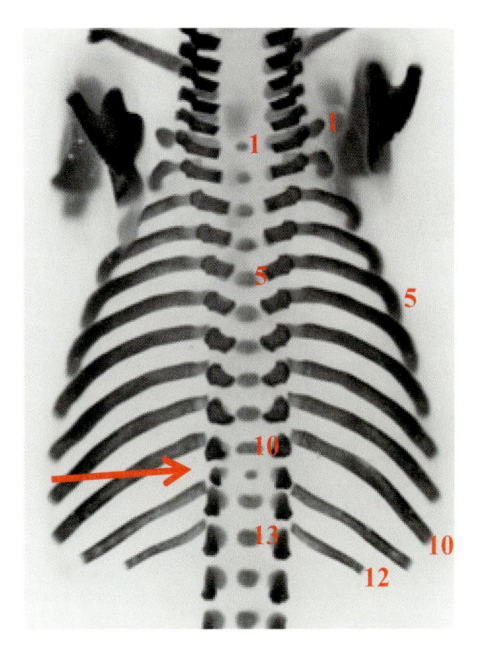

Species	Rat
Memo	Absent rib with Small thoracic vertebral arch (red arrow, 10677): The number of ribs is reduced to 12 pairs without reduced number of thoracic vertebrae. The left 11th thoracic vertebral arch and the 11th thoracic vertebral centrum are small (10677 and New, respectively, red arrow), and both 11th ribs are absent.
	肋骨欠損：左右 12 対。胸椎数は正常であるが、左第 11 胸椎弓が小型（赤矢印、10677）及び第 11 胸椎体が小型（New）であり、左右の第 11 肋骨が欠損している。

7-1 Continued

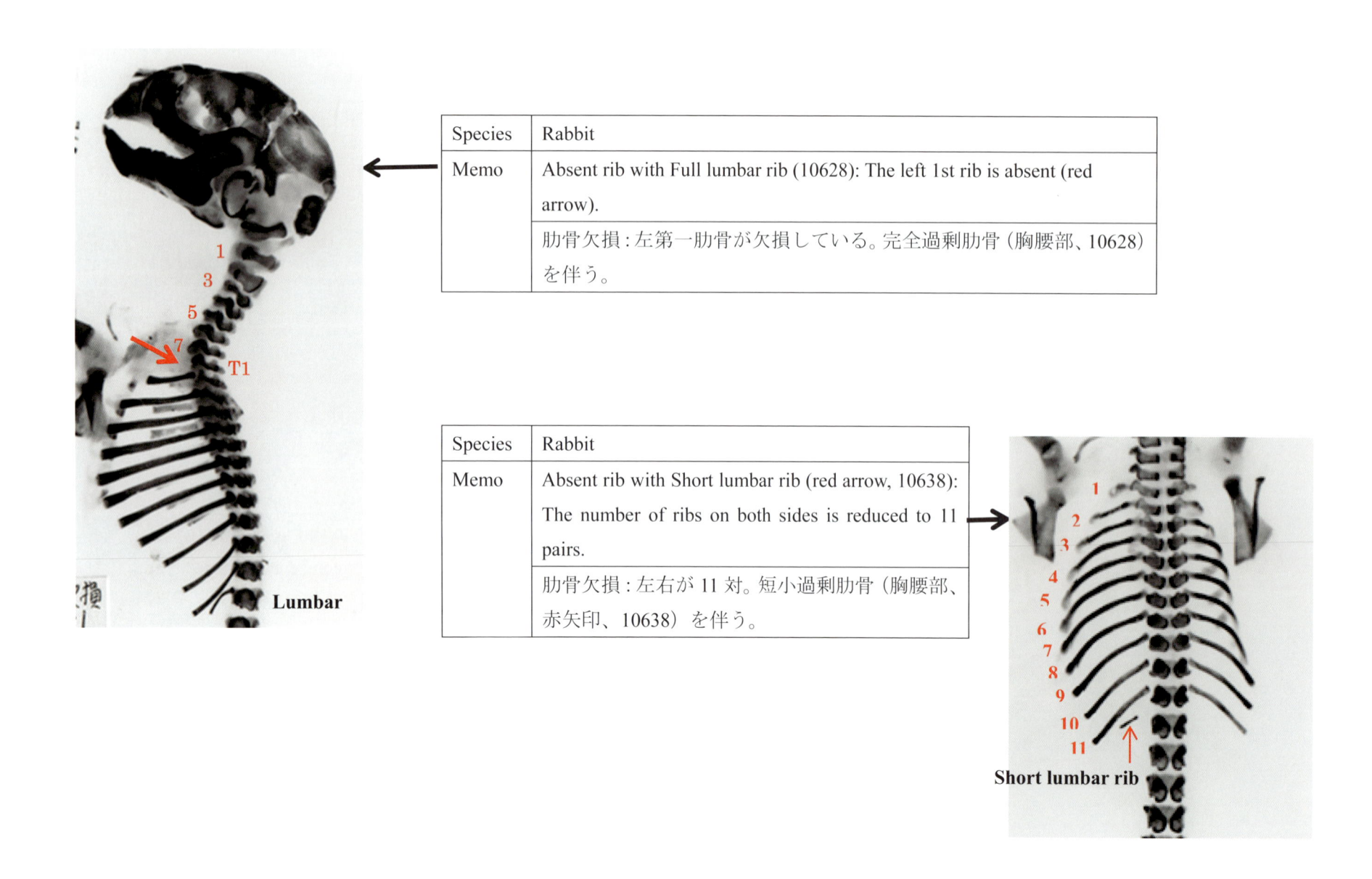

Species	Rabbit
Memo	Absent rib with Full lumbar rib (10628): The left 1st rib is absent (red arrow).
	肋骨欠損：左第一肋骨が欠損している。完全過剰肋骨（胸腰部、10628）を伴う。

Species	Rabbit
Memo	Absent rib with Short lumbar rib (red arrow, 10638): The number of ribs on both sides is reduced to 11 pairs.
	肋骨欠損：左右が11対。短小過剰肋骨（胸腰部、赤矢印、10638）を伴う。

7-1 Continued

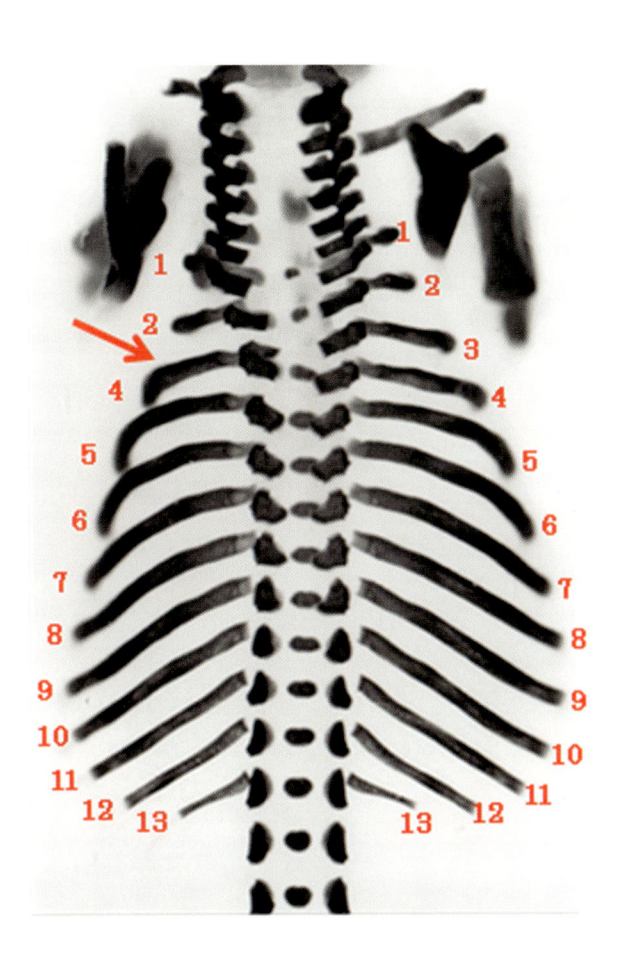

Species	Rat
Memo	Absent rib: The left 3rd rib is absent (red arrow). Right ribs are normal. This may be considered as "Thoracic hemivertebra (10696)" at the 3rd and 4th thoracic vertebrae.
	肋骨欠損：左第三肋骨が欠損している（赤矢印）。右肋骨は正常。第3、4胸椎部分が半椎（10696）である。

7-2　Branched rib　　肋骨分岐　(10623)

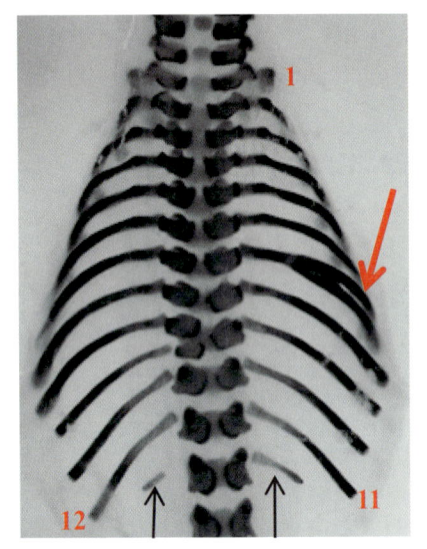

Species	Rabbit
Memo	Branched rib (red arrow) with Thoracic hemivertebra (10696), Absent rib (right side, 10621), and Supernumerary thoracolumbar rib (black arrow), (Full, 10628 and Short, 10638). This is considered a "Branched rib" because it is attached to a single thoracic vertebra.
	肋骨分岐（赤矢印）：胸椎半椎（10696）、肋骨欠損（10621）及び過剰肋骨（10628 及び 10638）を伴う。肋骨癒合（10629）との区分であるが、本例は当該肋骨が1椎骨に接続していることから、「分岐」が望ましいと考える。

Supernumerary rib

Species	Rabbit
Memo	Branched rib (red arrow) with Absent thoracic vertebra (10694) and Absent rib (10621) or Reduced number of ribs and thoracic vertebrae
	肋骨分岐（赤矢印）：胸椎欠損（10694）及び肋骨欠損（10621）あるいは胸椎及び肋骨数の減少を伴う。

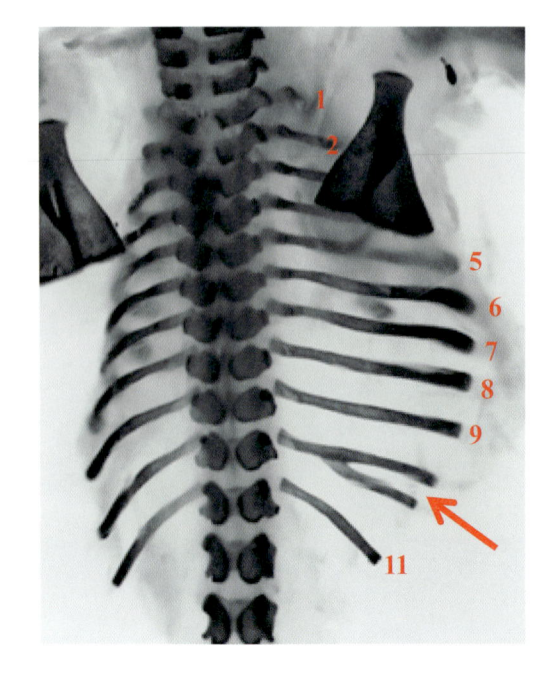

7-2 Continued

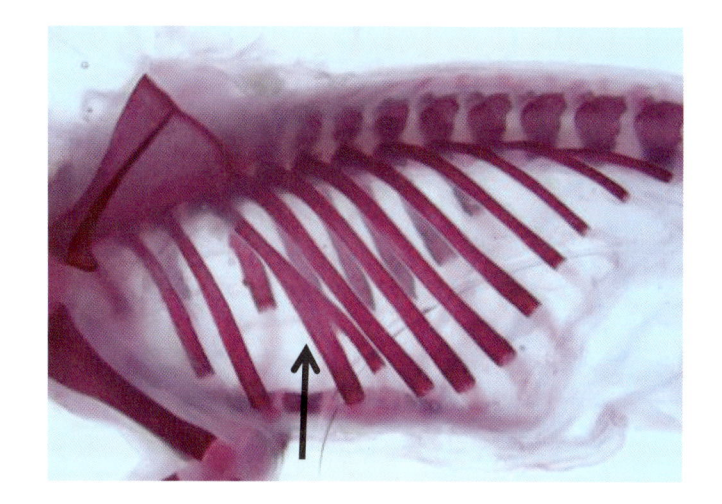

Species	Rabbit
Memo	Branched rib (black arrow)
	肋骨分岐（矢印）

7-3   Detached rib   肋骨分離   (10626)

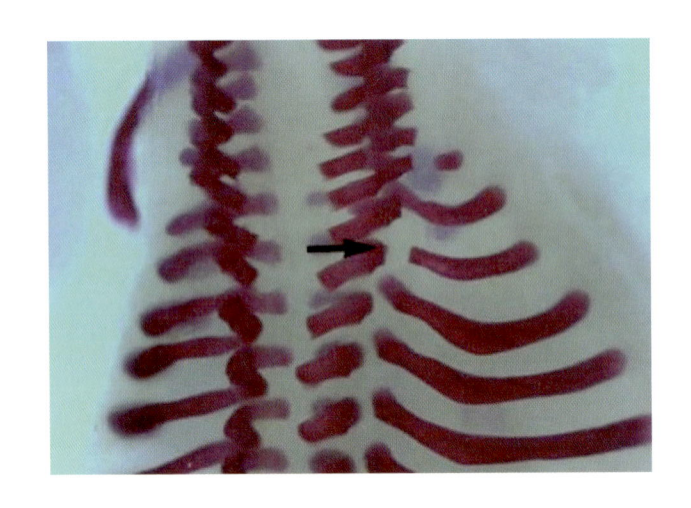

Species	Rat
Memo	Detached rib: The 3rd right rib does not articulate with vertebral column (arrow).
	肋骨分離：右第3肋骨が関節結合していない（矢印）。

7-4   Fused rib   肋骨癒合   (10629)

Species	Rat
Memo	Fused rib: The 4 specimens below show various types of "Fused rib" (arrow).
	肋骨癒合：以下の4写真は肋骨癒合であるが、色々なパターンが見られる（矢印）。

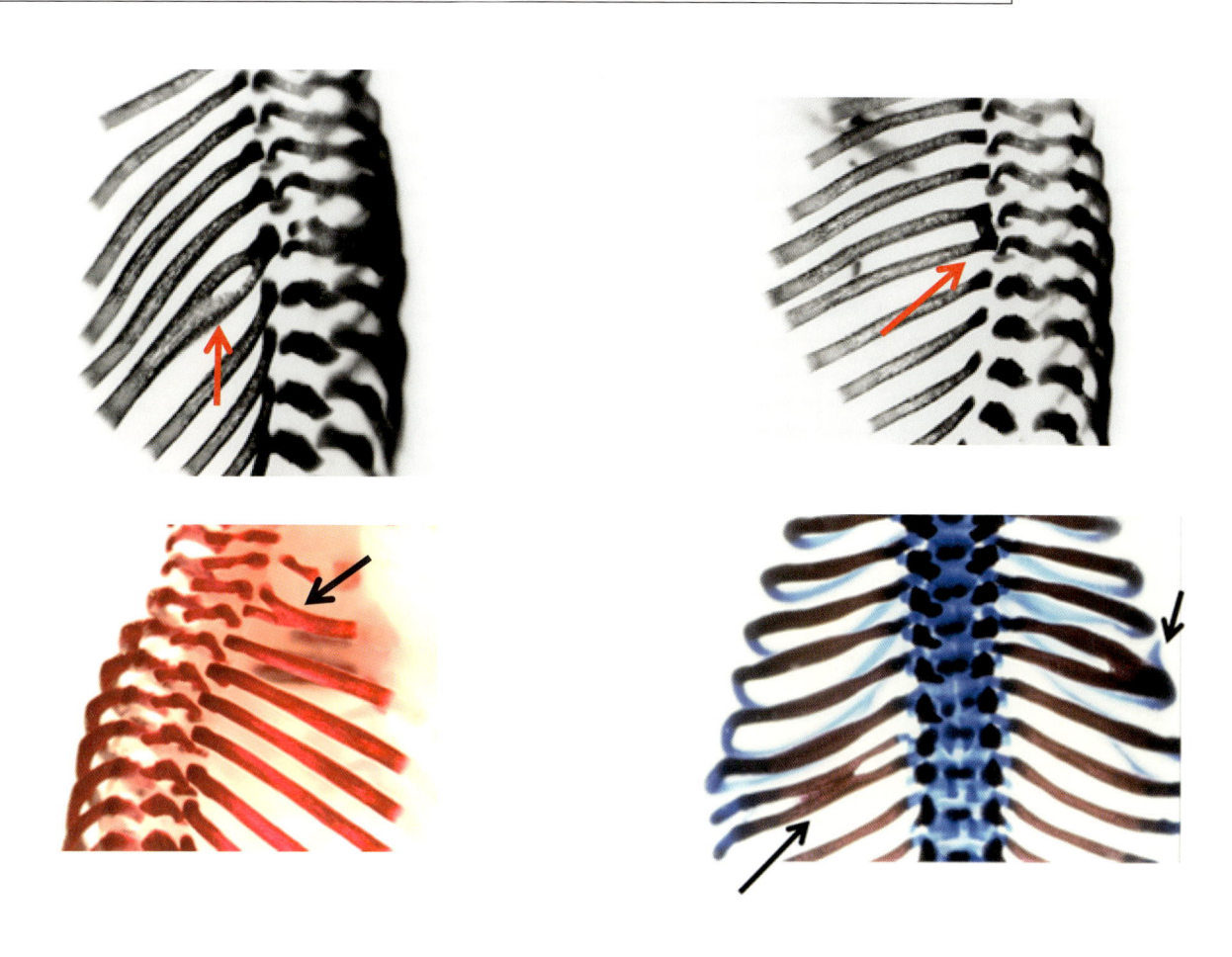

7-4 Continued

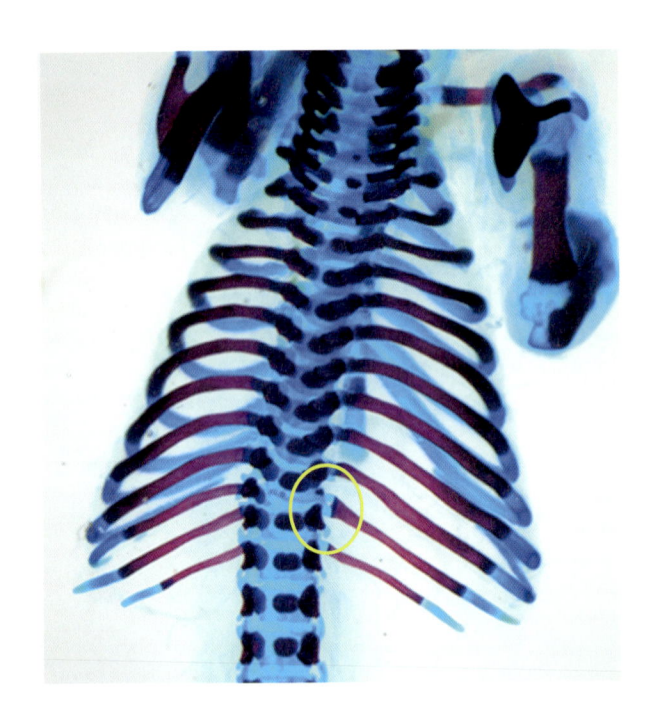

Species	Rat, SD
Memo	Fused rib: The 11th and 12th ribs are fused. This fetus is double-stained to show the fusion of ribs at the joint region although the ossified ribs look very much like a normal rib (circle). The 11th right thoracic vertebral arch is small.
	肋骨癒合：右第11と12肋骨が癒合している。骨化している肋骨は正常とほぼ同様の形態であるが、関節部（軟骨）は一部癒合しているものの2個存在する（楕円）。第11右椎弓が小型化（10677）である。

Species	Rabbit
Memo	Fused rib: The 2 specimens on the right show different types of "Fused rib" (arrow).
	肋骨癒合：右2写真はウサギの肋骨癒合

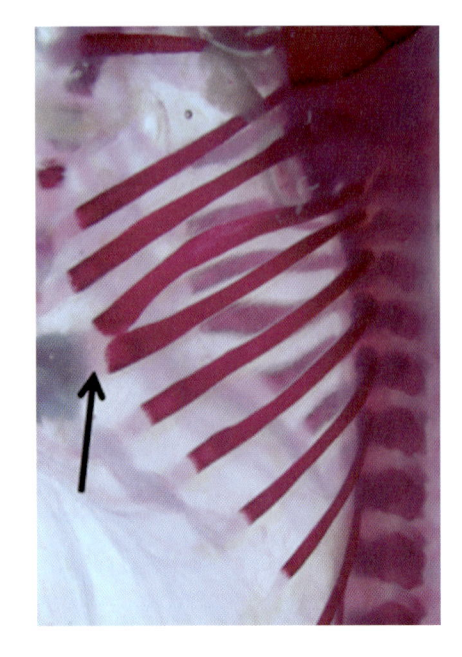

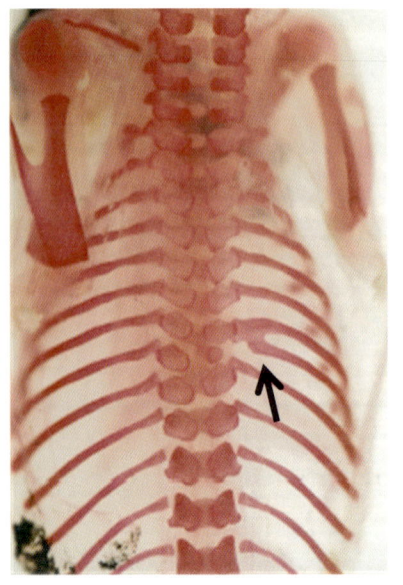

7-5   Intercostal rib   肋間肋骨   (10632)

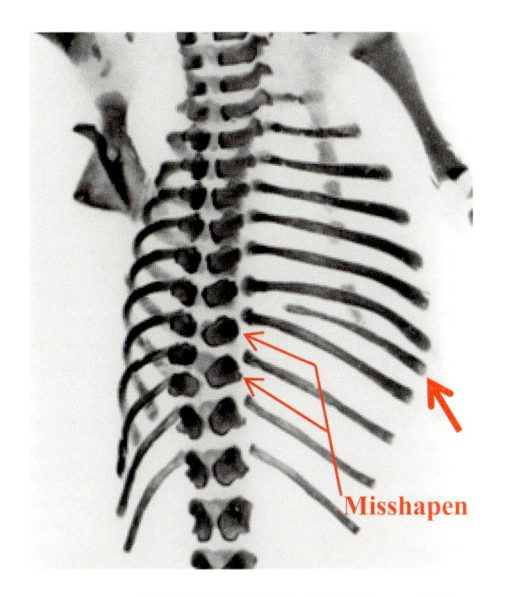

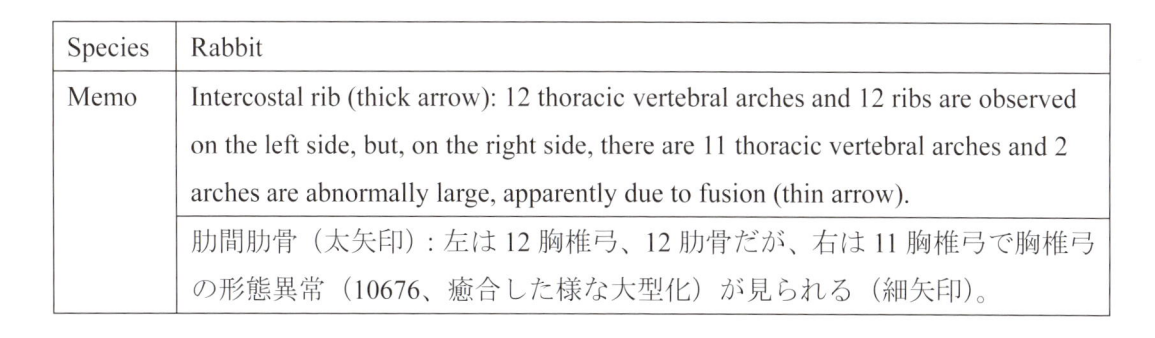

Species	Rabbit
Memo	Intercostal rib (thick arrow): 12 thoracic vertebral arches and 12 ribs are observed on the left side, but, on the right side, there are 11 thoracic vertebral arches and 2 arches are abnormally large, apparently due to fusion (thin arrow).
	肋間肋骨（太矢印）：左は 12 胸椎弓、12 肋骨だが、右は 11 胸椎弓で胸椎弓の形態異常（10676、癒合した様な大型化）が見られる（細矢印）。

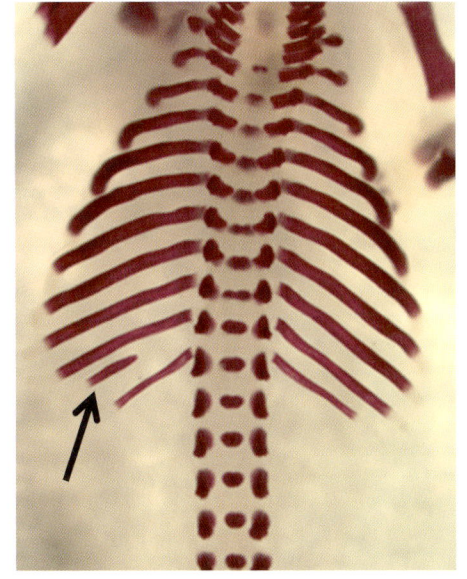

Species	Rat
Memo	Intercostal rib (arrow) with Absent thoracic vertebra (10694) and Absent rib (10621) or Reduced number of ribs and thoracic vertebrae
	肋間肋骨（矢印）：胸椎欠損（10694）及び肋骨欠損（10621）あるいは肋骨及び胸椎数の減少を伴う。

7-5 Continued

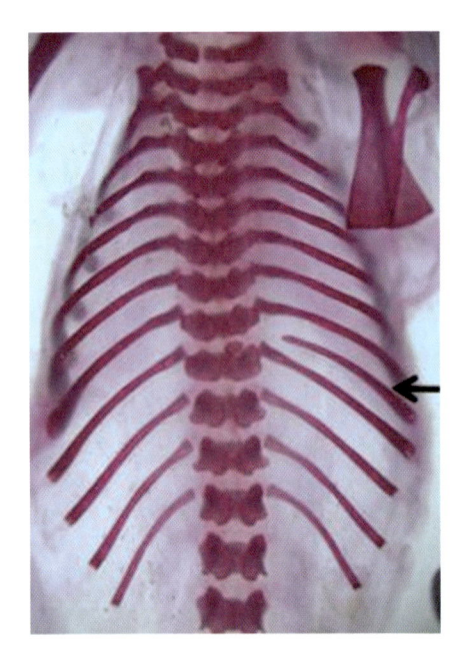

Species	Rabbit
Memo	Intercostal rib: An additional rib-like structure between the 8th and 9th right ribs does not articulate with a thoracic vertebra (arrow).
	肋間肋骨：右第8と9肋骨の間に過剰な肋骨様の構造物がみられるが、胸椎と関節結合していない（矢印）。

Species	Rat, SD
Memo	Intercostal rib (red arrow) with Thoracic hemivertebra (10696), Small thoracic vertebral centrum (New), and Misshapen thoracic vertebral arch (10676): The 9th right rib does not articulate with vertebral column (red arrow). The left thoracic vertebra arch and centrum of the 9th thoracic vertebra are small, and its right arch is absent (circle). The 12th and 13th thoracic vertebra centrum are small, and the shape of the right 13th thoracic vertebra arch is abnormal (black arrow).
	肋間肋骨：右第9肋骨の椎骨端が欠損し、関節結合していない（赤矢印）。胸椎半椎（10696、第9胸椎の左椎弓と椎体が小型化し、右椎弓は欠損している。）と関連した異常である（楕円）。第12、13椎体は小型化（New）し、右第13椎弓は形態異常（10676）である（黒矢印）。

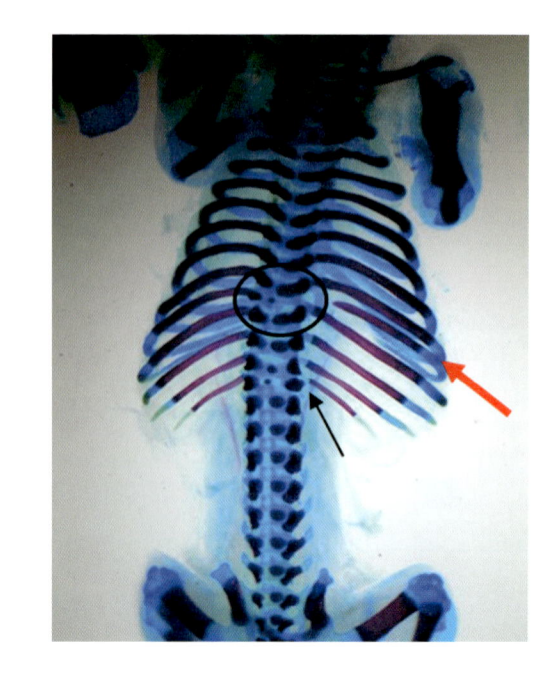

7-6 Interrupted rib 肋骨不連続 (10627)

Species	Rat
Memo	Interrupted rib (arrow): Although the ribs in the specimens below are also Short supernumerary thoracolumbar rib (10638) on the left and Full supernumerary thoracolumbar rib (10628) on the right, these ribs are also interrupted.
	肋骨不連続（矢印）：過剰（胸腰部）肋骨であるが、所見名がないため、「肋骨」に登録する。

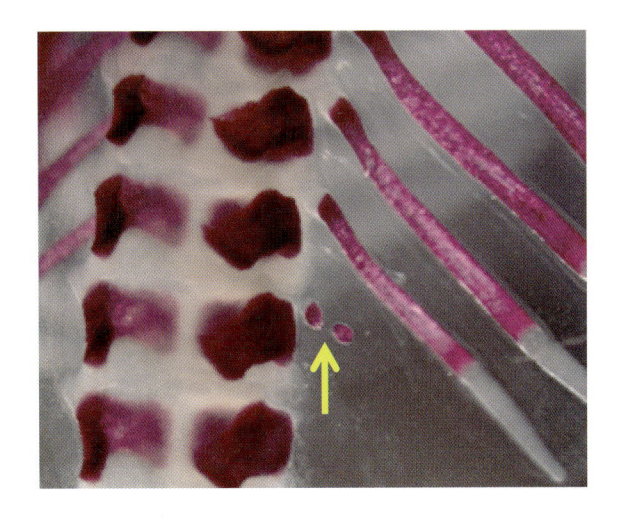

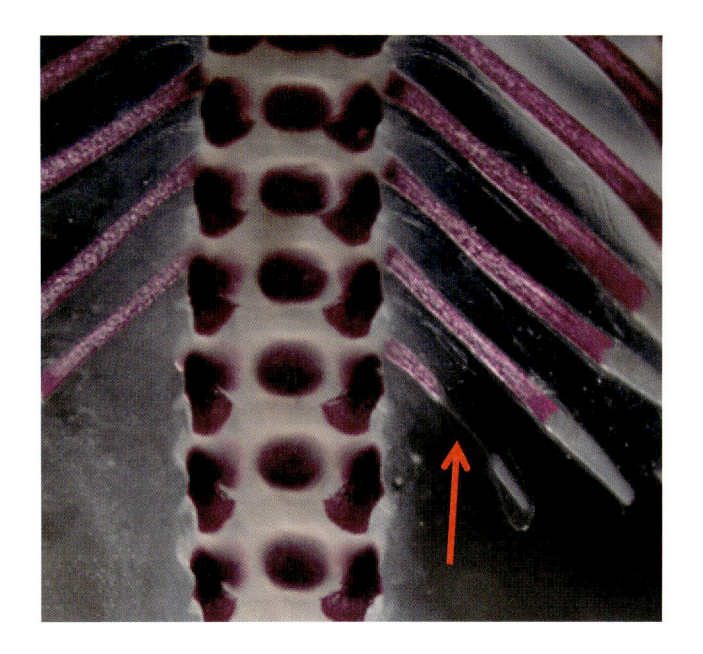

7-7　**Misaligned ribs**　　肋骨配列異常　（10635）

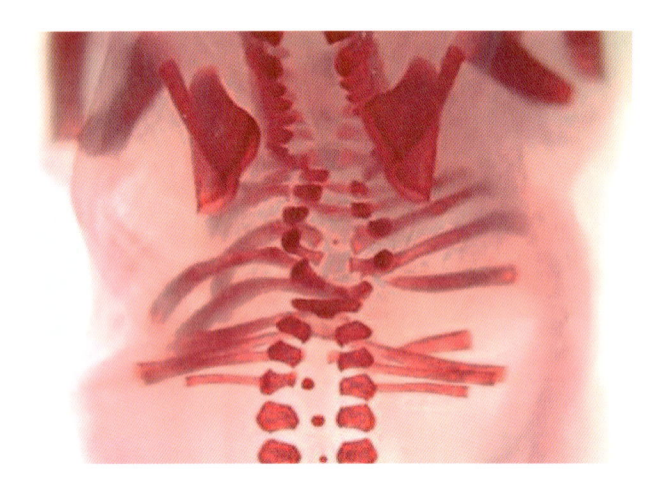

Species	Rat
Memo	Misaligned ribs: This fetus has complex anomalies such as Absent rib (10621), Misshapen rib (10636), and Absent thoracic vertebrae (10694).
	肋骨配列異常：本例は肋骨欠損（10621）、肋骨形態異常（10636）、胸椎欠損（10694）を伴った複合異常。

7-8 Misshapen rib 肋骨形態異常 (10636)

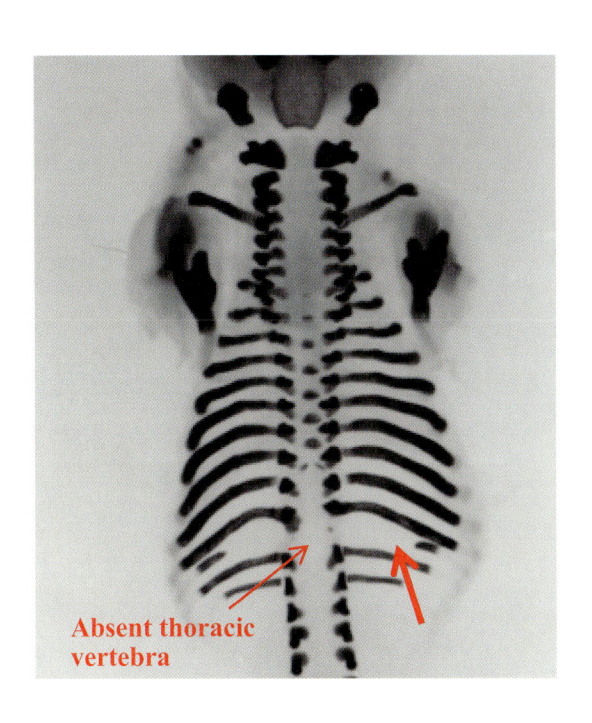

Absent thoracic vertebra

Species	Rat
Memo	Misshapen rib (thick arrow) with Absent thoracic vertebra (thin arrow, 10694) and Absent thoracic and lumbar vertebral centra (10680 and 10707): The vertebral site of the rib is partially absent.
	肋骨形態異常（太矢印）：胸椎が欠損し（細矢印、10694）、肋骨の椎骨側が部分的に欠損している。椎体の欠損（10680 と 10707）も伴っている。胸椎の欠損は「未骨化」あるいは「不完全骨化」かもしれない。

7-9　Nodulated rib　　肋骨結節状　(10633)

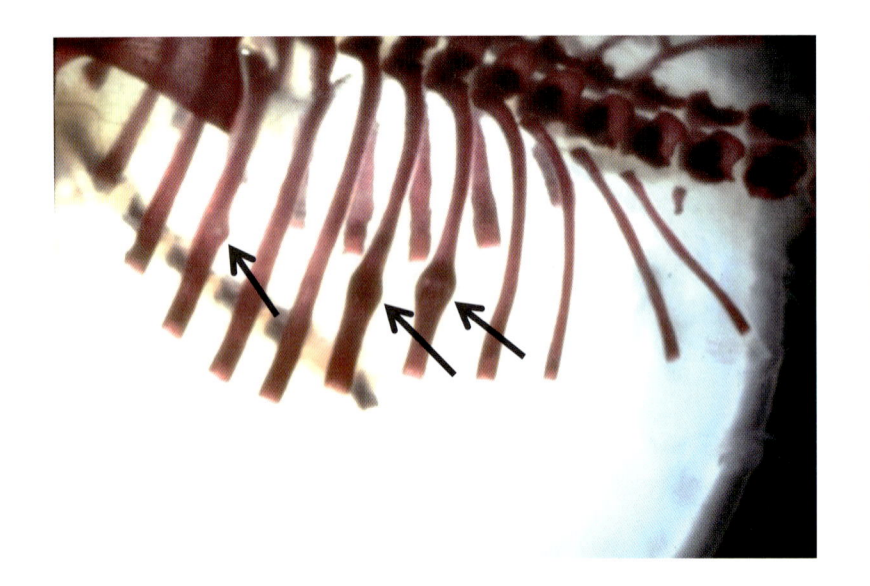

Species	Rabbit
Memo	Nodulated rib (arrow): Both focal enlargement and knobby are observed in this fetus.
	肋骨結節状（矢印）：円形状（局所肥大）とノブ状が見られる。

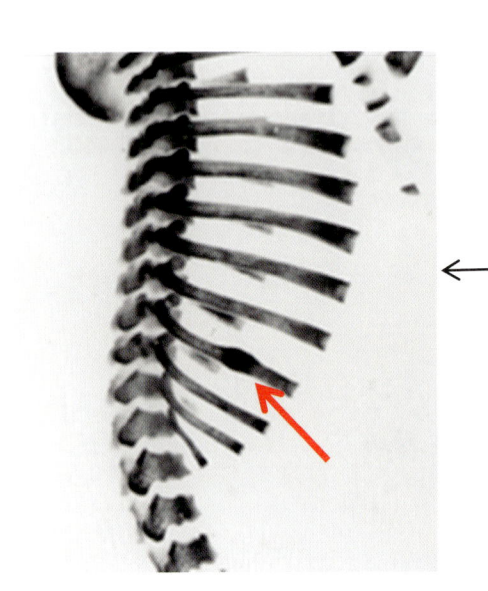

Species	Rabbit
Memo	Nodulated rib (arrow): The knobby type is observed in these specimens.
	肋骨結節状（矢印）：ノブ状の結節が見られる。

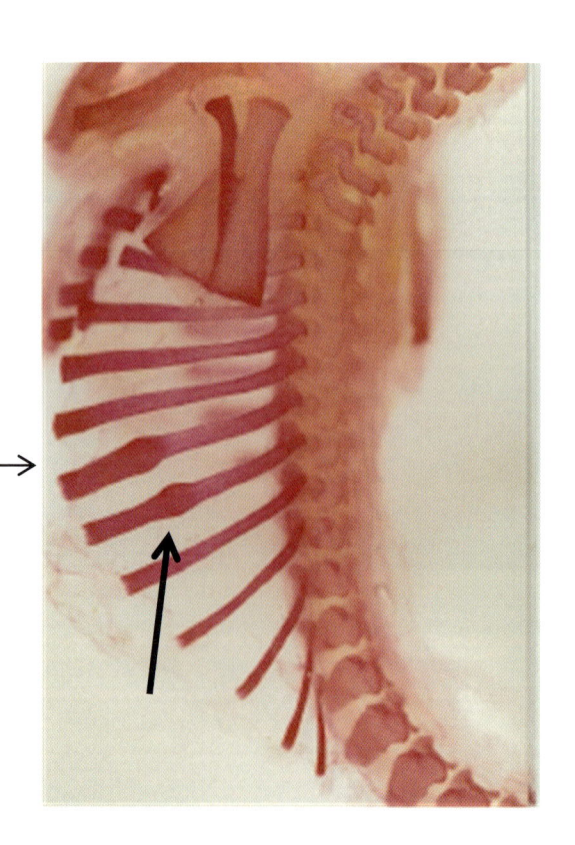

7-9　Continued

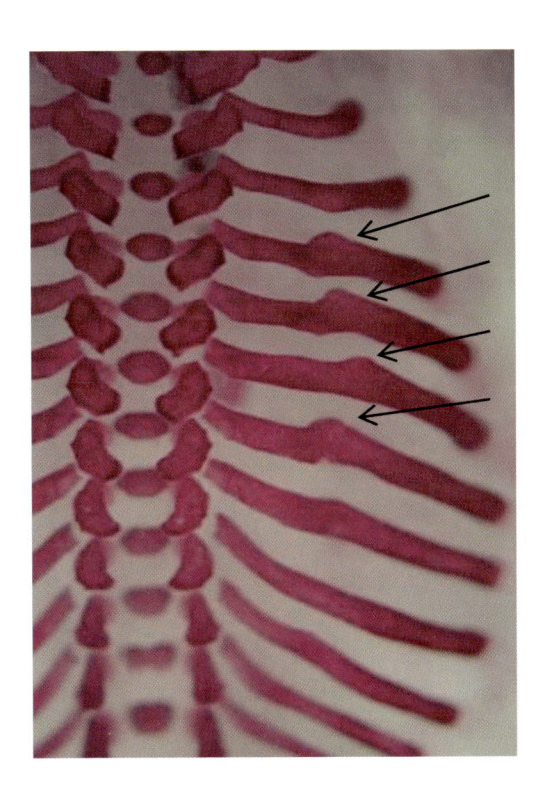

Species	Rat
Memo	Nodulated rib (arrow): This may also be considered as "Wavy rib (10641)".
	肋骨結節状：波状肋骨（10641）でも良い。

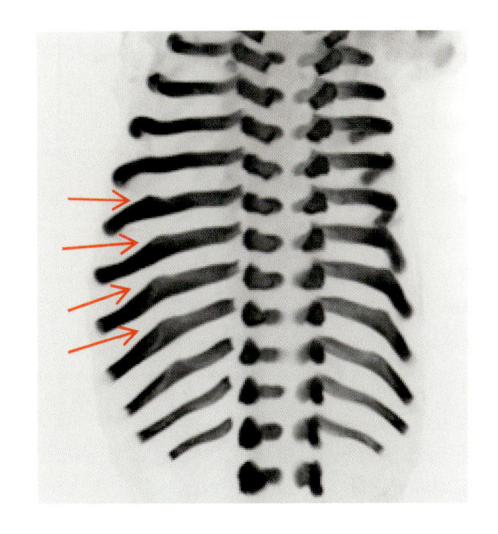

Species	Rat
Memo	Nodulated rib (arrow)
	肋骨結節状（矢印）

7-10　　Short rib　　肋骨短小（化）　　(10637)

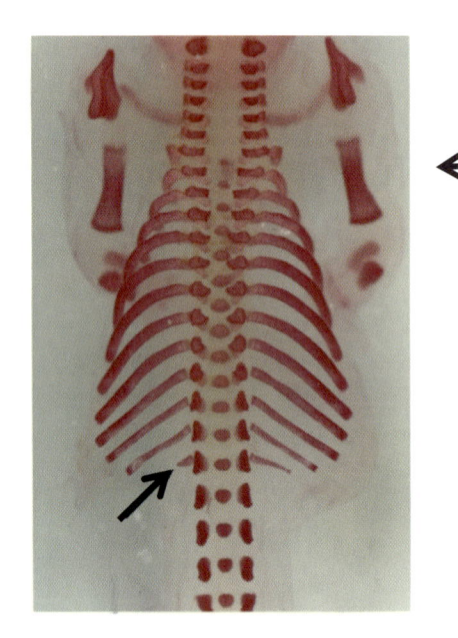

Species	Rat, SD
Memo	Short rib: The 13th rib is short (arrow in photo).
	肋骨短小（化）：第 13 肋骨が短小（矢印）

Species	Rat
Memo	Short rib: The 13th rib is short (arrow in photo).
	肋骨短小（化）：第 13 肋骨が短小（矢印）

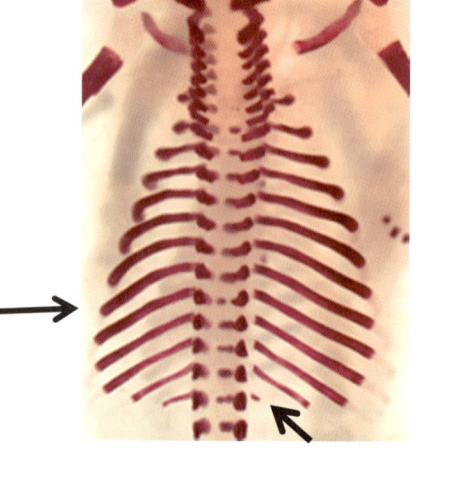

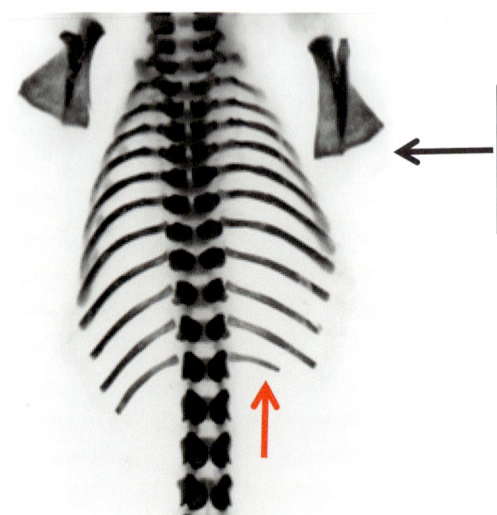

Species	Rabbit
Memo	Short rib: The 12th rib is short (arrow in photo).
	肋骨短小（化）：第 12 肋骨が短小（矢印）

Species	Rabbit
Memo	Short rib: The 1st rib is short (arrow in photo).
	肋骨短小（化）：第 1 肋骨が短小（矢印）

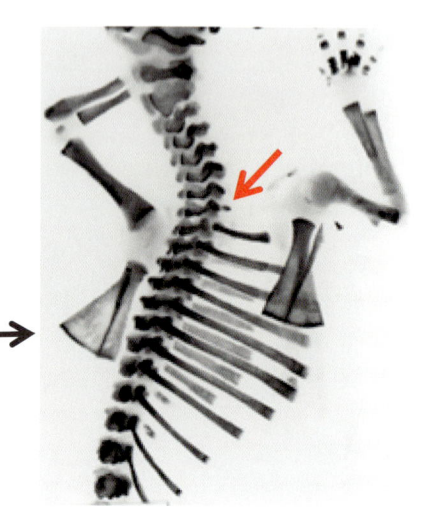

7-11 Supernumerary articulated rib   肋骨過剰   (New)

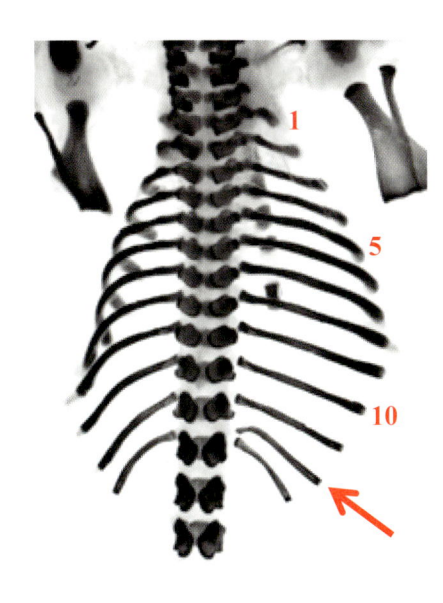

Species	Rabbit
Memo	Supernumerary articulated rib (arrow): An additional full and articulated rib is observed at the right 12th thoracic vertebra.
	肋骨過剰（矢印）：第 12 胸椎部右側に過剰な肋骨があり、脊柱と関節結合している。

7-12　**Thick rib**　　肋骨肥厚（化）　　**(10639)**

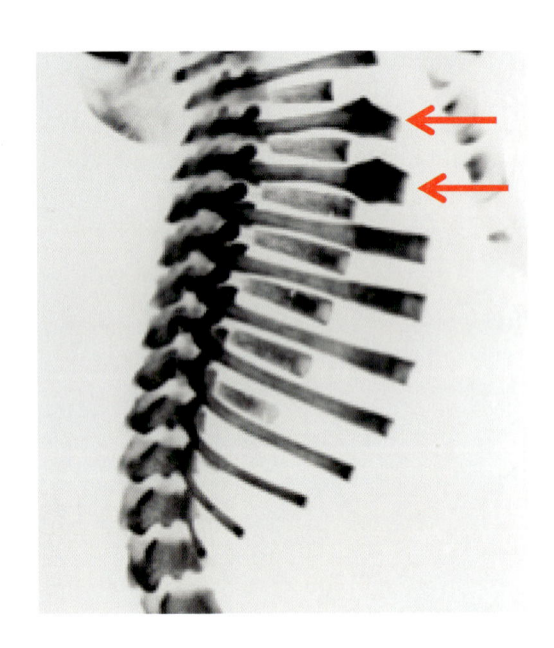

Species	Rabbit
Memo	Thick rib (arrow): A localized thickening is observed in 2 ribs. This may also be considered as "Nodulated rib (10633)".
	肋骨肥厚（化）（矢印）：肋骨が部分的に肥厚している。結節状肋骨（10633）でも良いかも知れない。

7-13　Wavy rib　　波状肋骨　(10641)

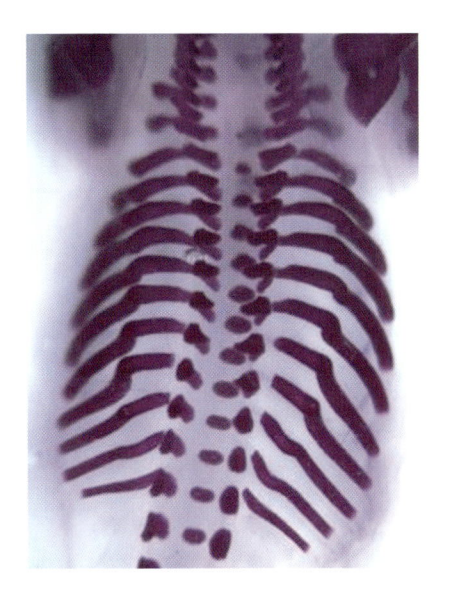

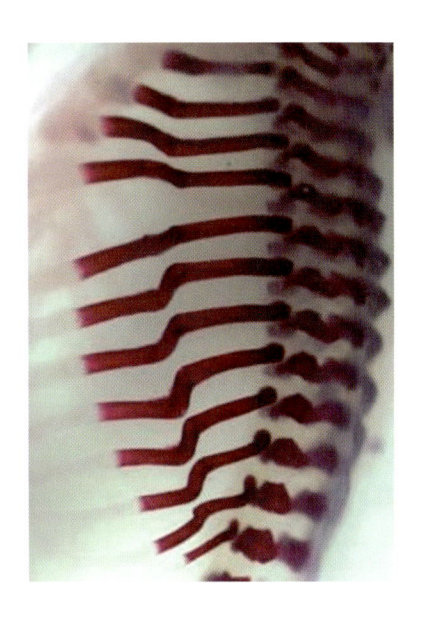

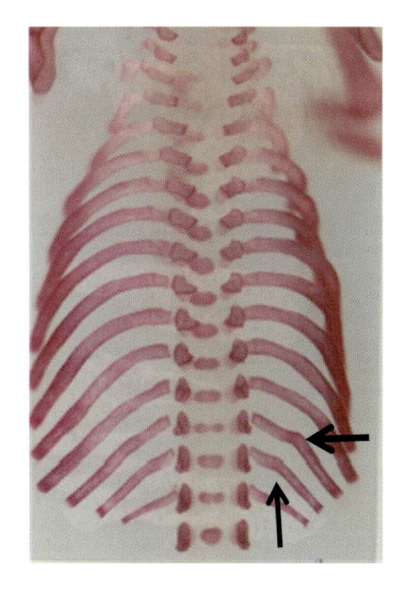

Species	Rat
Memo	Wavy rib
	波状肋骨

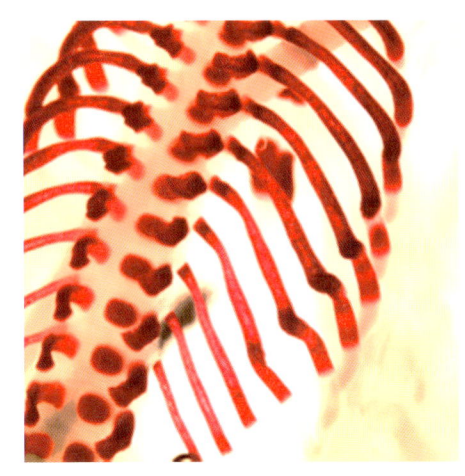

Species	Mouse
Memo	Wavy rib
	波状肋骨

7-14　**Branched costal cartilage**　　肋軟骨分岐　　(10624)

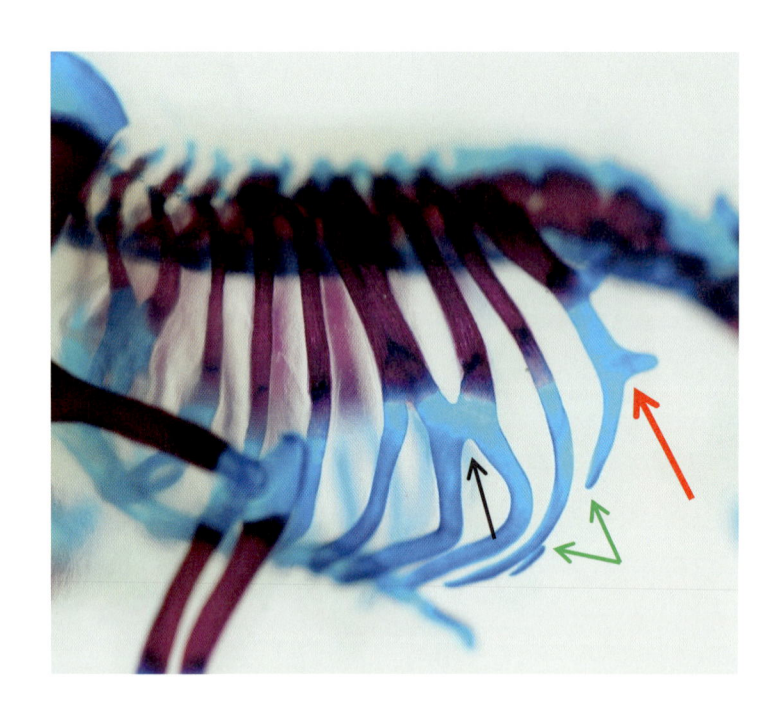

Species	Rat
Memo	Branched costal cartilage (red arrow) with Fused costal cartilage (black arrow, 10630), Interrupted costal cartilage (green arrow, New) and Fused rib (10629)
	肋軟骨分岐（赤矢印）：肋軟骨癒合（黒矢印、10630）、肋軟骨不連続（緑矢印、New）及び肋骨癒合（10629）を伴う。

7-15　Interrupted costal cartilage　　肋軟骨不連続　(New)

Species	Rat
Memo	Interrupted costal cartilage (arrow)
	肋軟骨不連続（矢印）

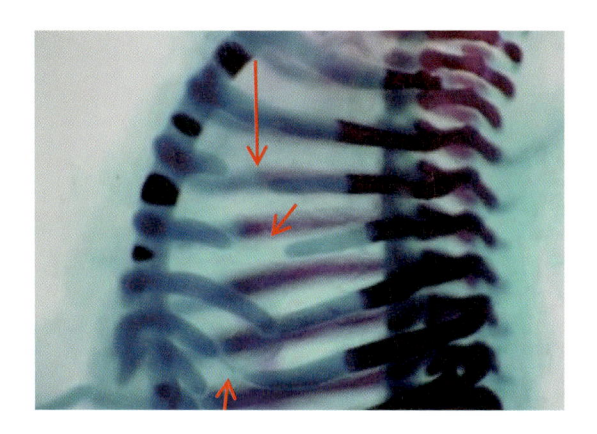

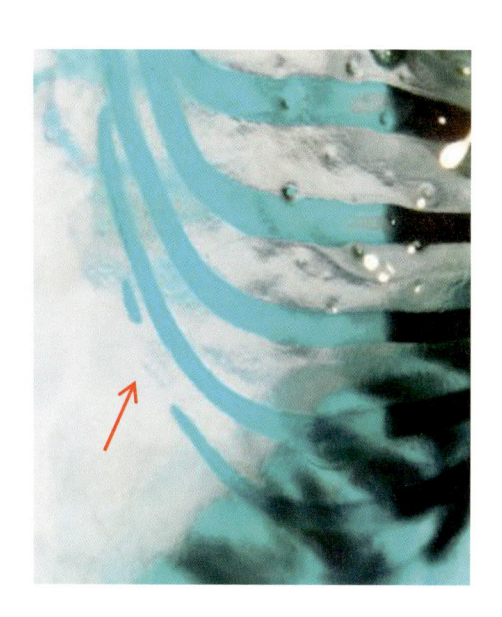

7-16 Fused costal cartilage 肋軟骨癒合 (10630)

Species	Rat
Memo	Fused costal cartilage (arrow)
	肋軟骨癒合（矢印）

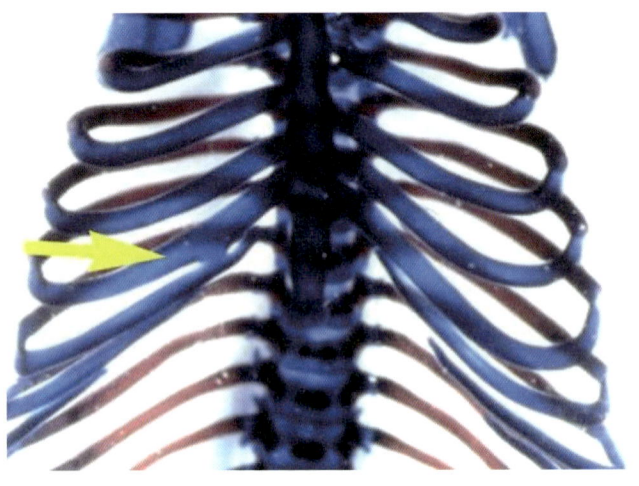

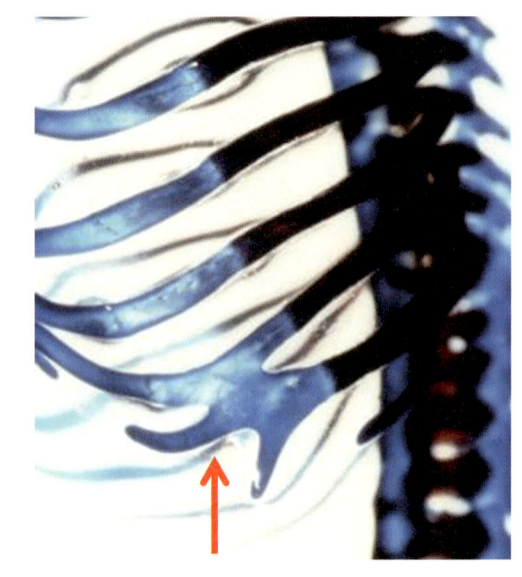

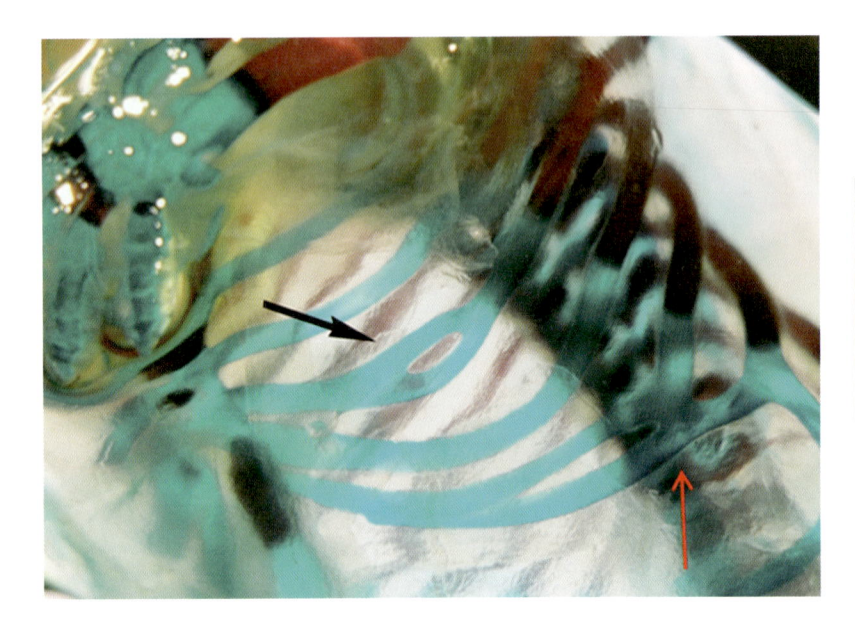

Species	Rat
Memo	Fused costal cartilage (red arrow) with Partially duplicated costal cartilage (black arrow, New)
	肋軟骨癒合（赤矢印）：肋軟骨部分重複（黒矢印、New）を伴う。

7-16　Continued

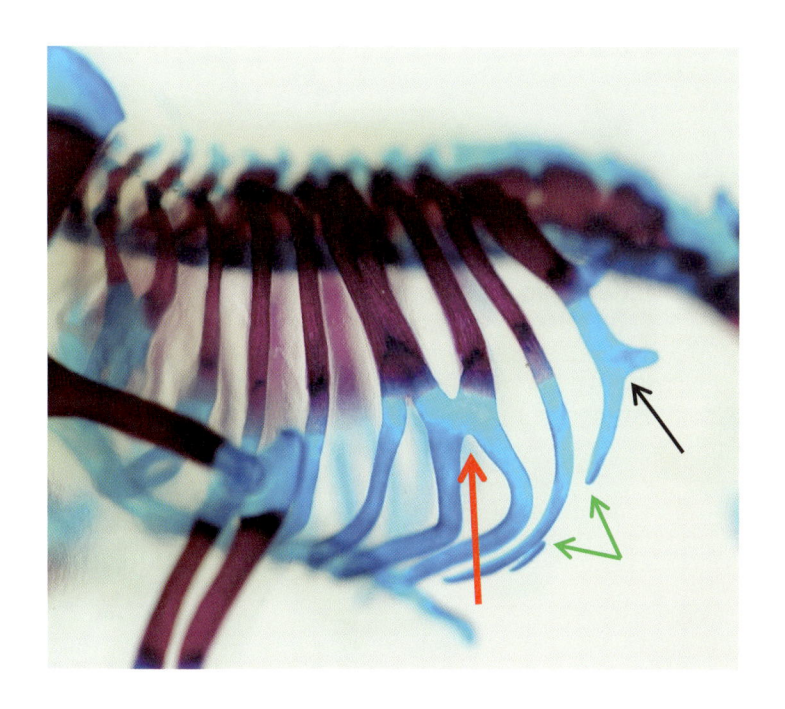

Species	Rat
Memo	Fused costal cartilage (red arrow) with Branched costal cartilage (black arrow, 10624), Interrupted costal cartilage (green arrow, New) and Fused rib (10629)
	肋軟骨癒合（赤矢印）：肋軟骨分岐（黒矢印、10624）、肋軟骨不連続（緑矢印、New）及び肋骨癒合（10629）を伴う。

7-17 **Costal cartilage not fused to sternum**　　肋軟骨胸骨不接続　(New)

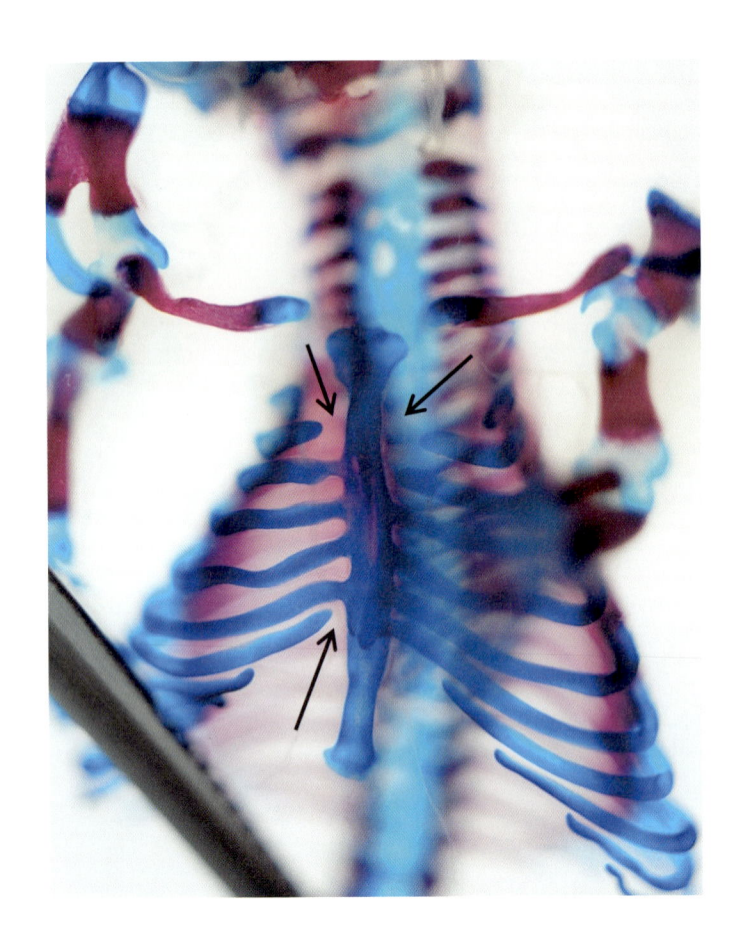

Species	Rat
Memo	Costal cartilage not fused to sternum (arrow) with Unossified sternebra (10620)
	肋軟骨胸骨不接続（矢印）：胸骨分節未骨化（10620）を伴う。

7-18 Partially duplicated costal cartilage 肋軟骨部分重複 (New)

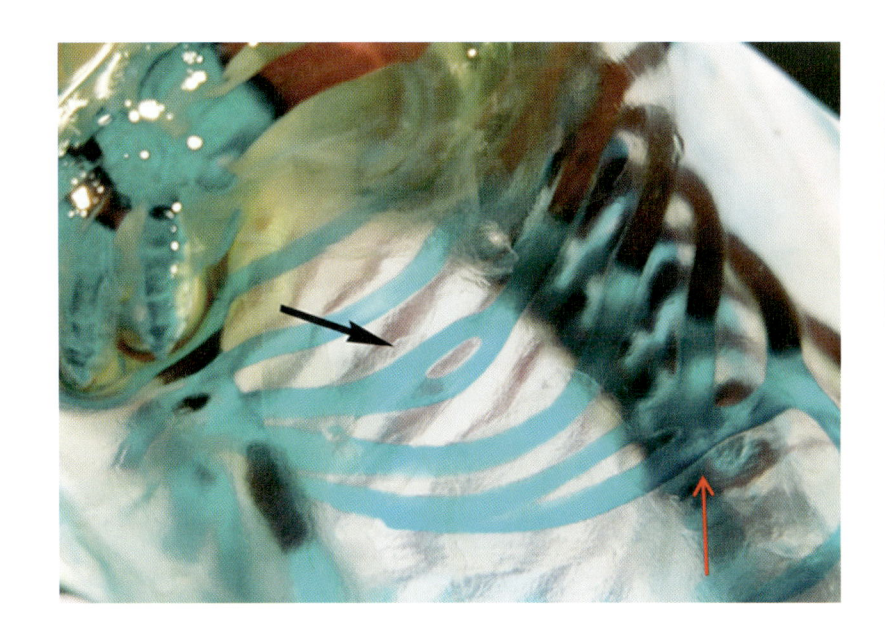

Species	Rat
Memo	Partially duplicated costal cartilage (black arrow) with Fused costal cartilage (red arrow, New)
	肋軟骨部分重複（黒矢印）：肋軟骨癒合（赤矢印、New）を伴う。

7-19 Full cervical supernumerary rib   頸部完全過剰肋骨   (New)

Species	Rat and Rabbit
Memo	Full cervical supernumerary rib (arrow)
	頸部完全過剰肋骨（矢印）

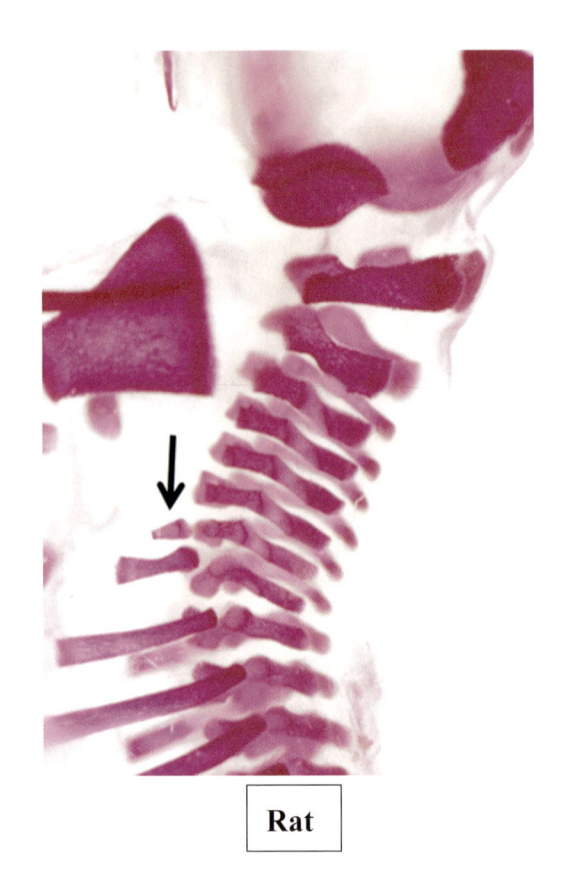

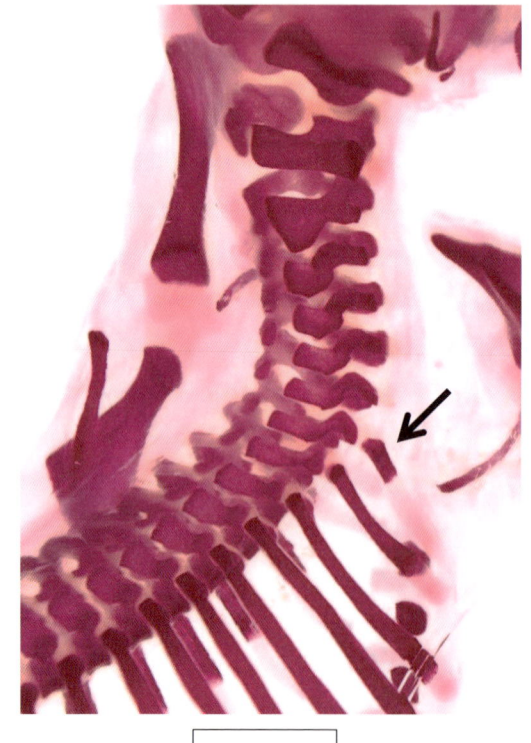

Rat

Rabbit

7-20 Short cervical supernumerary rib　頸部短小過剰肋骨　(10625)

Species	Rabbit and mouse
Memo	Short cervical supernumerary rib or Rudimentary cervical rib (arrow)
	頸部短小過剰肋骨、頸肋（痕跡）（矢印）

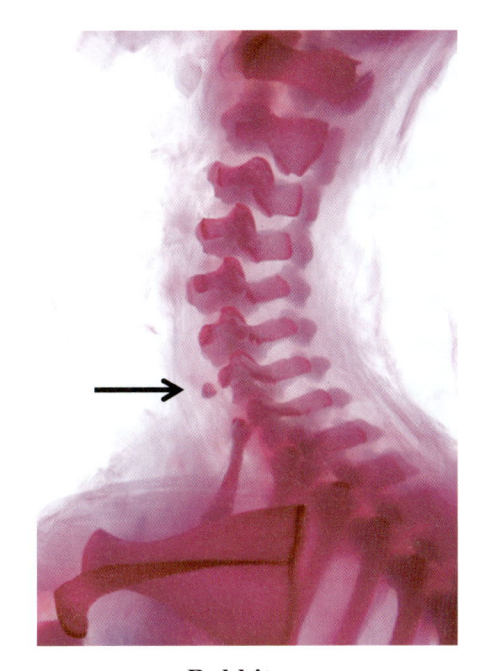

Rabbit

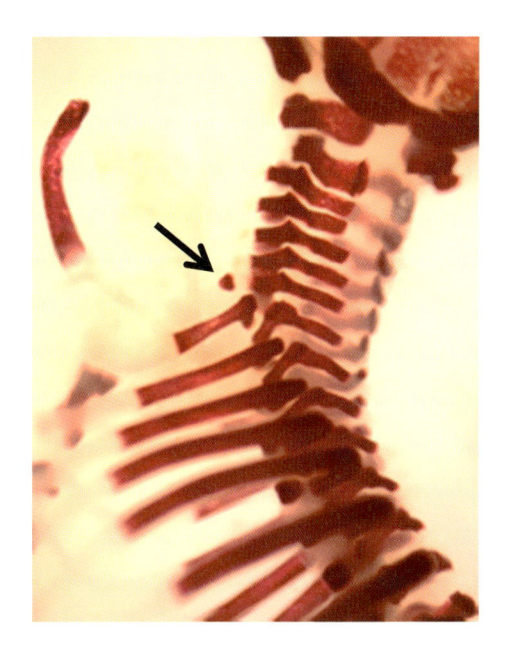

Mouse

7-21　Full thoracolumbar supernumerary rib　　胸腰部完全過剰肋骨　（10628）

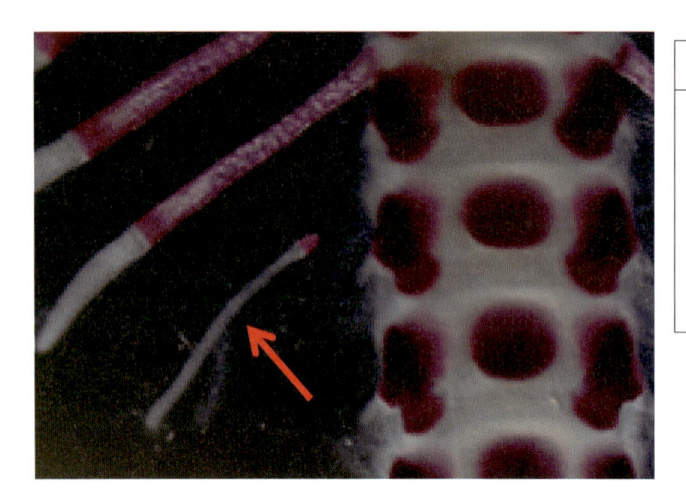

Species	Rat
Memo	Full thoracolumbar supernumerary rib (arrow): Although the ossified part is small, this is judged to be a full lumbar rib because of the presence of a long unossified section.
	胸腰部完全過剰肋骨（矢印）：骨化部分は小さいが、未骨化部分から「完全」とする。

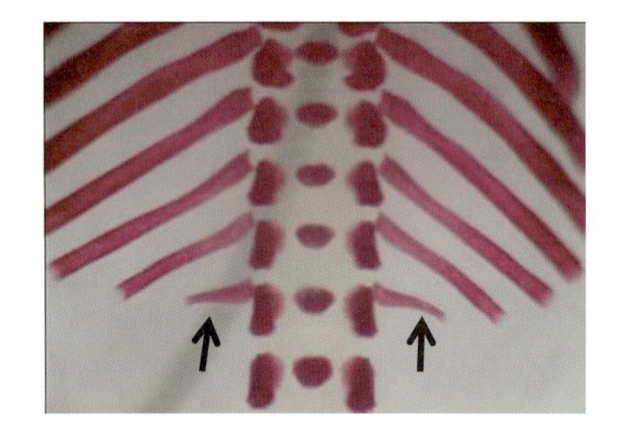

Species	Rat
Memo	Full thoracolumbar supernumerary rib (arrow)
	胸腰部完全過剰肋骨（矢印）

7-21 continued

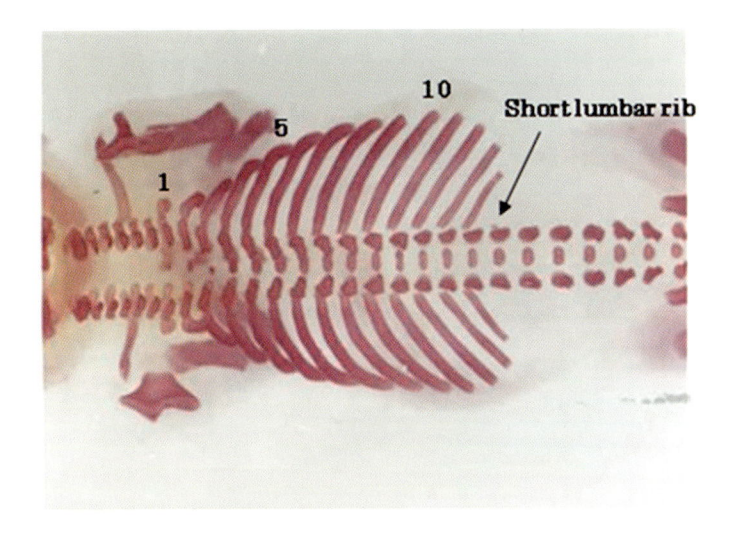

Species	Rat, SD
Memo	Full thoracolumbar supernumerary rib with Increased presacral vertebrae (10643) and Short thoracolumbar rib (10638):
	完全胸腰部過剰肋骨：仙椎前椎骨数増加（10643）及び痕跡程度の短小過剰肋骨（右側、10638）を伴う。

7-22 Short thoracolumbar supernumerary rib 胸腰部短小過剰肋骨 (10638)

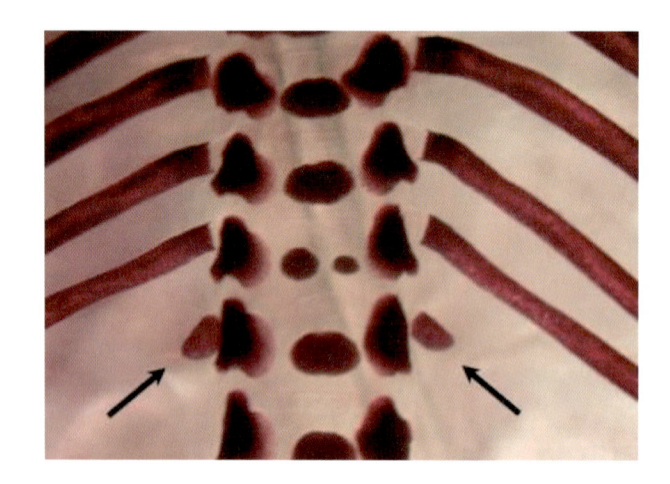

Species	Rat
Memo	Short thoracolumbar supernumerary rib or Rudimentary lumbar rib (arrow)
	胸腰部短小過剰肋骨、腰肋（痕跡）（矢印）

Photographs of Skeletal Anomalies

8. Vertebral canal and Cervical vertebra

8-1 Supernumerary vertebrae 椎骨過剰 (10643)

Species	Rat, SD
Memo	Increased number of presacral vertebrae with Full supernumerary thoracolumbar rib (10628) and Short supernumerary thoracolumbar rib (10638): This fetus is judged to have "Supernumeray vertebrae (presacral) (10643)" because it is difficult to distinguish between thoracic vertebra and lumbar vertebra. But, this fetus may also be considered to have "Supernumerary thoracic vertebrae (10697)" and "Supernumerary ribs (New)" because a complete set of 14th rib is present and an additional 15th short rib (arrow) is observed, and number of lumbar vertebrae is normal (6 vertebrae).
	仙椎前椎骨数増加：胸腰部の両側に完全過剰肋骨（10628）、右側には更に痕跡程度の短小過剰肋骨（10638）を伴う。本標本において胸腰椎の識別は不確実であるため、椎弓の形態並びに腸骨との位置関係から腰仙椎を識別し、「仙椎前椎骨数増加」とする。過剰肋骨が完成された形態であり、また、腰椎数は正常（6椎）と思われることから、「胸椎数増加（10697）」及び「肋骨過剰（New）」とも考えられる。

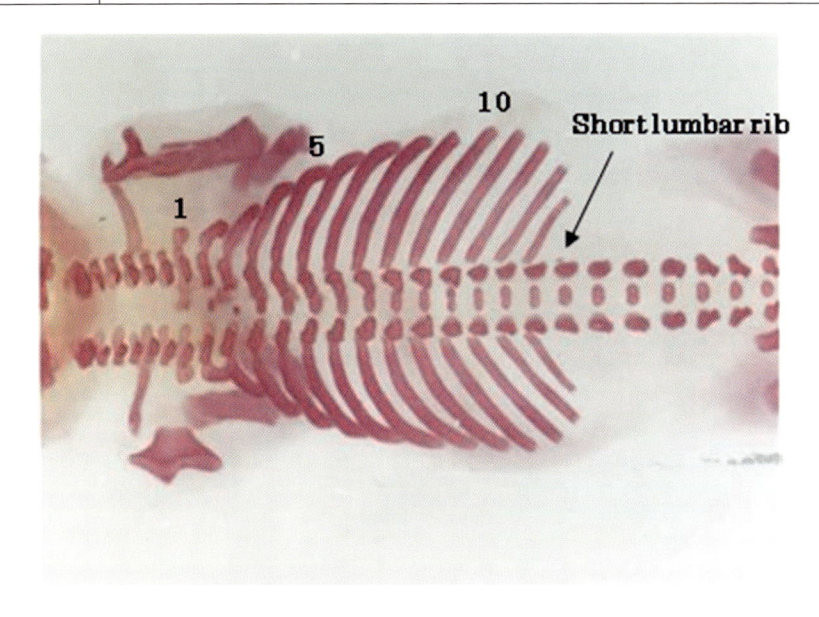

8-2　Interrupted vertebral canal　脊柱管不連続　(New)

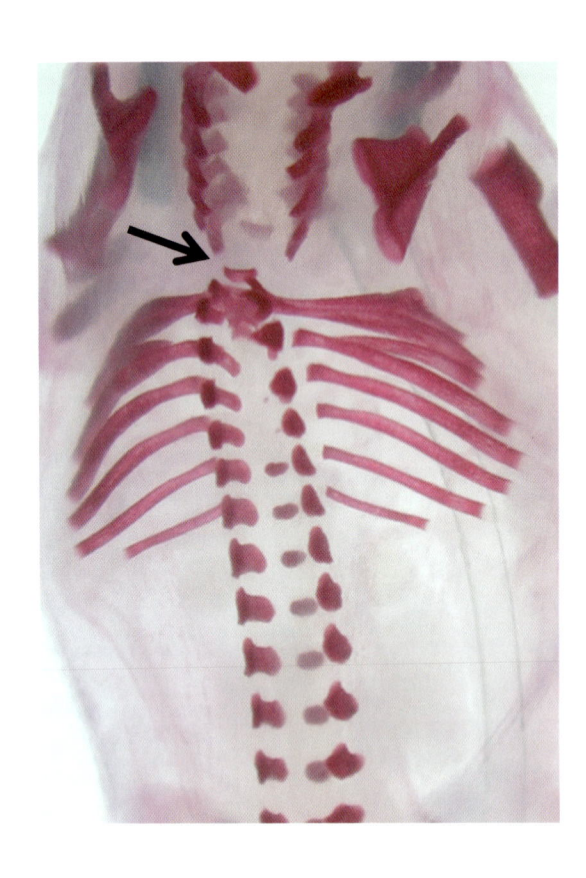

Species	Rat
Memo	Interrupted vertebral canal with Absent thoracic vertebra (10694), Absent rib (10621) and Fused rib (10629) or Branched rib (10623)
	脊柱管不連続：胸椎欠損（10694）、肋骨欠損（10621）、肋骨癒合（10629）あるいは肋骨分岐（10623）を伴う。

8-3 Double vertebral canal   脊柱管二重   (New)

Species	Rat
Memo	Double vertebral canal: A form of conjoined twins; The dorsal region of this fetus appears normal in external observation. The right photograph shows external feature of this fetus demonstrating Exencephaly (10013) and Bifurcated tail (10097).
	脊柱管二重：二重体の一種。外表観察では二重体の所見はなかった。右写真は本胎児の外表写真で、外脳（10013）及び二又尾（10097）が見られる。

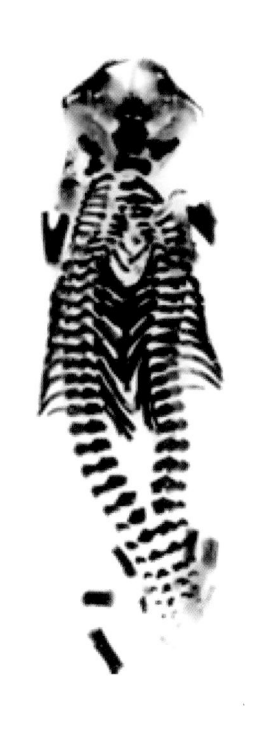

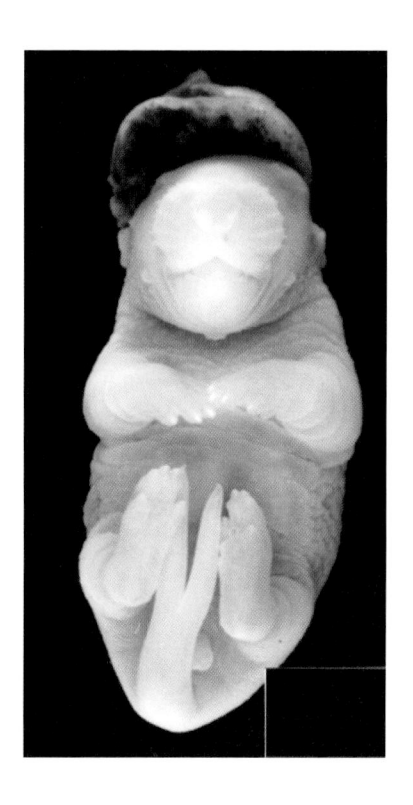

8-3 Continued

Species	Rat
Memo	Double vertebral canal: This fetus is considered to be cranio-thoraco-omphalopagus, symmetrical monozygotic twins, or conjoined twins (10002) (see photograph of external feature).
	脊柱管二重：外表では対称性二重体のうち、頭胸腹部接合体と思われる（写真添付）。

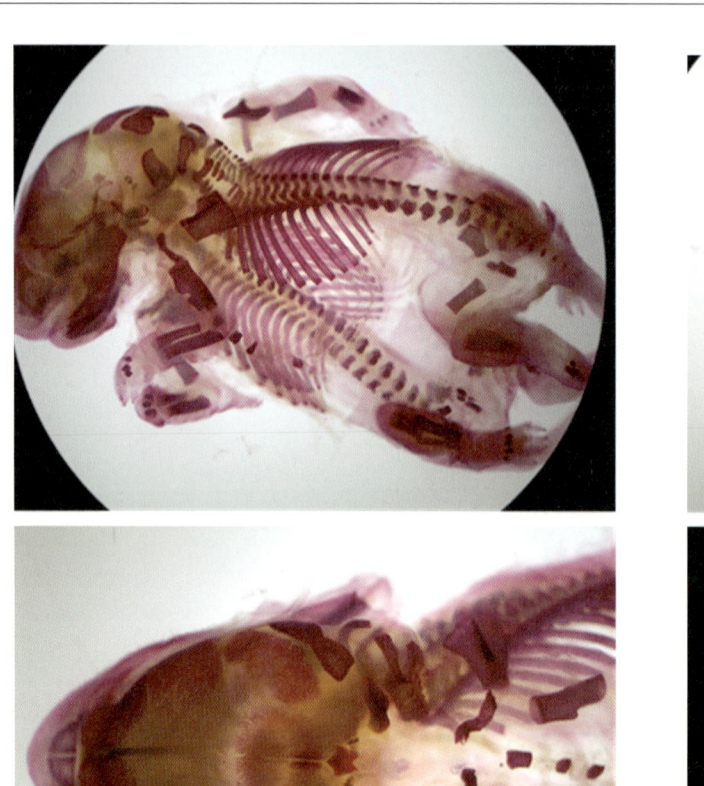

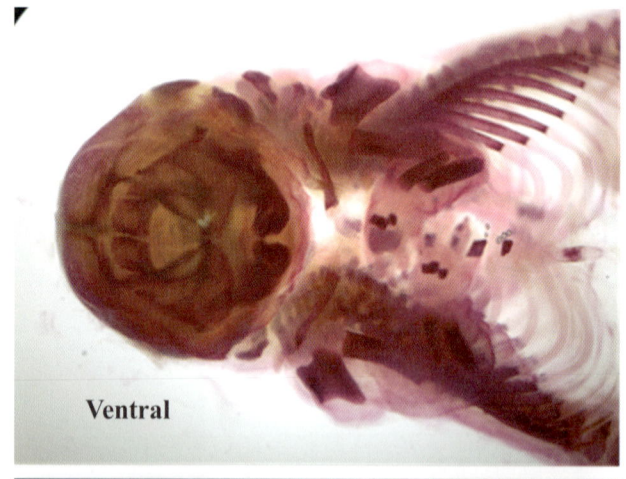

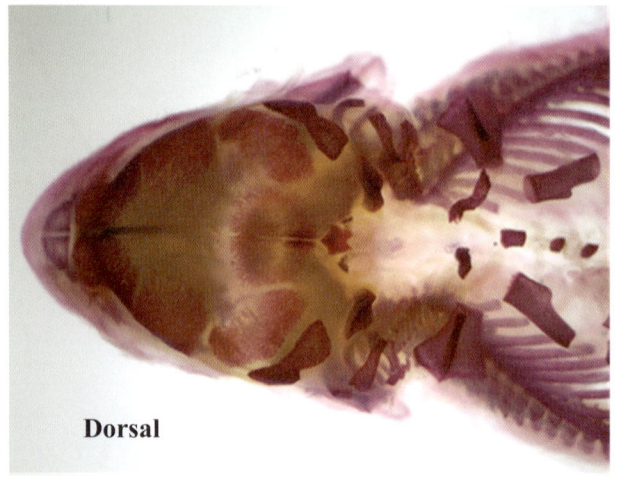

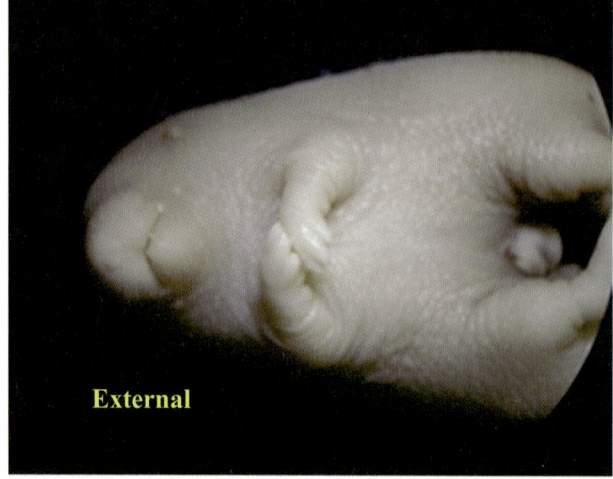

Ventral

Dorsal

External

8-4 Absent atlas　　環椎欠損　(New)

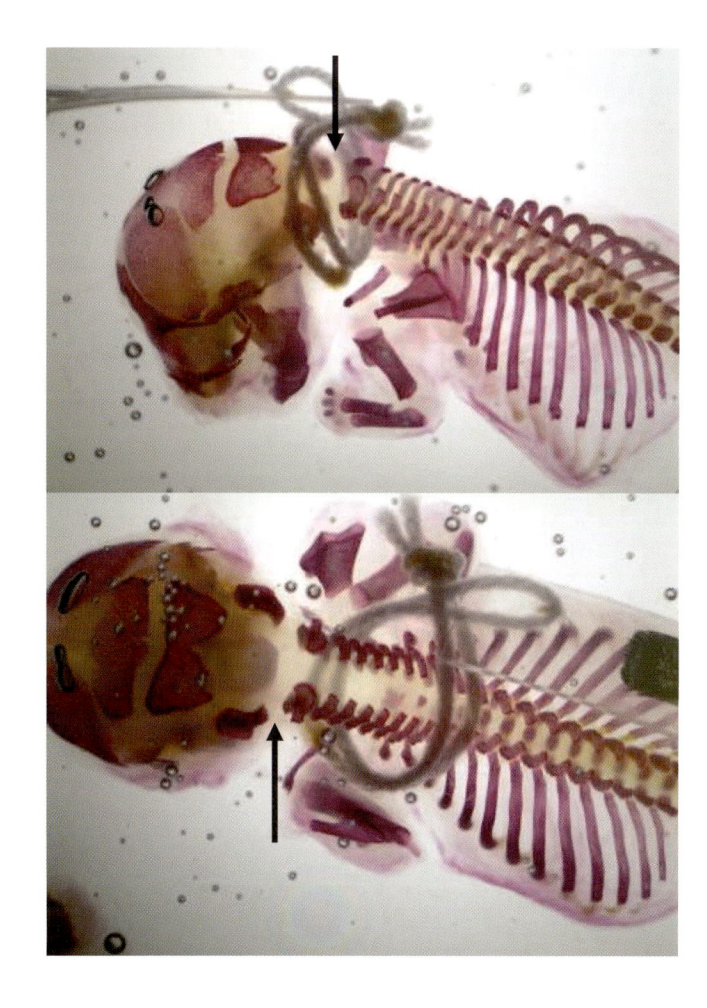

Species	Rat, SD
Memo	Absent atlas (arrow): The 1st cervical vertebra (Atlas) is absent, and there are only 6 cervical vertebrae in this fetus.
	環椎欠損（矢印）：第1頸椎が欠損し、頸椎数は6対

8-5 Fused atlas 環椎癒合 (New)

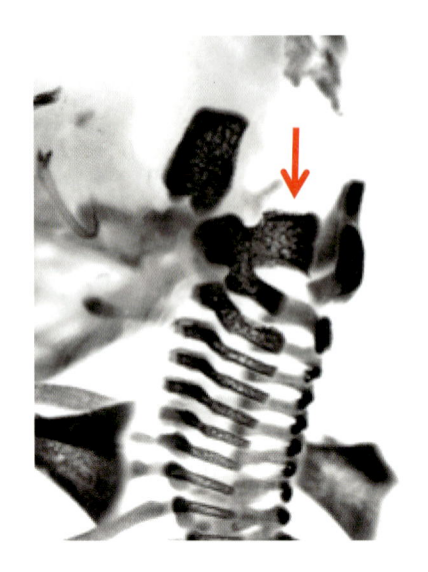

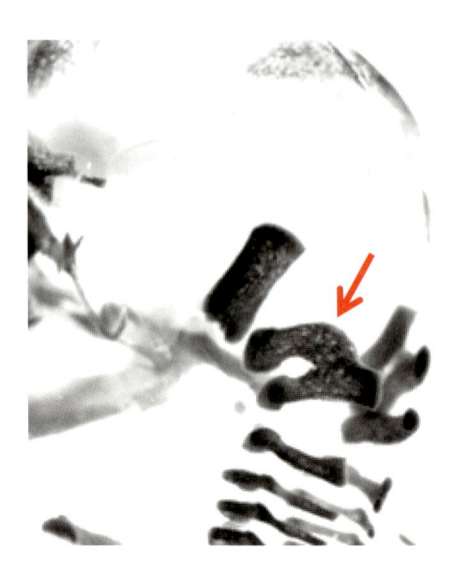

Species	Mouse
Memo	Fused atlas: Atlas fused with the 2nd cervical arch (arrow).
	環椎癒合：環椎と第2頸椎弓が癒合している（矢印）。

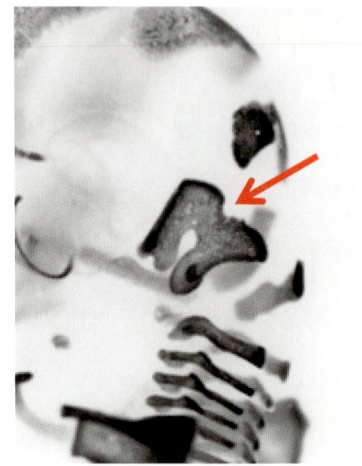

Species	Mouse
Memo	Atlas fused with exoccipital bone (arrow).
	環椎弓外後頭骨癒合：環椎と外後頭骨が癒合している（矢印）。

8-6 Misshapen atlas 環椎形態異常 (New)

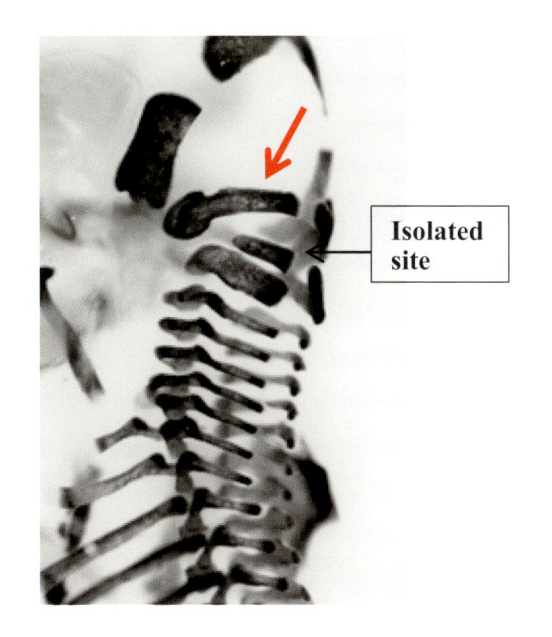

Species	Mouse
Memo	Misshapen atlas with Isolated ossification site (New). Atlas arch is narrow (red arrow).
	環椎形態異常：幅が狭くなっている（矢印）。頸椎弓分離骨化部位（New）も伴う。

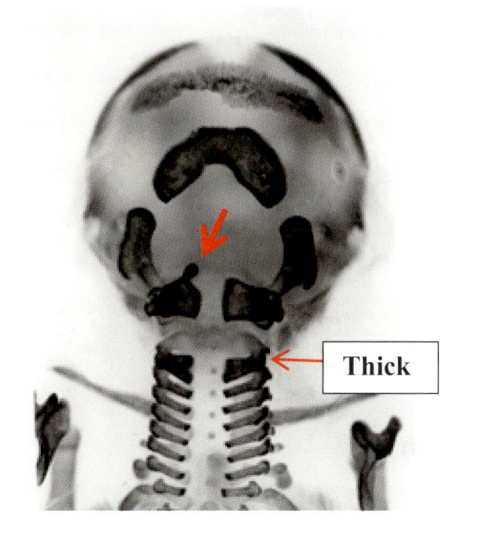

Species	Mouse
Memo	Misshapen atlas with Thick cervical arch (2nd, New): The atlas is abnormally shaped (thick arrow)
	環椎形態異常：環椎に過剰部位が見られる（矢印）。頸椎弓の肥厚（New）を伴う。

8-7 Small atlas 環椎小型（化） (New)

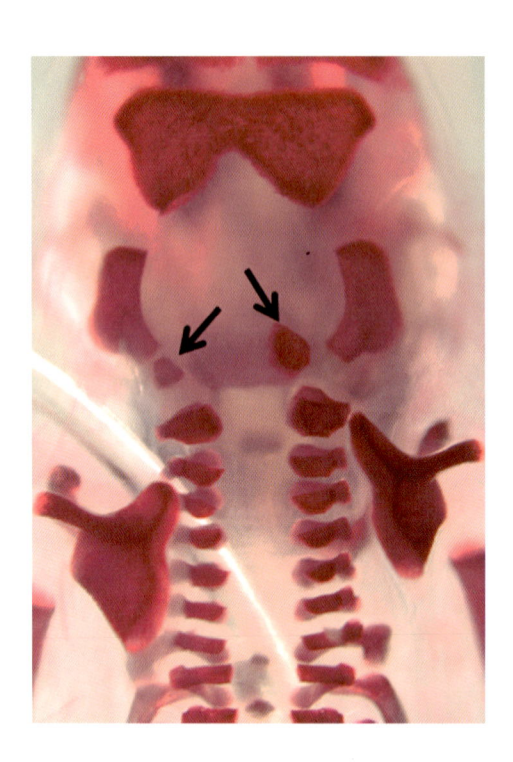

Species	Rat
Memo	Small atlas: The atlases are small bilaterally (arrow).
	環椎小型（化）：左右の環椎が小型（矢印）

8-8　Fused cervical arch　　頸椎弓癒合　　(10645)

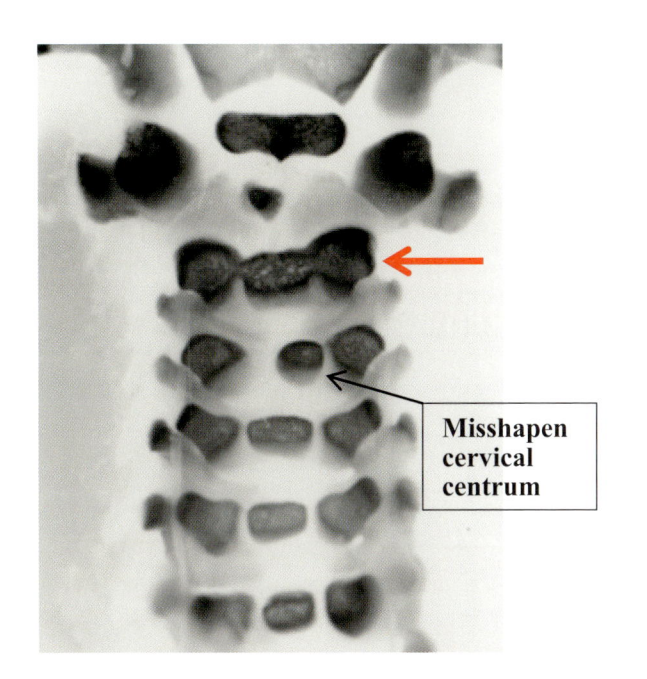

Species	Rabbit
Memo	Fused cervical arch and body with Misshapen cervical vertebral centrum or Unilateral ossification of cervical vertebral centrum (thin black arrow, 10662 or New, respectively): Cervical vertebral arch fuses with cervical vertebral centrum (red arrow).
	頸椎弓癒合：椎弓と椎体の癒合（赤矢印）。頸椎体形態異常あるいは頸椎体片側性骨化（細黒矢印、10662 あるいは New）を伴う。

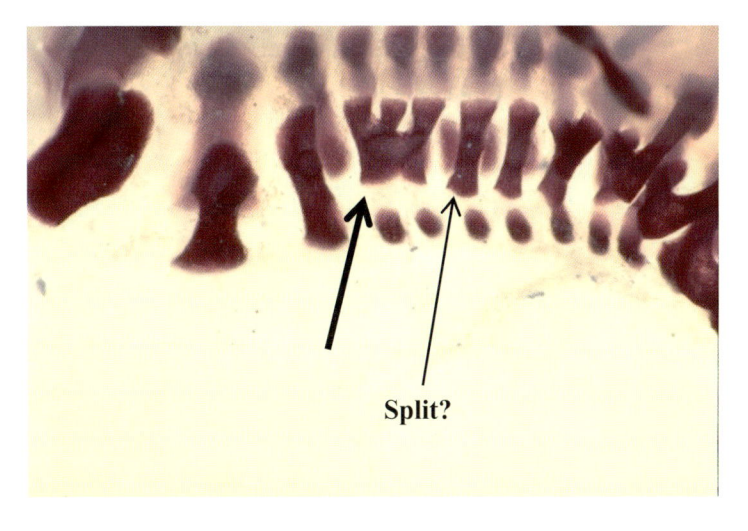

Misshapen cervical centrum

Species	Rat
Memo	Fused cervical vertebral arches: Shapes as same as "split arches" are observed (arrow). However, they are considered to be normal because they are seen usually in retarded rat fetuses.
	頸椎弓癒合：頸椎弓の腹側部に分離の様な部分（矢印）が見られるが、ラットの場合、発育抑制で良く見られるものであり、所見としないのが通常。

Split?

8-8 Continued

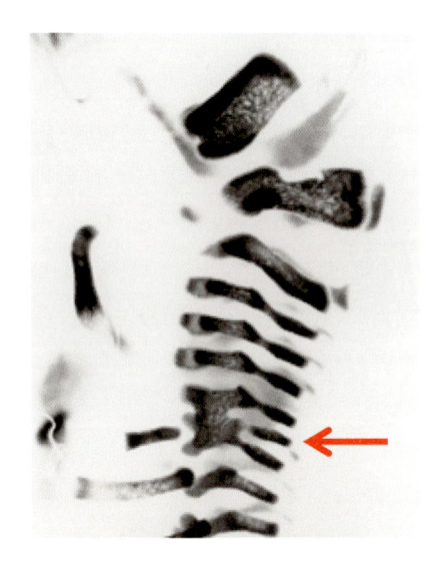

Species	Mouse
Memo	Fusion of thoracic and cervical vertebral arches: Thoracic arch fuses with cervical arch (arrow).
	胸椎弓頸椎弓癒合：胸椎弓と頸椎弓の癒合（矢印）

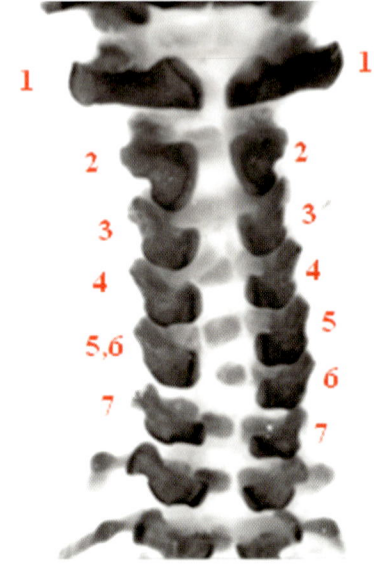

Species	Rabbit
Memo	Fused cervical vertebral arches (5th and 6th).
	頸椎弓癒合：第5と第6頸椎弓の癒合

8-8 Continued

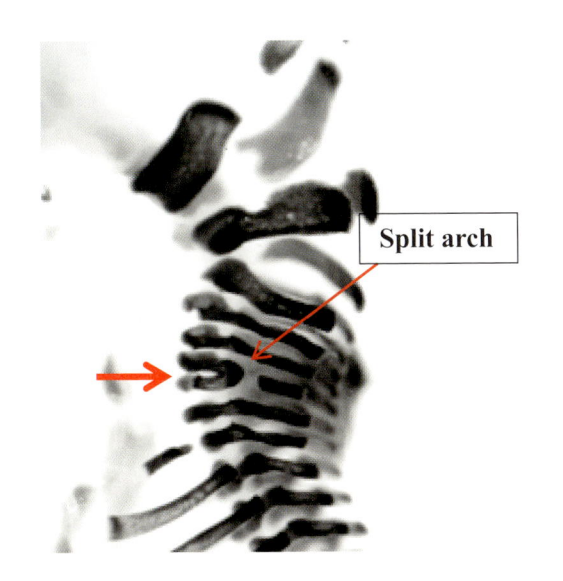

Species	Mouse
Memo	Fused cervical vertebral arches with Split arch (thin arrow, New): Fusion of the 5th and 6th cervical vertebral arches is observed (thick red arrow).
	頸椎弓癒合：第5頸椎弓と第6頸椎弓が癒合（太赤矢印）。頸椎弓分離（細矢印、New）を伴う。

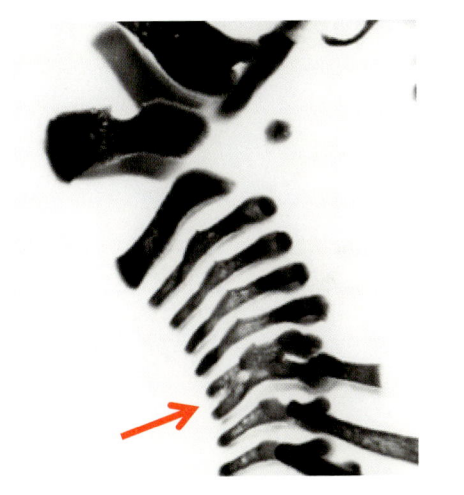

Species	Mouse
Memo	Fusion of cervical and thoracic vertebral arches: Cervical arch fuses to thoracic arch (red arrow).
	頸椎弓胸椎弓癒合：頸椎弓と胸椎弓の癒合（赤矢印）

8-8 Continued

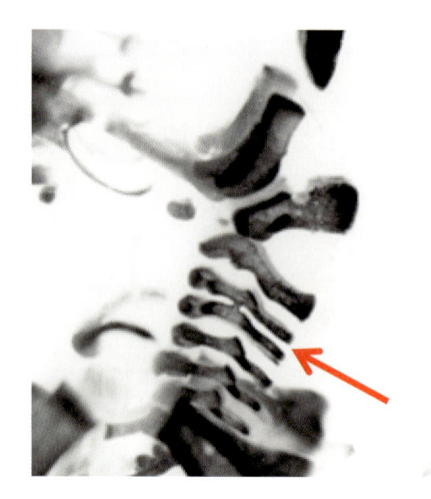

Species	Mouse
Memo	Fused cervical arches: Fusion of the 3rd and 4th cervical vertebral arches is observed (red arrow).
	頸椎弓癒合：第3頸椎弓と第4頸椎弓が癒合（赤矢印）

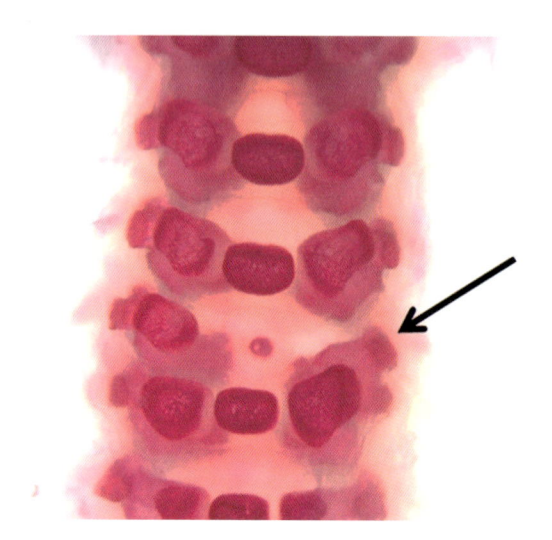

Species	Rabbit
Memo	Fused cervical arches with Small cervical centrum (New)
	頸椎弓癒合：癒合した椎弓部分の椎体が小さい（New）

8-9　Misshapen cervical arch　頸椎弓形態異常　(10649)

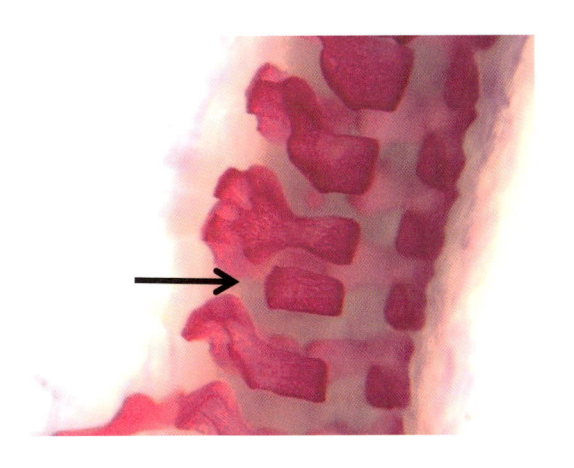

Species	Rabbit
Memo	Misshapen cervical arch: The 5th cervical arch is abnormal shape, and the 6th cervical arch is short (arrow).
	頸椎弓形態異常：左側第 5 及び 6 頸椎弓の形態異常（矢印）

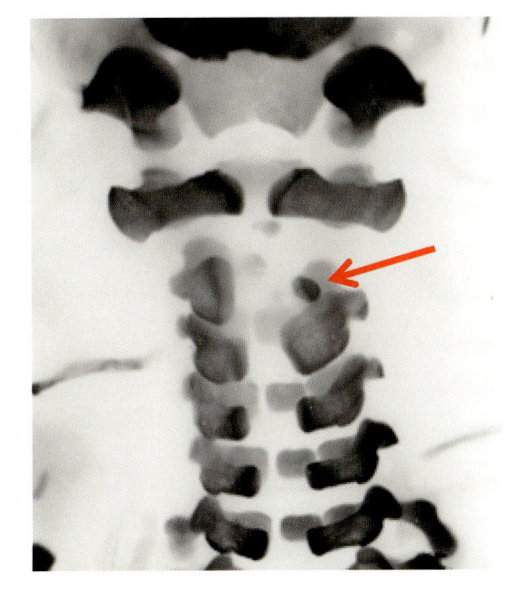

Species	Rabbit
Memo	Misshapen cervical vertebral arch (red arrow) with Absent cervical vertebrae (10667): The right 2nd arch is rudimental, so, this finding may be considered to be "small cervical vertebral arch (10650)". The number of cervical vertebrae reduces to 5 pairs.
	頸椎弓形態異常（矢印）：痕跡状で「小型化（10650）」でも良いかも知れない。頸椎の欠損（5 対、10667）を伴う。

8-10 Split cervical vertebral arch　　頚椎弓分離　(New)

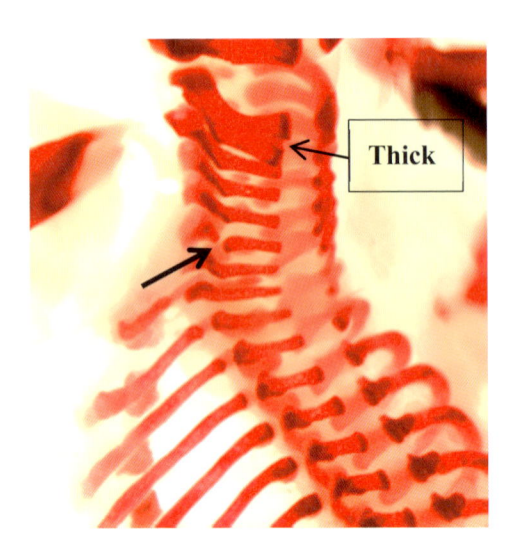

Species	Mouse
Memo	Split cervical vertebral arch, Interrupted cervical vertebral arch: The 6th cervical vertebral arch is interrupted at the middle position (thick arrow). The 2nd arch is thick (thin arrow, New).
	頸椎弓分離・不連続：第6頸椎弓が中央で分離（不連続）している（太矢印）。第2頸椎弓は肥厚（細矢印、New）が見られる。

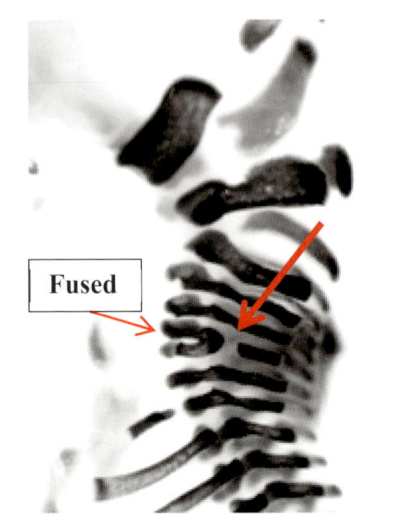

Species	Mouse
Memo	Split cervical vertebral arch with Fused cervical vertebral arches (10645): Fusion of the 5th and 6th cervical vertebral arches is observed (thin arrow), and these arches interrupted (thick arrow).
	頸椎弓分離：第5頸椎弓と第6頸椎弓が癒合（細矢印、10645）し、その頸椎弓が分離している（太矢印）。

8-11 Thick cervical vertebral arch　頸椎弓肥厚（化）　(New)

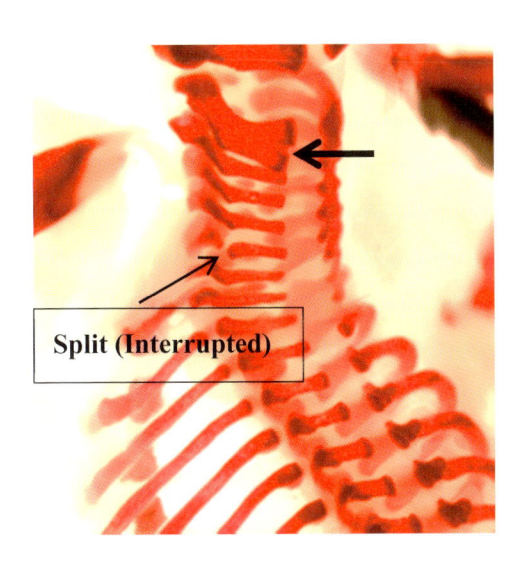

Split (Interrupted)

Species	Mouse
Memo	Thick cervical vertebral arch: The 2nd arch is split at the dorsal tip (thick arrow; New, bifurcated). The 6th cervical vertebral arch is interrupted at the middle position (thin arrow; split or interrupted).
	頸椎弓肥厚（化）：第2頸椎弓の幅は広くなっている（太矢印）。第6頸椎弓が中央で分離（不連続）している（細矢印）。

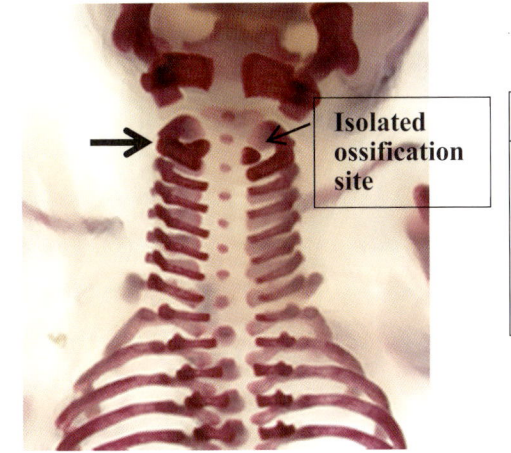

Isolated ossification site

Species	Mouse
Memo	Thick cervical vertebral arch: The left 2nd cervical arch (dorsal site) is thick (thick arrow), and the right arch has isolated ossification site (thin arrow, New).
	頸椎弓肥厚（化）：左第2頸椎弓の背側が肥厚している（太矢印）。右第2頸椎弓は分離骨化部位（細矢印、New）。

8-12   **Thin cervical vertebral arch**   頸椎弓菲薄（化）   **(New)**

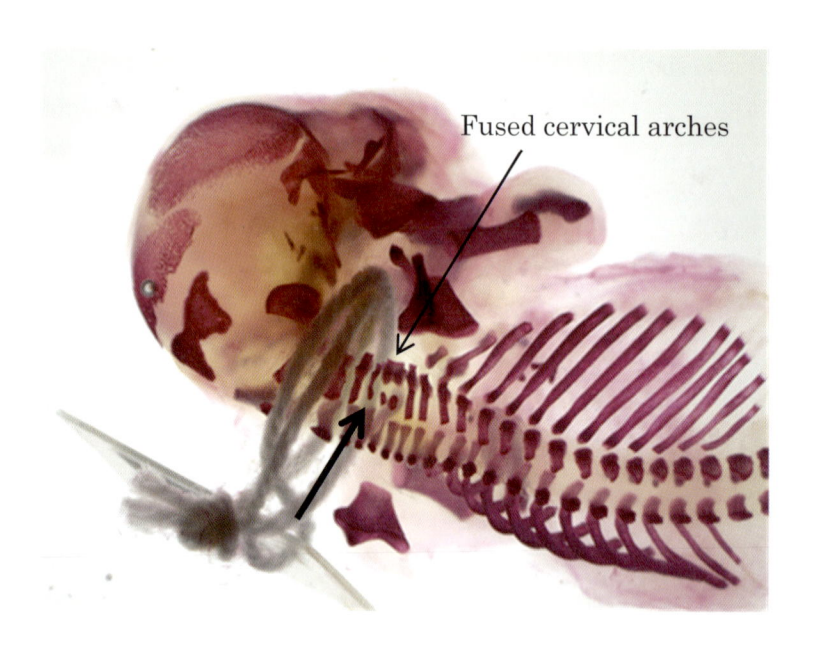

Species	Rat, SD
Memo	Thin cervical vertebral arch (thick arrow) with Fused cervical vertebral arches (10645, thin arrow): The right 4th cervical vertebral arch is thin and the 5th and 6th cervical vertebral arches are fused.
	頸椎弓菲薄（化）（太矢印）：右第4椎弓が細い。第5及び6頸椎の頸椎弓癒合（10645、細矢印）を伴う。

8-13 Isolated ossification site of the cervical vertebral arch　頸椎弓分離骨化部位　(New)

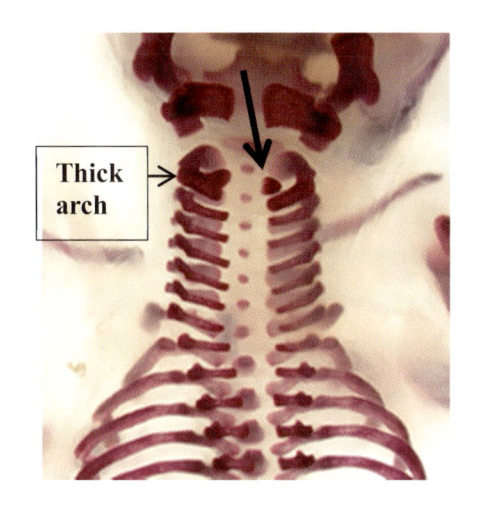

Species	Mouse
Memo	Isolated ossification site of the cervical vertebral arch: The left 2nd cervical vertebral arch (dorsal site) is thick (thin arrow, New), and the right arch has isolated ossification site (thick arrow).
	頸椎弓分離骨化部位：右第2頸椎弓は分離骨化部位（太矢印、New）。左第2頸椎弓の背側が肥厚している（細矢印、New）。

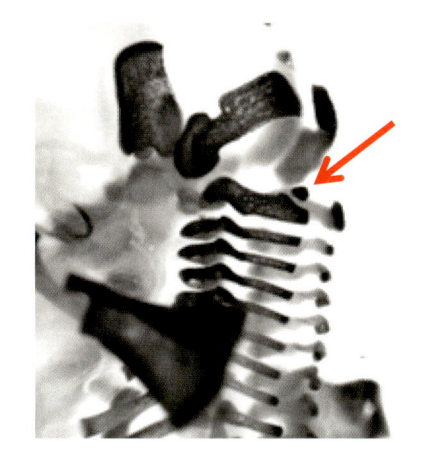

Species	Mouse
Memo	Isolated ossification site of the cervical vertebral arch: The left 2nd cervical arch (dorsal site) has isolated ossification site (arrow).
	頸椎弓分離骨化部位：第2頸椎弓は骨化部位が分離している（矢印）。

8-13 Continued

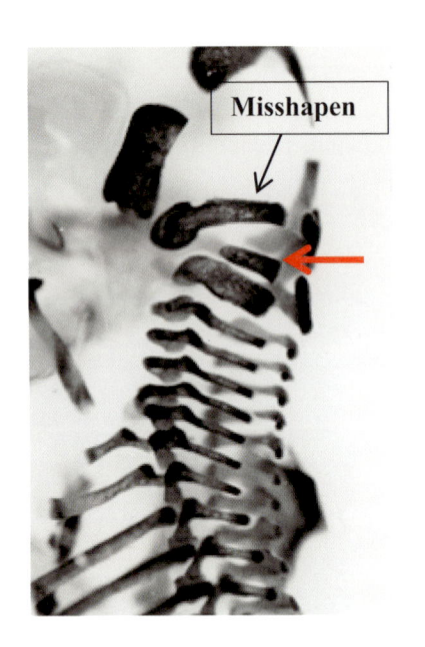

Species	Mouse
Memo	Isolated ossification site of the cervical vertebral arch: The left 2nd cervical vertebral arch (dorsal site) has isolated ossification site (red arrow). Thick cervical vertebral arch may be recommended for this arch. The first arch (atlas) is "Misshapen" because its narrow shape (black arrow, New).
	頸椎弓分離骨化部位：第2頸椎弓は骨化部位が分離している（赤矢印）。頸椎弓の肥厚も所見として良いかもしれない。第1頸椎（Atlas）は幅が狭く、形態異常（黒矢印、New）である。

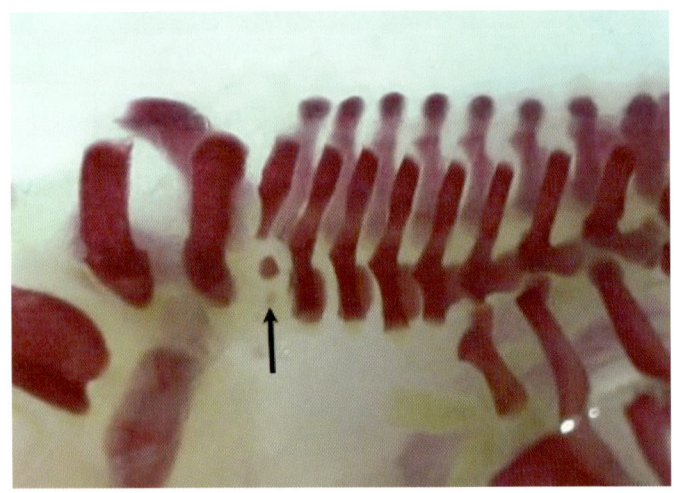

Species	Rat
Memo	Isolated ossification site of the cervical vertebral arch: The left 3rd cervical vertebral arch (dorsal site) has isolated ossification site (arrow).
	頸椎弓分離骨化部位：第3頸椎弓は骨化部位が分離している（矢印）。

8-14　Absent cervical vertebral centrum　　頸椎体欠損　(10653)

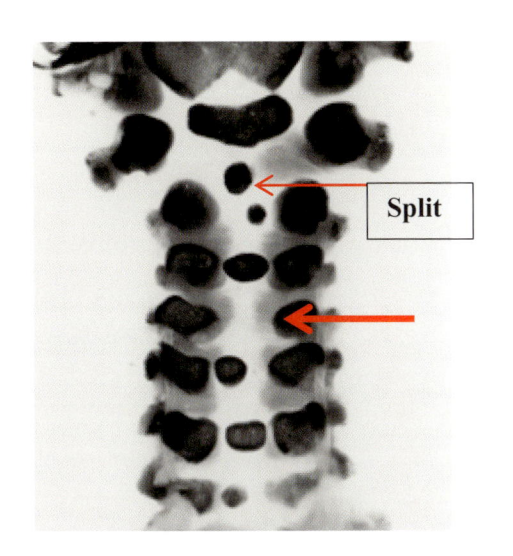

Species	Rabbit
Memo	Absent cervical vertebral centrum (thick arrow) with Split cervical vertebral centrum (thin arrow, 10663)
	頸椎体欠損：第4頸椎体が欠損（太矢印）。頸椎体分離（細矢印、10663）を伴う。

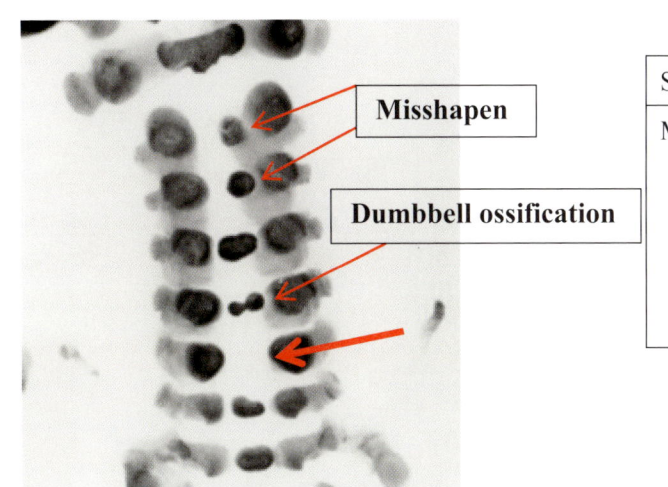

Species	Rabbit
Memo	Absent cervical vertebral centrum with Dumbbell-shaped cervical vertebral centrum (thin arrow, 10656) and Misshapen cervical vertebral centrum (thin arrow, 10662): The 6th vertebral centrum is absent (thick arrow).
	頸椎体欠損：第6頸椎体が欠損している（太矢印）。頸椎体ダンベル状骨化（10655）及び頸椎体形態異常（10662）を伴う（細矢印）。

8-15 Fused cervical vertebral centrum　頸椎体癒合　(10657)

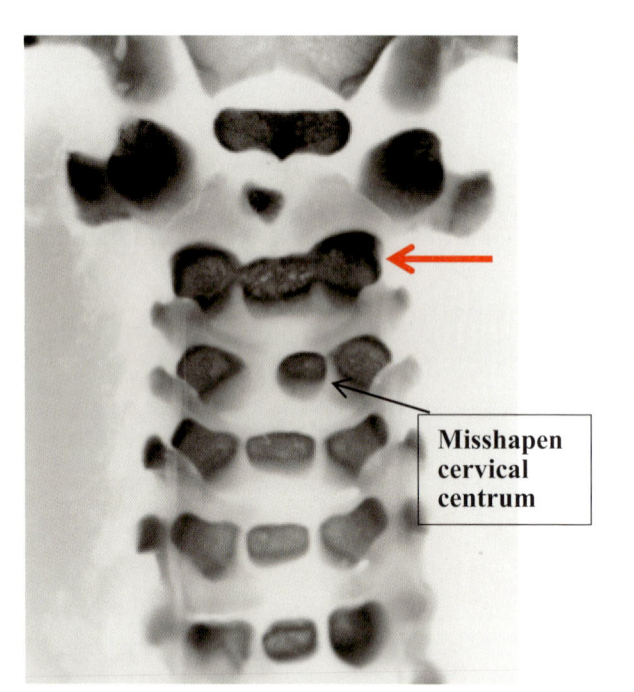

Species	Rabbit
Memo	Fused cervical vertebral arch and centrum with Misshapen cervical vertebral centrum or Unilateral ossification of cervical vertebral centrum (thin black arrow, 10662 or New, respectively): Cervical vertebral arch fused with cervical vertebral centrum.
	頸椎体癒合：椎弓と椎体の癒合。頸椎体形態異常あるいは頸椎体片側性骨化（細黒矢印、10662 あるいは New）を伴う。

Misshapen cervical centrum

Species	Rat
Memo	Fused cervical vertebral centra (thick arrow) with Unossified sternebrae (thin arrow, 10620) and Unossified cervical vertebral centrum (10666): Cervical vertebral centra from #2 to #7 are fused.
	頸椎体癒合：第2から第7頸椎体が癒合している（太矢印）。胸骨分節未骨化（細矢印、10620）及び頸椎体未骨化（10666）を伴う。

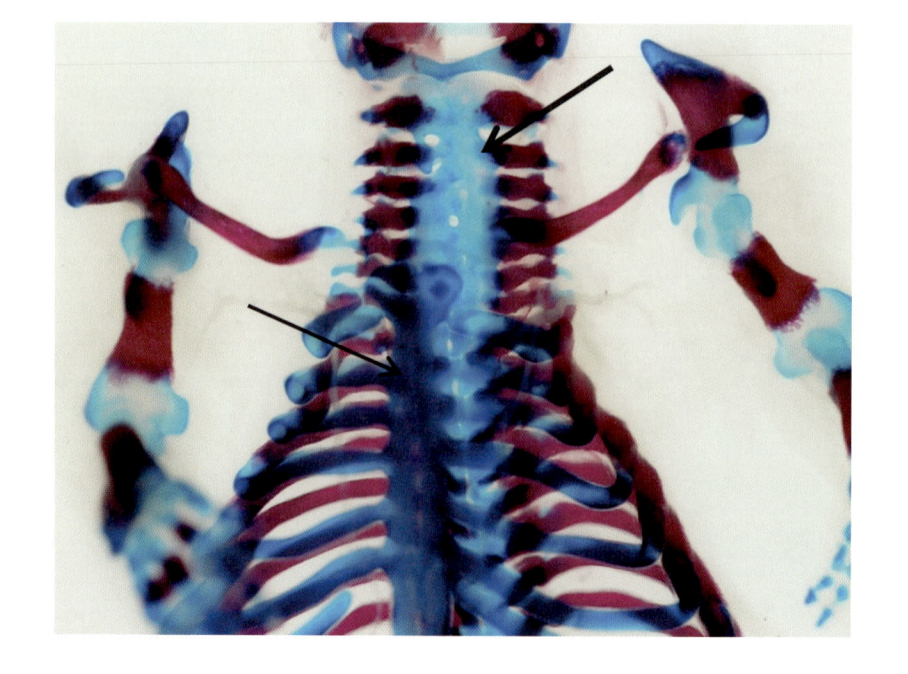

8-16 Misshapen cervical vertebral centrum　　頸椎体形態異常　(10662)

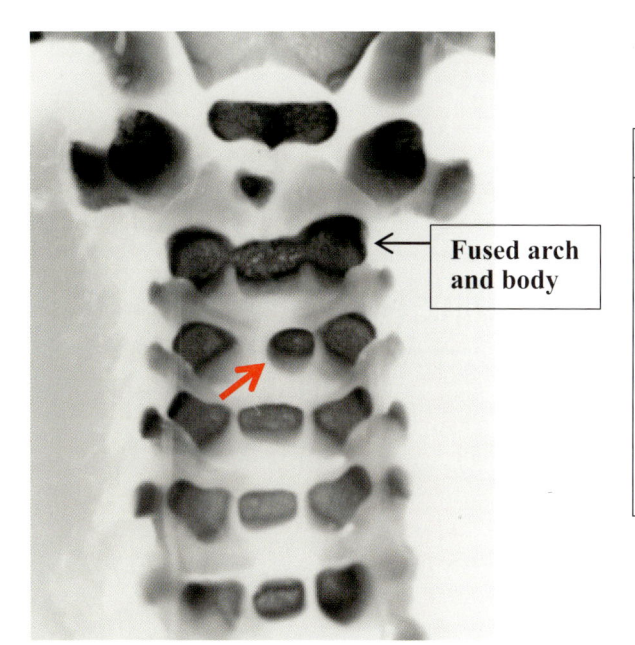

Fused arch and body

Species	Rabbit
Memo	Misshapen cervical vertebral centrum with Fused cervical vertebral arch and centrum (10645 and 10657, respectively): The 3rd cervical vertebral centrum is small and malpositioned (red arrow). This may be considered as "Small cervical vertebral centrum (New)".
	頸椎体形態異常：第3頸椎体が小さく、位置は片側化している（赤矢印）。椎体の小型化（New）でも良いかも。頸椎弓椎体癒合（10645及び10657）を伴う。

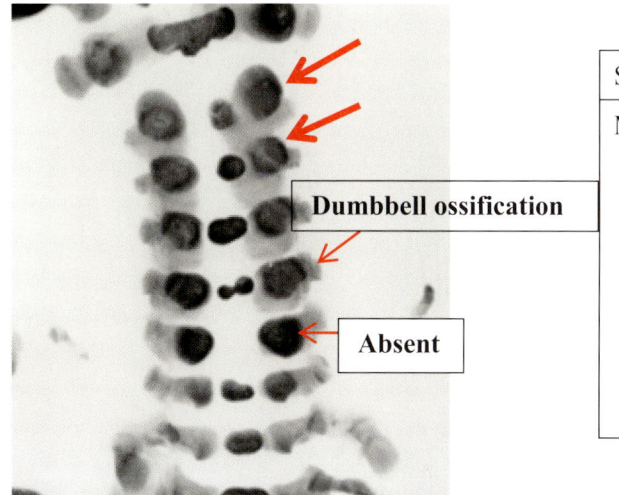

Dumbbell ossification

Absent

Species	Rabbit
Memo	Misshapen cervical vertebral centrum with Dumbbell-shaped cervical vertebral centrum (10656) and Absent cervical vertebral centrum (10653): The 2nd and 3rd cervical vertebral centra are small and located off-center (red thick arrow). They may be considered as "Small cervical vertebral centrum (New)".
	頸椎体形態異常：椎体が小さく、位置は片側化している（赤太矢印）。椎体の小型化（New）でも良いかも。頸椎体ダンベル状骨化（10655）及び頸椎体欠損（10653）を伴う。

8-17 Split cervical vertebral centrum   頸椎体分離 (10663)

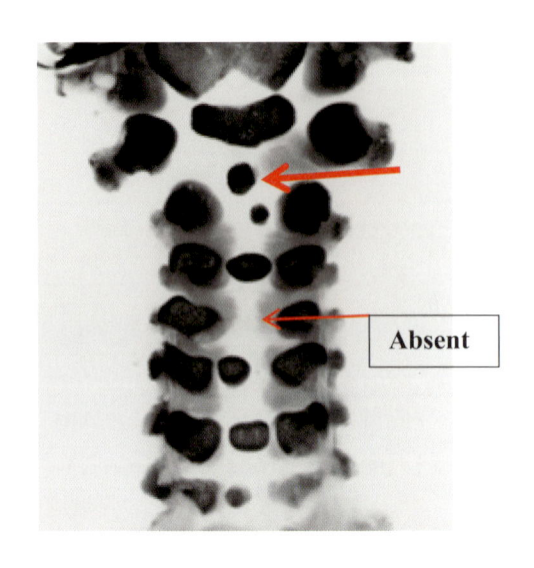

Species	Rabbit
Memo	Split cervical vertebral centrum (red thick arrow) with Absent cervical vertebral centrumy (10653)
	頸椎体分離：第2頸椎体が分離（赤太矢印）。頸椎体欠損（10653）を伴う。

8-18　Dumbbell ossification of cervical vertebral centrum　　頸椎体ダンベル状骨化　(10655)

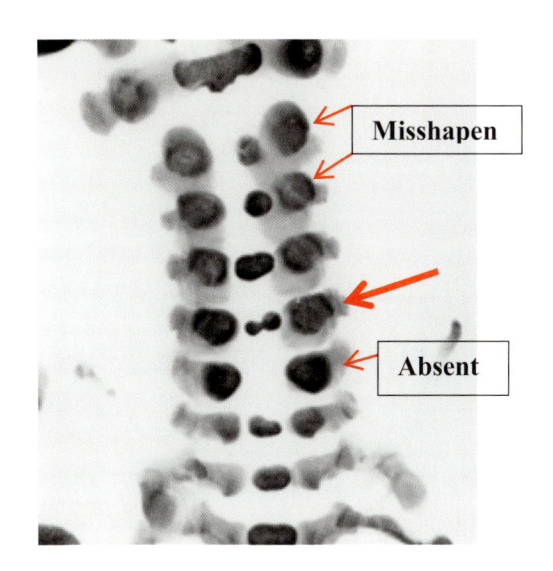

Species	Rabbit
Memo	Dumbbell ossification of cervical vertebral centrum (red thick arrow) with Misshapen cervical vertebral centrum (10662) and Absent cervical vertebral centrum (10653)
	頸椎体ダンベル状骨化（赤太矢印）：頸椎体形態異常（10662）及び頸椎体欠損（10653）を伴う。

8-19　Absent cervical vertebra　頸椎欠損　(10667)

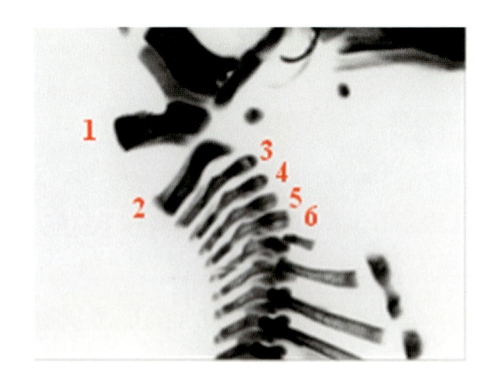

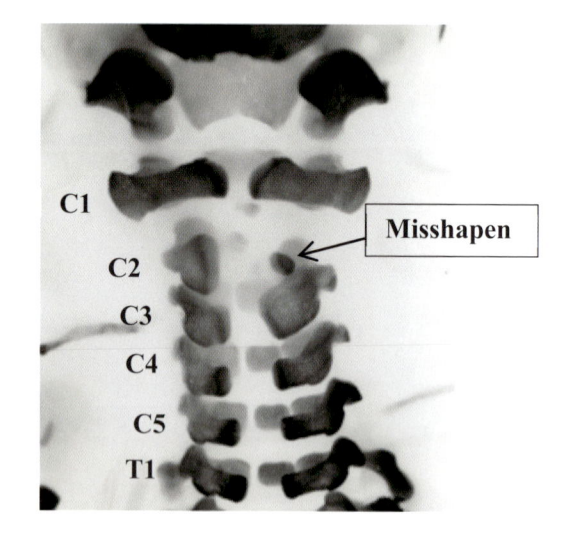

Species	Mouse
Memo	Absent cervical vertebra: There are only 6 cervical vertebrae.
	頸椎欠損：頸椎が 6 対

Species	Rabbit
Memo	Absent cervical vertebrae with Misshapen cervical vertebral arch (10649): There are only 5 cervical vertebrae.
	頸椎欠損：頸椎が 5 対のみ。頸椎弓形態異常（10649）を伴う。

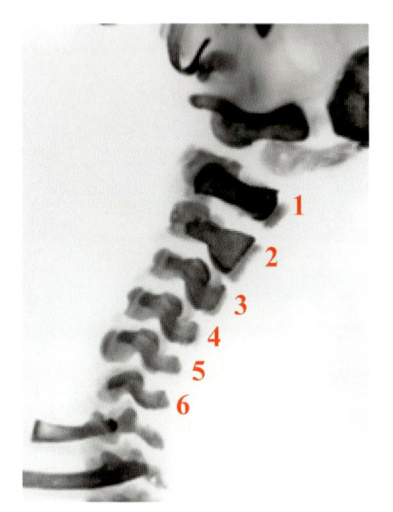

Species	Rabbit
Memo	Absent cervical vertebra: There are only 6 cervical vertebrae.
	頸椎欠損：頸椎が 6 対

Photographs of Skeletal Anomalies

9. Thoracic vertebra

9-1　Absent thoracic vertebral arch　胸椎弓欠損　(10671)

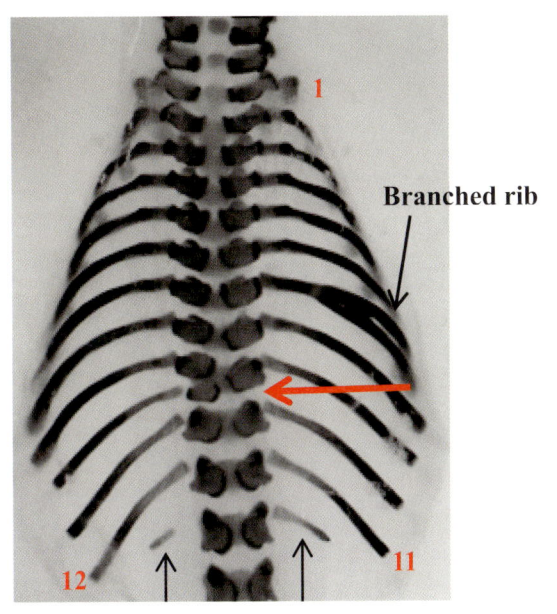

Species	Rabbit
Memo	Absent thoracic vertebral arch (red arrow) with Branched rib (10623), Absent rib (10621), and supernumerary thoracolumbar rib (10628 and 10638). 11 thoracic arches and 11 ribs at the right side and 12 thoracic arches and 12 ribs at the left side are confirmed. Although this may be considered to be "Hemivertebra", this is recommended to be "Absent thoracic arch" because of shape of arches and number of ribs at the right side.
	胸椎弓欠損：肋骨分岐（10623）、肋骨欠損（10621）及び過剰肋骨（10628及び10638）を伴う。右側は11個の椎弓と11本の肋骨が、左側は12個の椎弓と12本の肋骨が見られる。胸椎半椎（10696）と言う所見とも考えられるが、右側の椎弓の形態や肋骨数から「胸椎弓欠損」とした。

Species	Rat, SD
Memo	Absent thoracic vertebral arch (circle) without absent rib (10628): The left arch and body of the 11th thoracic vertebra are absent.
	胸椎弓欠損（円）：第11胸椎の左椎弓及び椎体が欠損している。肋骨の欠損は見られない。

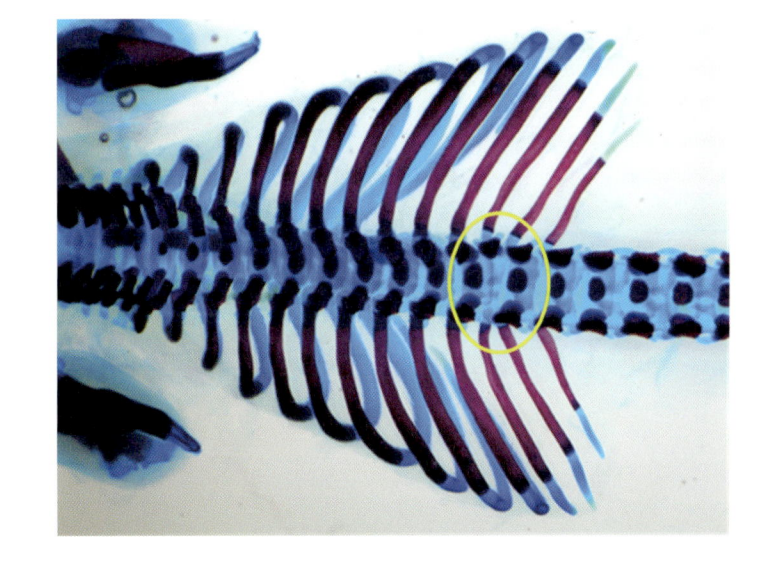

9-2 Fused thoracic vertebral arches　　胸椎弓癒合　(10672)

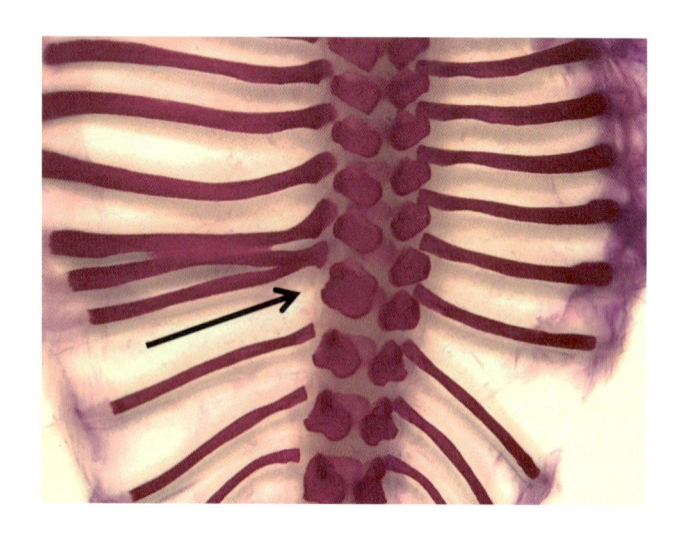

Species	Rabbit
Memo	Fused thoracic vertebral arches with Fused ribs (10629): Arches fused and this arch is large (arrow).
	胸椎弓癒合：椎弓が癒合し、大型化している（矢印）。肋骨癒合（10629、癒合した椎弓に対応する肋骨の近位部癒合も含め）も伴う。

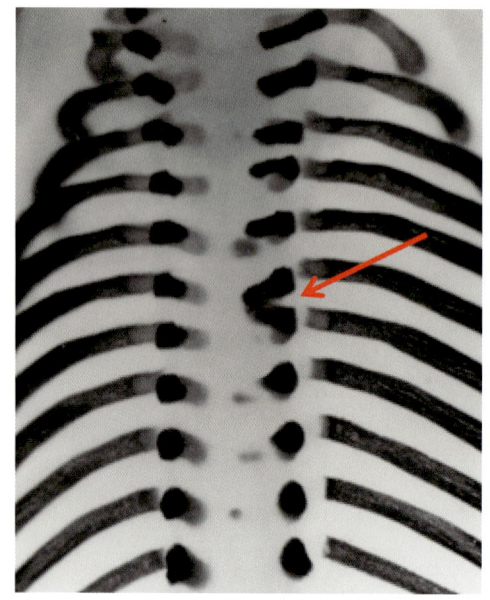

Species	Rat
Memo	Fused thoracic vertebral arches (arrow)
	胸椎弓癒合（矢印）

9-2 Continued

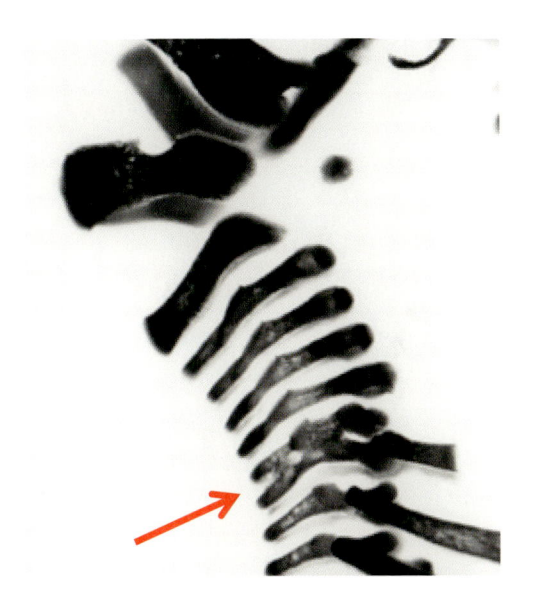

Species	Mouse
Memo	Fused thoracic and cervical vertebral arches: The first thoracic arch fuses with the 7th cervical arch (arrow).
	胸椎弓頸椎弓癒合：第1胸椎弓と第7頸椎弓の癒合（矢印）

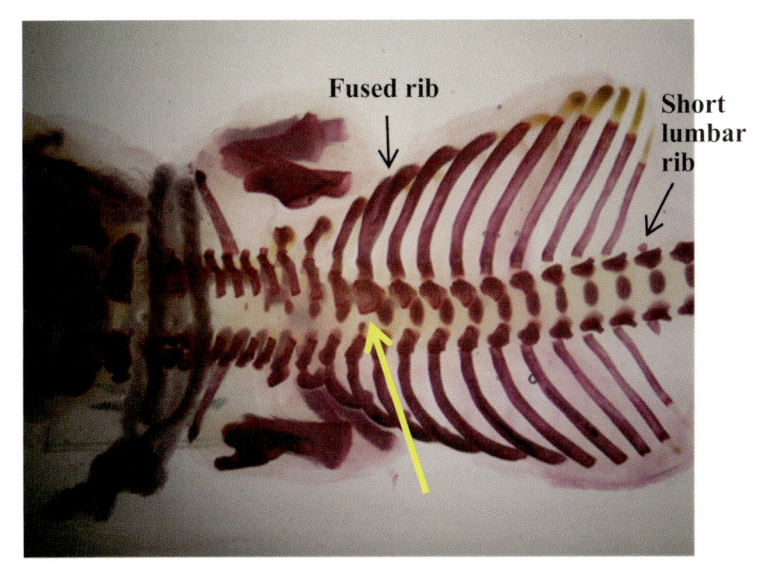

Species	Rat, SD
Memo	Fused thoracic vertebral arch with Fused rib (10629) and Short thoracolumbar rib (10638): The right 4th and 5th arches fused (yellow arrow).
	胸椎弓癒合：右第4、5胸椎弓が癒合している（黄矢印）。肋骨癒合（10629、癒合した椎弓に対応する肋骨の近位部の癒合）及び過剰肋骨（胸腰部、短小、10638）を伴う。

9-2 Continued

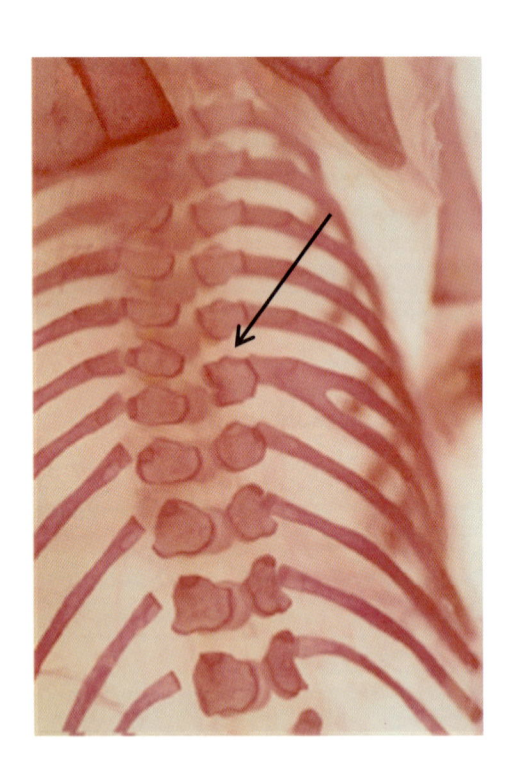

Species	Rabbit
Memo	Fused thoracic vertebral arches with Fused ribs (10629): The right 7th and 8th arches fused (arrow).
	胸椎弓癒合：右第7、8胸椎弓が癒合している（矢印）。肋骨（右第7、8）の癒合（10629）もみられる。

9-3　Large thoracic vertebral arch　　胸椎弓大型（化）　　(New)

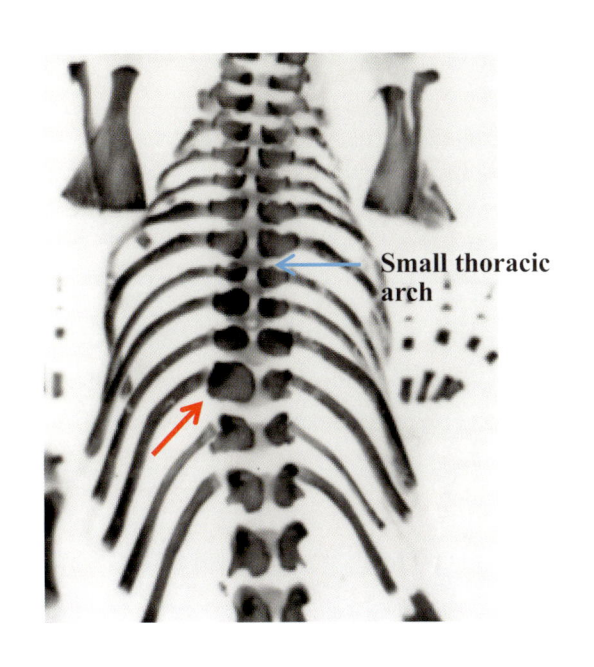

Small thoracic arch

Species	Rabbit
Memo	Large thoracic vertebral arch (red arrow) with Small thoracic arch (blue arrow, 10677)
	胸椎弓大型（化）（赤矢印）:胸椎弓小型（化）（青矢印、10677）を伴う。

9-4　Misshapen thoracic vertebral arch　　胸椎弓形態異常　(10676)

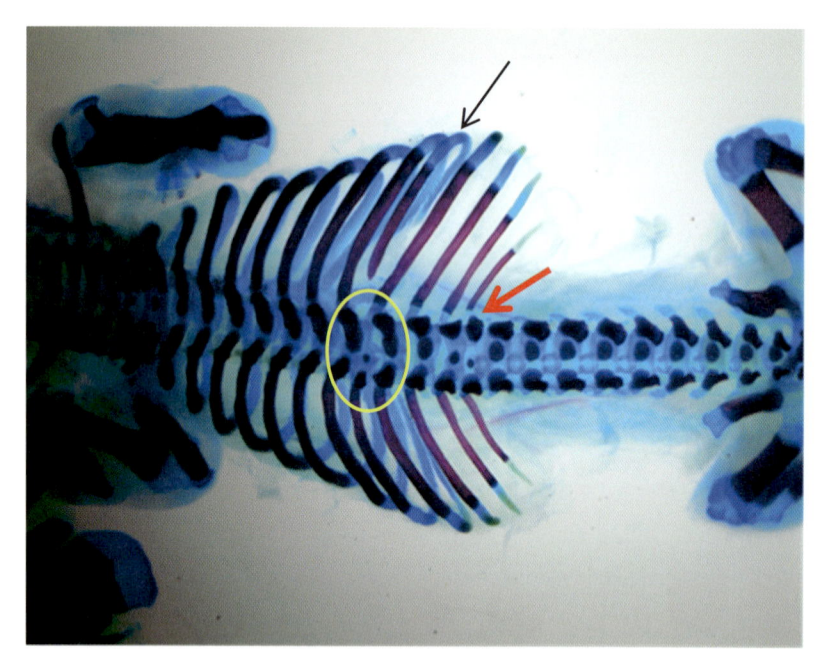

Species	Rat, SD
Memo	Misshapen thoracic vertebral arch with Thoracic hemivertebra (10696), Detached rib (10626), and Small thoracic vertebral centra (New): The shape of the right 13th arch is abnormal (red arrow), and the 12th and 13th thoracic vertebral centra are small. The left arch and centrum of the 9th thoracic vertebra are small, and its right arch is absent (circle, Thoracic hemivertebra, 10696). The 9th right rib does not articulate with vertebral column (black arrow, Detached rib, 10626).
	胸椎弓形態異常：右第13椎弓は形態異常であり（赤矢印）、第12、13椎体は小型化（New）している。胸椎半椎（楕円、10696、第9胸椎の左椎弓と椎体が小型化し、右椎弓は欠損している。）及び右第9肋骨の分離（黒矢印、10626）が見られる。

9-5 Small thoracic vertebral arch　　胸椎弓小型（化）　　(10677)

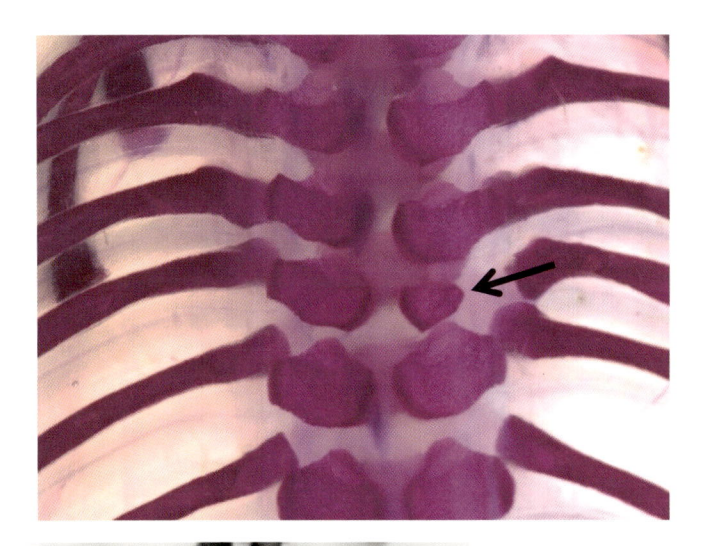

Species	Rabbit
Memo	Small thoracic vertebral arch (arrow): Ribs may be fused at the joint region. It is clear if this is a double-stained specimen.
	胸椎弓小型（化）（矢印）：肋骨関節部が癒合している（二重染色であれば明確）

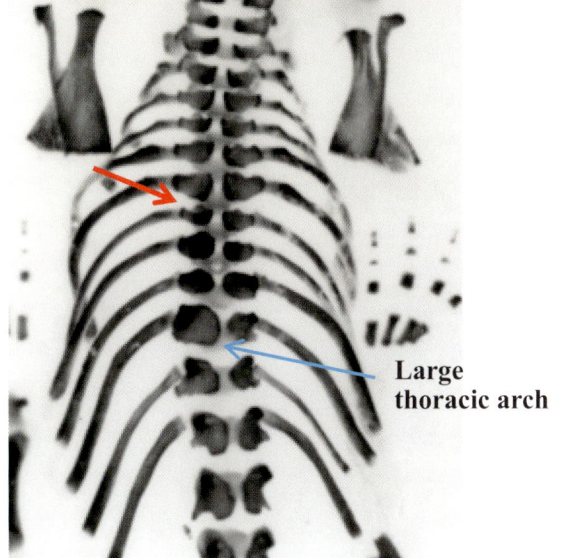

Large thoracic arch

Species	Rabbit
Memo	Small thoracic vertebral arch (red arrow) with Large thoracic arch (New)
	胸椎弓小型（化）（赤矢印）：胸椎弓大型（化）（New）を伴う。

9-5 Continued

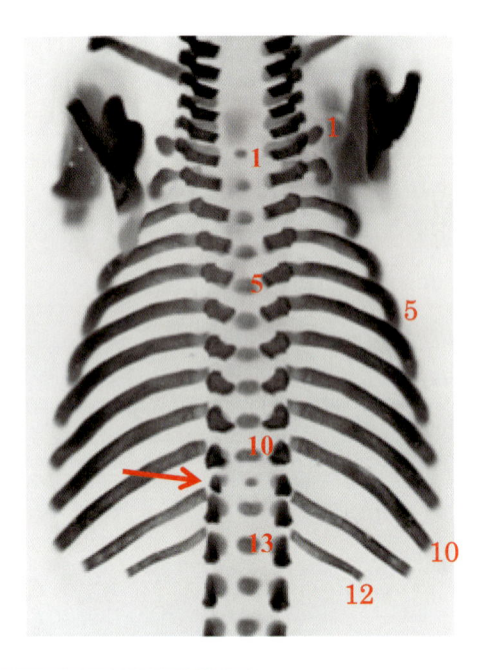

Species	Rat
Memo	Small thoracic vertebral arch (arrow) with Absent rib (10621; 12 pairs) and Small thoracic vertebral centrum (New): The left 11th thoracic arch is small (red arrow), and both 11th ribs are absent.
	胸椎弓小型（化）（矢印）：肋骨欠損（10621、左右12対）、胸椎体小型（化）（New）を伴う。左第11胸椎弓が小型（赤矢印、10677）であり、左右の第11肋骨が欠損している。

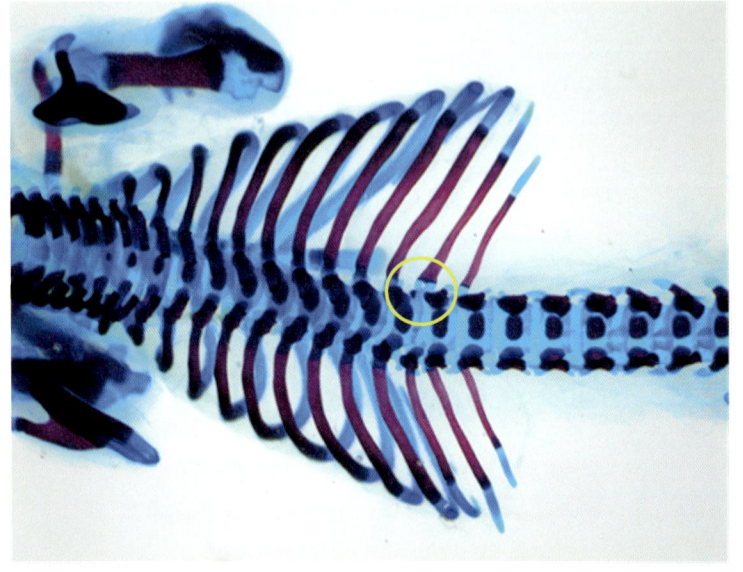

Species	Rat, SD
Memo	Small thoracic vertebral arch: The 11th right thoracic vertebral arch is small (circle). The left arch is slightly small. The 11th and 12th ribs fused. This fetus is double-stained, then, Fused ribs is clear.
	胸椎弓小型（化）：第11右椎弓が小型化している（楕円）。左椎弓もやや小さい。右第11、12肋骨が癒合している。肋骨関節端の軟骨部分は一部癒合しているが、2個の関節部が確認できる。

9-6 Isolated ossification site of the thoracic vertebral arch　　胸椎弓分離骨化部位　(New)

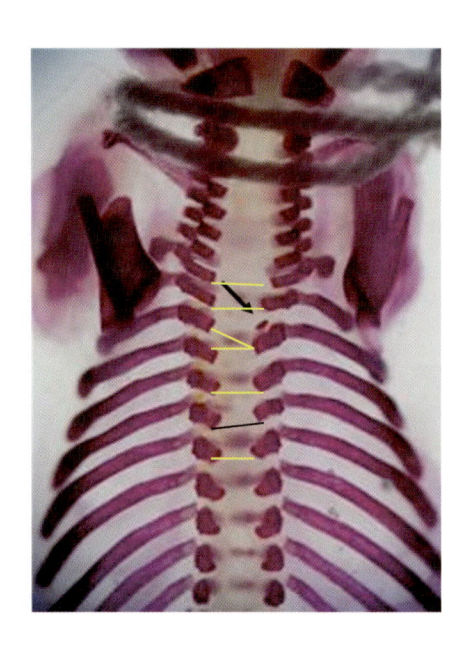

Species	Rat, SD
Memo	Isolated ossification site of the thoracic vertebral arch (black arrow): The numbers of thoracic vertebral arches and ribs are differ from side to side (R:12, L:13). So, It is possible that hemivertebra or absent arch is present at the 3rd or 4th thoracic region.
	胸椎弓分離骨化部位（黒矢印）：左右の椎弓数及び肋骨数が異なり（右12、左13）、第3あるいは4胸椎で半椎あるいは椎弓の欠損があると思われる。

9-7　**Absent thoracic vertebral centrum**　　胸椎体欠損　（10680）

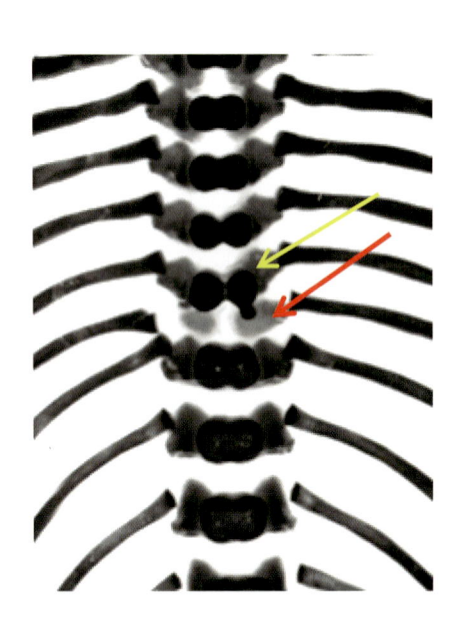

Species	Rabbit
Memo	Absent thoracic vertebral centrum with Misshappen thoracic vertebral centrum (yellow arrow): This fetus has misshapen thoracic vertebral arch (10676), and absence of its corresponding vertebral centrum (red arrow).
	胸椎体欠損：椎弓の形態異常（10676）に伴い、該当する椎体が欠損している（赤矢印）。胸椎体形態異常（10689）を伴う（黄矢印）。

9-8 Fused thoracic vertebral centra   胸椎体癒合   (10684)

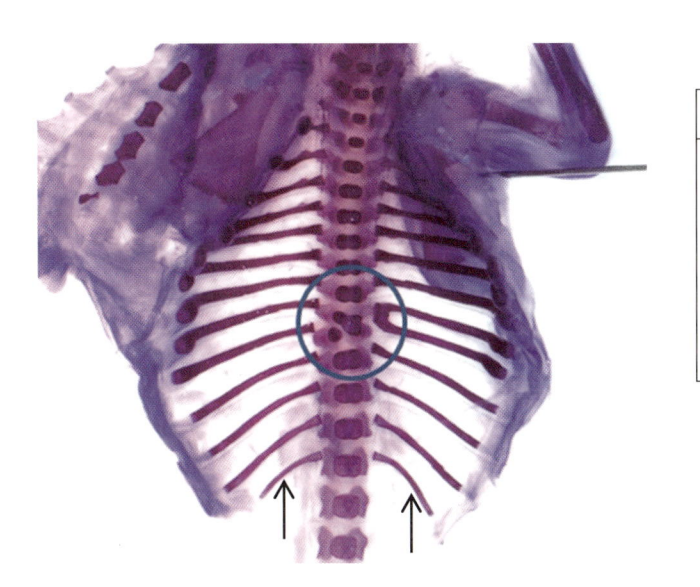

Species	Rabbit
Memo	Fused thoracic vertebral centra (circle) with Fused ribs (circle, 10629), Split thoracic vertebral centra (circle, 10690) and Full supernumerary thoracolumbar rib (arrow, bilateral, 10628)
	胸椎体癒合（円）：肋骨癒合及び胸椎体分離（円、10629 及び 10690）、胸腰部完全過剰肋骨（矢印、両側、10628）を伴っている。

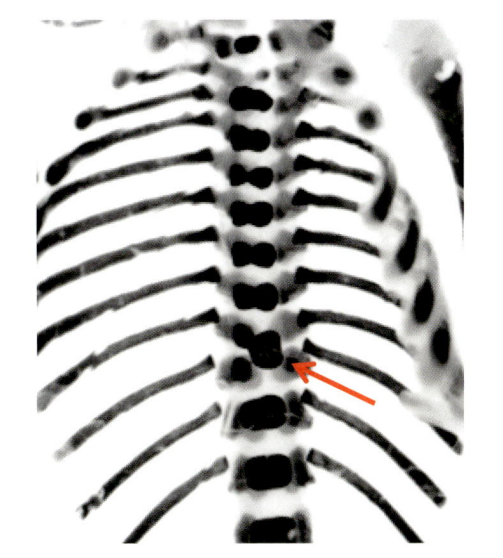

Species	Rabbit
Memo	Fused thoracic vertebral centra: The 9th and 10th thoracic vertebral centra fused (arrow).
	胸椎体癒合：第 9 と 10 の椎体が癒合している（矢印）。

9-8 Continued

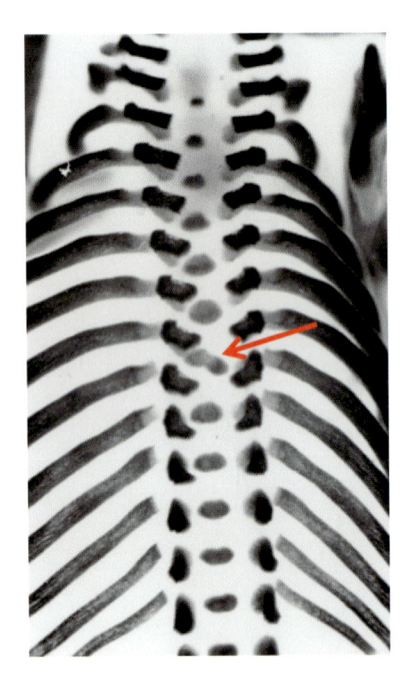

Species	Rat
Memo	Fused thoracic vertebral centra: The 7th and 8th thoracic vertebral centra fused (arrow).
	胸椎体癒合：第7と8の椎体が癒合している（矢印）。

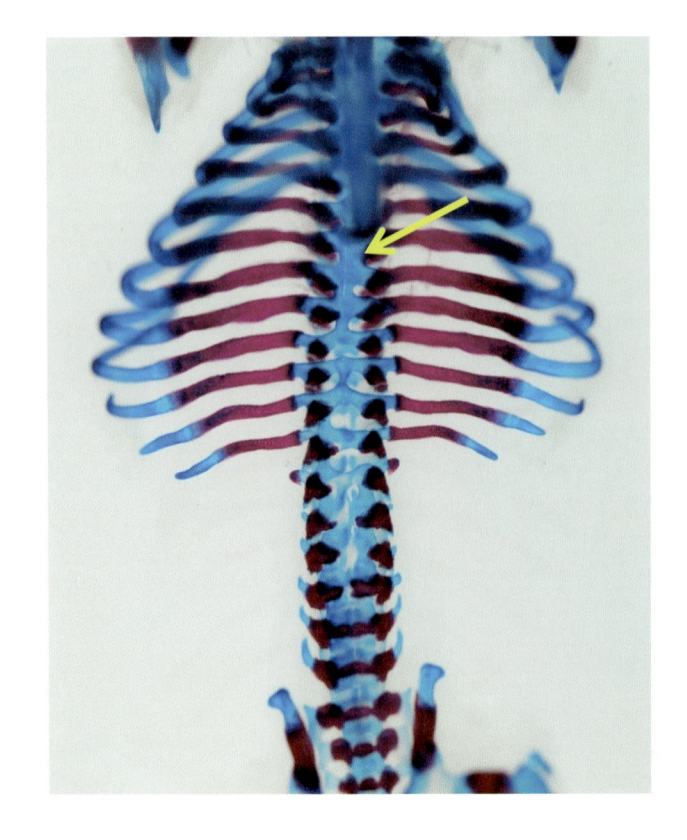

Species	Rat
Memo	Fused thoracic vertebral centra with Misshapen lumbar vertebral centra (10716): Several cartilaginous centra fused and their ossification centers are absent (arrow).
	胸椎体癒合：複数の椎体が軟骨で癒合し、骨化中心が認められない（矢印）。腰椎体形態異常（10716）を伴う。

9-9 Small thoracic vertebral centrum   胸椎体小型（化）   (New)

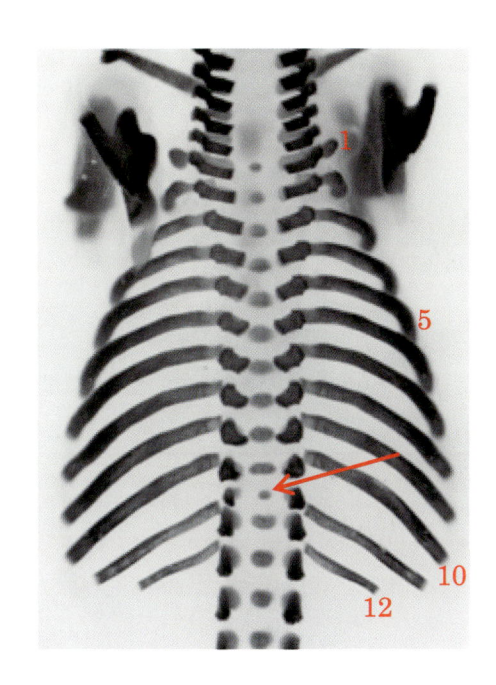

Species	Rat
Memo	Small thoracic vertebral centrum (arrow) with Absent 11th rib (10621; 12 pairs), and Small thoracic vertebral arch (10677)
	胸椎体小型（化）（矢印）：肋骨欠損（10621、左右 12 対、第 11 肋骨の欠損）、胸椎弓小型（化）（10677）を伴う。

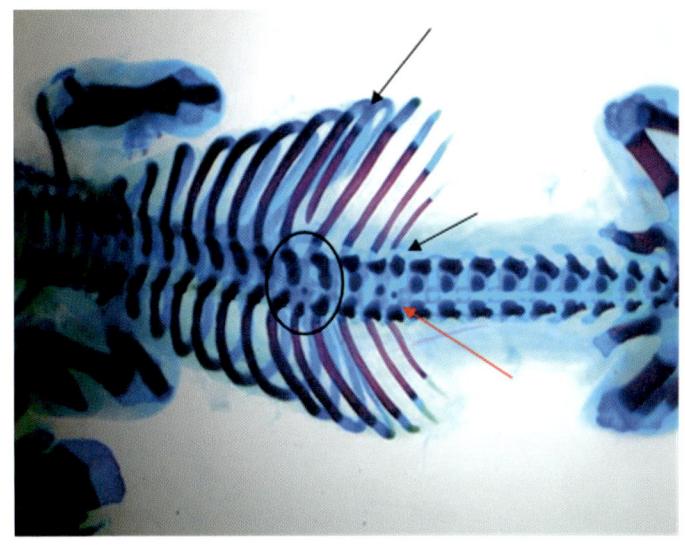

Species	Rat, SD
Memo	Small thoracic vertebral centrum with Thoracic hemivertebra (10696) Detached rib (10626), and Misshapen thoracic vertebral arch (10676): The 12th and 13th thoracic vertebral centra are small (red arrow), and the right 13th thoracic vertebral arch is abnormally shaped (black arrow). The left arch and centrum of the 9th thoracic vertebra are small, and its right arch is absent (circle, Thoracic hemivertebra, 10696). The 9th right rib does not articulate with thoracic vertebra (black arrow).
	胸椎体小型（化）：第 12、13 椎体は小型化している（赤矢印）。右第 13 椎弓の形態異常（黒矢印、10676）も見られる。胸椎半椎（円、10696、第 9 胸椎の左椎弓と椎体が小型化し、右椎弓は欠損している。）と右第 9 肋骨の分離（黒矢印、10626、椎骨との関節結合がない。）も見られる。

9-10　**Bipartite ossification of thoracic vertebral centrum**　　胸椎体二分骨化　(10681)

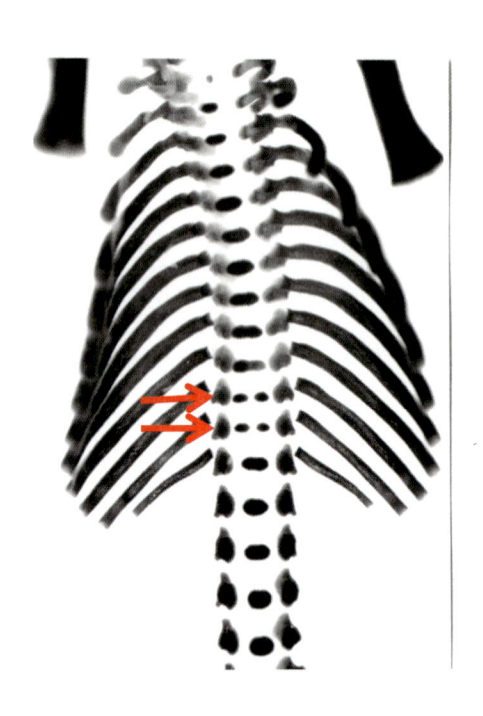

Species	Rat
Memo	Bipartite ossification of thoracic vertebral centrum (red arrow): This finding is frequently observed in fetuses with growth retardation.
	胸椎体二分骨化（赤矢印）：発育遅延胎児でよく見られる。

9-11 Dumbbell ossification of thoracic vertebral centrum　　胸椎体ダンベル状骨化　(10682)

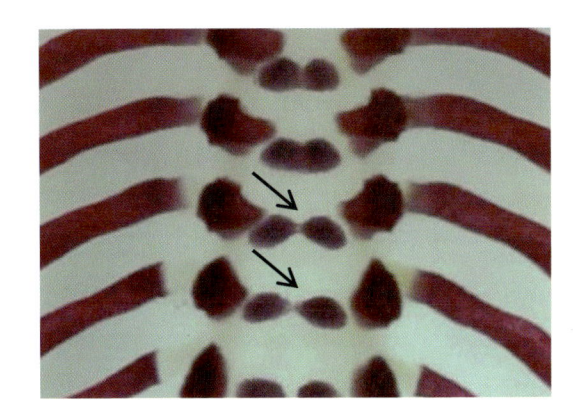

Species	Rat
Memo	Dumbbell ossification of thoracic vertebral centrum (arrow): This finding is frequently observed in fetuses with growth retardation.
	胸椎体ダンベル状骨化（黄矢印）：発育遅延胎児でよく見られる。

Species	Rat
Memo	Dumbbell ossification of thoracic vertebral centrum (thick arrow) with Small thoracic vertebral centrum (thin arrow, New)
	胸椎体ダンベル状骨化（太矢印）：胸椎体小型（細矢印、New）を伴う。

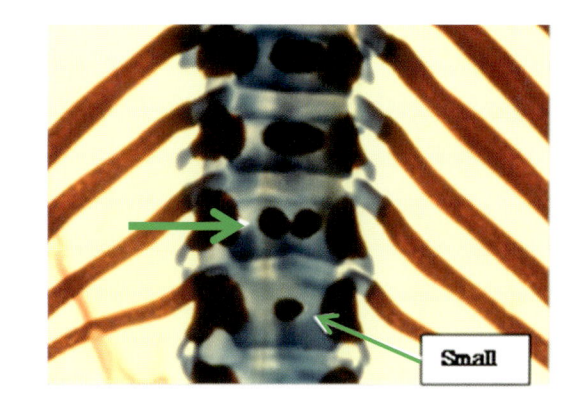

9-12　Unossified thoracic vertebral centrum　　胸椎体未骨化　(10693)

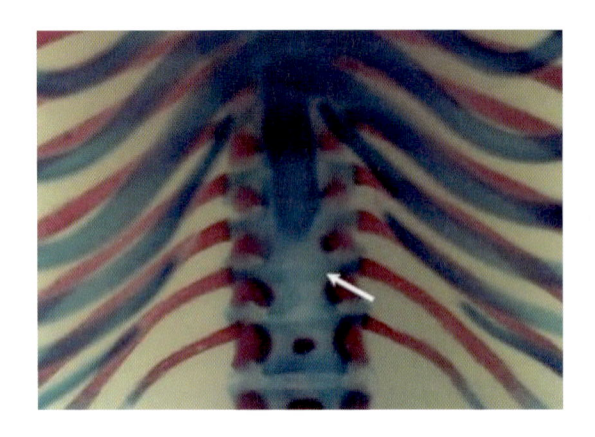

Species	Rat
Memo	Unossified thoracic vertebral centrum (arrow)
	胸椎体未骨化（矢印）

9-13　Absent thoracic vertebra　　胸椎欠損　(10694)

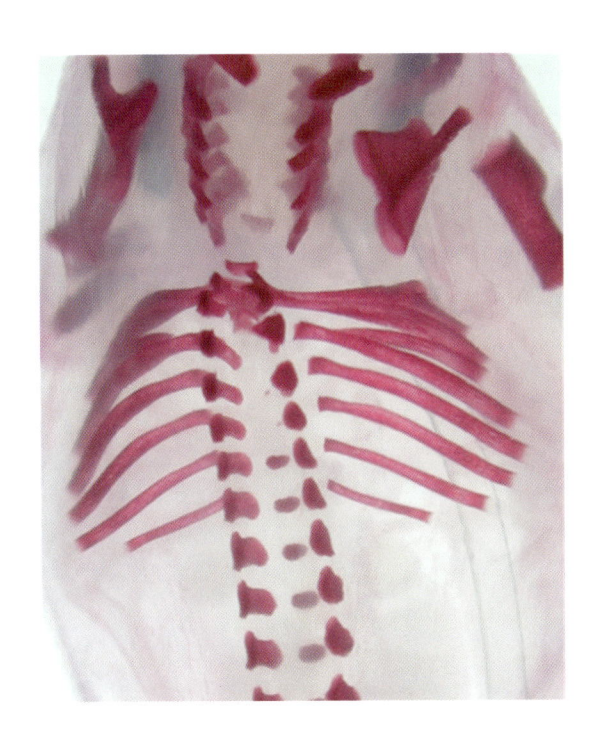

Species	Rat
Memo	Absent thoracic vertebra with Absent rib (10621), Fused rib (10629), and Interrupted vertebral canal (New)
	胸椎欠損：肋骨欠損（10621）、肋骨癒合（10629）、脊柱管不連続（New）を伴う。

9-14 Thoracic hemivertebra 胸椎半椎 (10696)

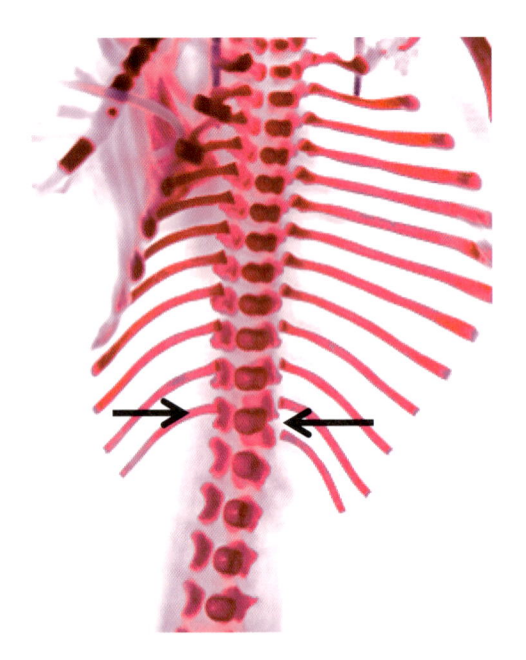

Species	Rabbit
Memo	Thoracic hemivertebra (arrow): The number of thoracic vertebral arches and ribs on the left and right are different.
	胸椎半椎（矢印）：左右の椎弓数が異なり、椎骨として三角状になっている。肋骨数も左右異なる。

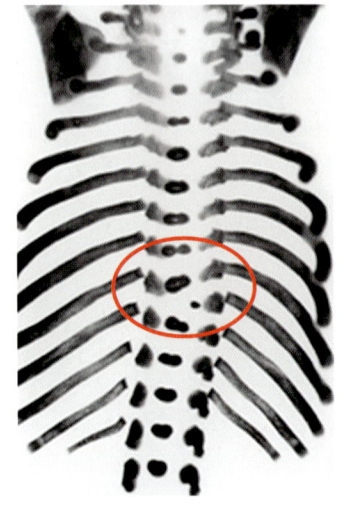

Species	Rat
Memo	Thoracic hemivertebra (circle): The number of thoracic vertebral arches and ribs on the left and right are different.
	胸椎半椎（円）：左右の椎弓数が異なり、椎骨として三角状になっている。肋骨数も左右異なる。

9-14 Continued

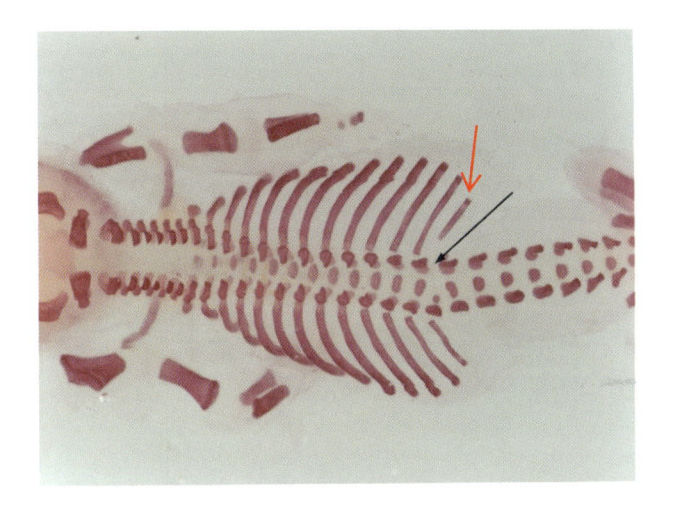

Species	Rat
Memo	Thoracic hemivertebra (black arrow) with Detached rib (red arrow, 10626) and Supernumerary lumbar vertebrae (10724)
	胸椎半椎（黒矢印）：第 13 胸椎の半椎で右椎弓が欠損している。肋骨分離（赤矢印、10626）及び腰椎過剰（10724）を伴う。

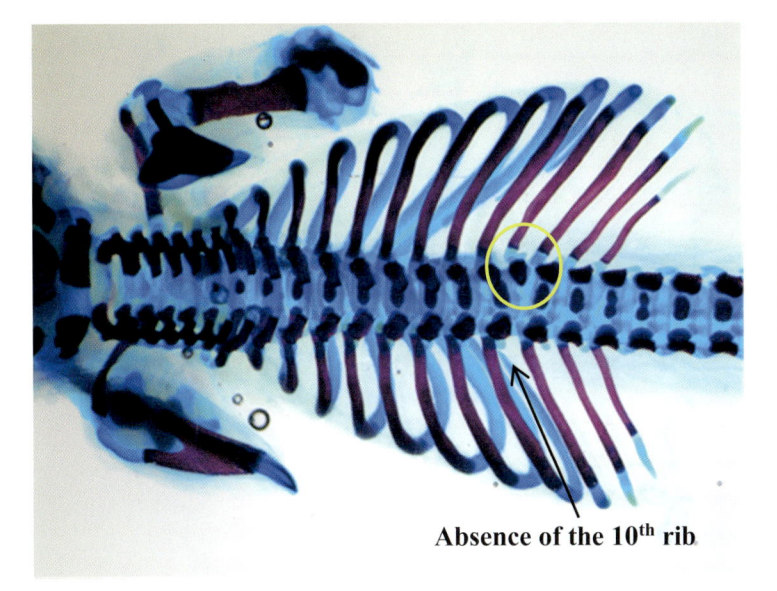

Species	Rat, SD
Memo	Thoracic hemivertebra (circle) with Absent rib (arrow, 10621): The left arch and centrum of the 10th thoracic vertebra are absent, and the 10th left rib is absent.
	胸椎半椎（円）：第 10 胸椎の左椎弓及び椎体が欠損している。左第 10 肋骨が欠損（矢印、10621）している。

Absence of the 10th rib

9-14 Continued

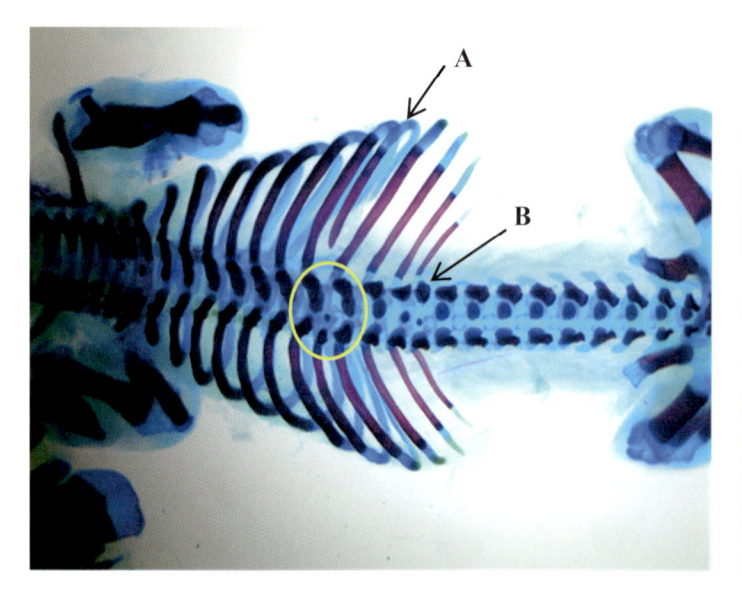

Species	Rat, SD
Memo	Thoracic hemivertebra (circle) with Intercostal rib (arrow A, 10632), Small thoracic vertebral centrum (arrow B, New), and Misshapen thoracic vertebral arch (arrow B, 10676): The left arch and centrum of the 9th thoracic vertebra are small, and its right arch is absent. The 9th right rib does not articulate with thoracic vertebra (arrow A). The 12th and 13th thoracic vertebral centra are small, and the shape of the right 13th arch is abnormal (arrow B).
	胸椎半椎（円）：第9胸椎の左椎弓と椎体が小型化し、右椎弓は欠損している。右第9肋骨は脊椎より分離し肋間肋骨（矢印A、10632）である。第12、13椎体は小型化（矢印B、New）し、右第13椎弓は形態異常（矢印B、10676）である。

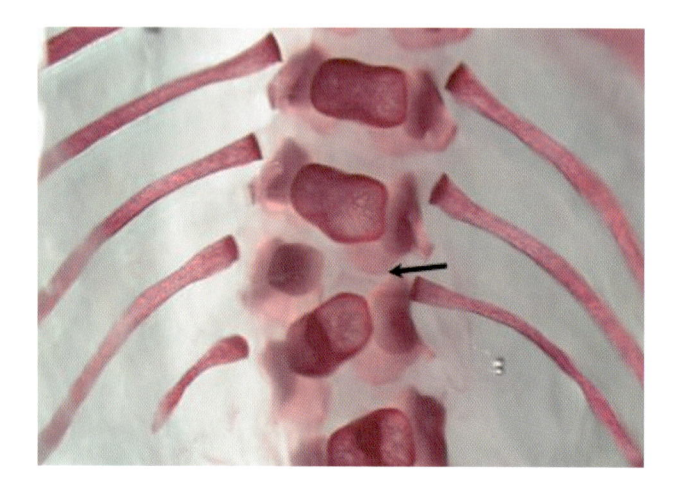

Species	Rabbit
Memo	Thoracic hemivertebra (arrow): The left 11th thoracic vertebral arch and rib are absent.
	胸椎半椎（矢印）：第11左椎弓及び肋骨が欠損している。

9-14 Continued

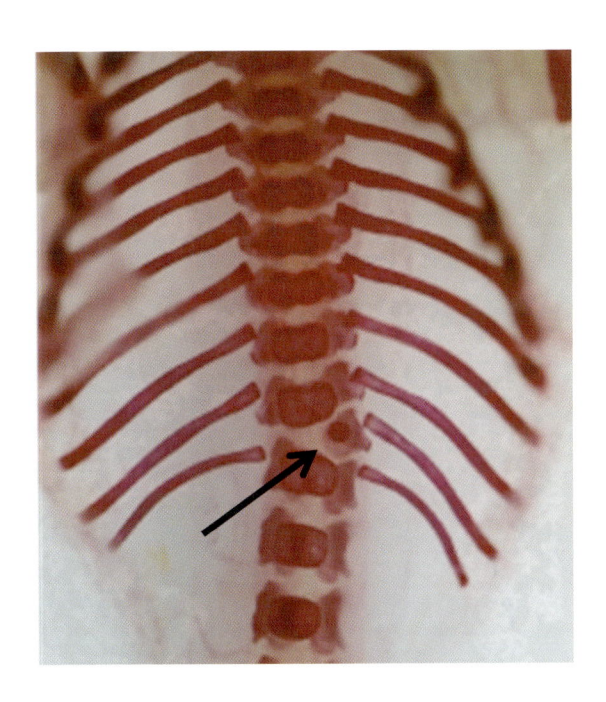

Species	Rabbit
Memo	Thoracic hemivertebra (arrow): The right 11th thoracic vertebral arch and rib are absent.
	胸椎半椎（矢印）：第11右椎弓及び肋骨が欠損している。

Photographs of Skeletal Anomalies

10. Lumbar vertebra

10-1 Fused lumbar vertebral arches　　腰椎弓癒合　(10699)

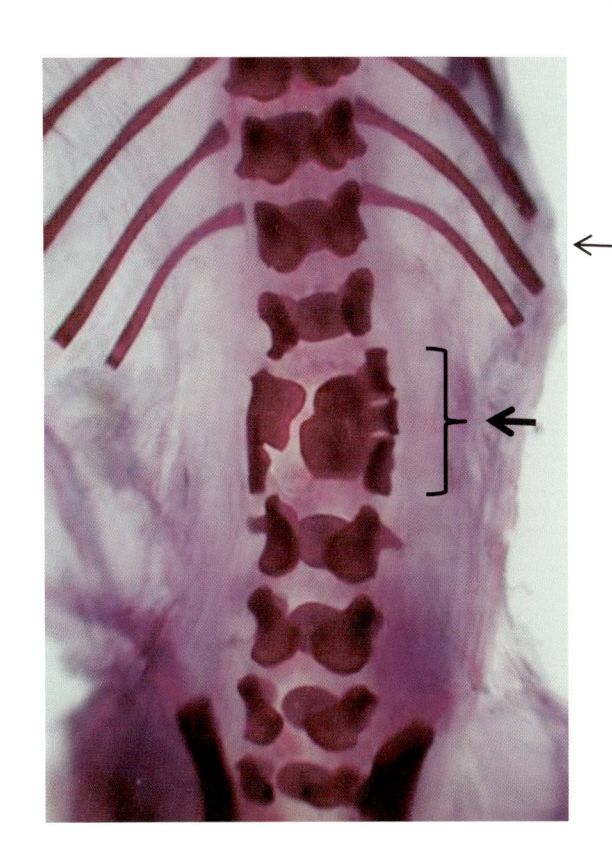

Species	Rabbit
Memo	Fused lumbar vertebral arches with Fused lumbar vertebral centra: The 2nd - 4th left arches fuse, and the 2nd – 4th right arches fuse to centra (arrow). The 2nd – 4th centras fuse (10711).
	腰椎弓癒合：第 2-4 左腰椎椎弓が癒合し、第 2-4 右腰椎椎弓が椎体と癒合している（矢印）。また、椎体どうしの癒合（10711）も見られる。

Species	Rat
Memo	Fused lumbar vertebral arches: The transverse processes of the 3rd and 4th lumbar vertebral arch fuse (arrow).
	腰椎弓癒合：第 3-4 腰椎椎弓横突起が癒合（矢印）。

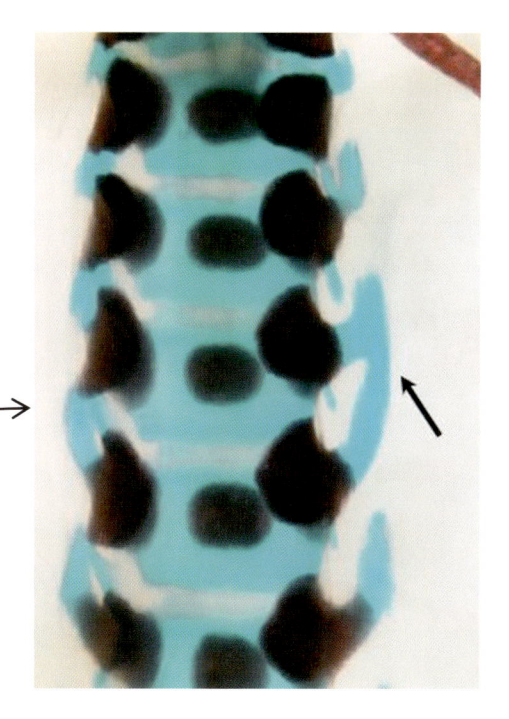

10-2　Misshapen lumbar vertebral arch　　腰椎弓形態異常　(10703)

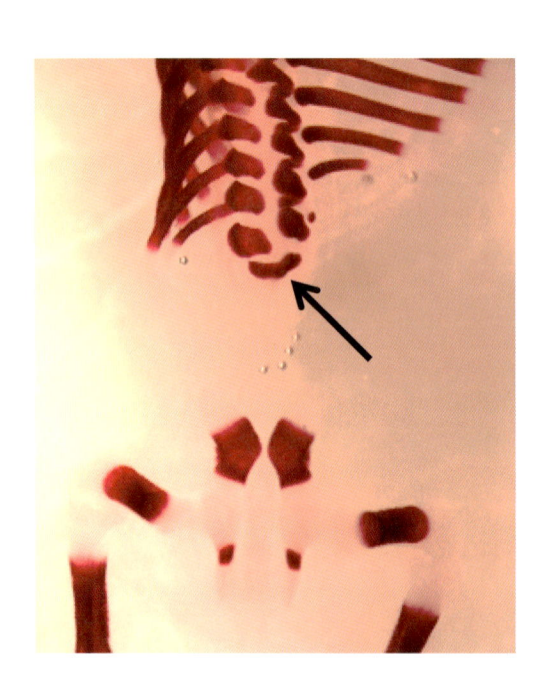

Species	Rat
Memo	Misshapen lumbar vertebral arch: Vertebral canal may be close (arrow). This fetus has also Absent lumbar vertebra (10721), Absent sacral vertebra (10748) and Absent caudal vertebra (10769).
	腰椎弓形態異常：脊柱管が閉鎖していると推測される（矢印）。腰椎欠損（10721）、仙椎欠損（10748）及び尾椎欠損（10769）を伴う。

10-3　Splayed lumbar vertebral arch　腰椎弓放散　(New)

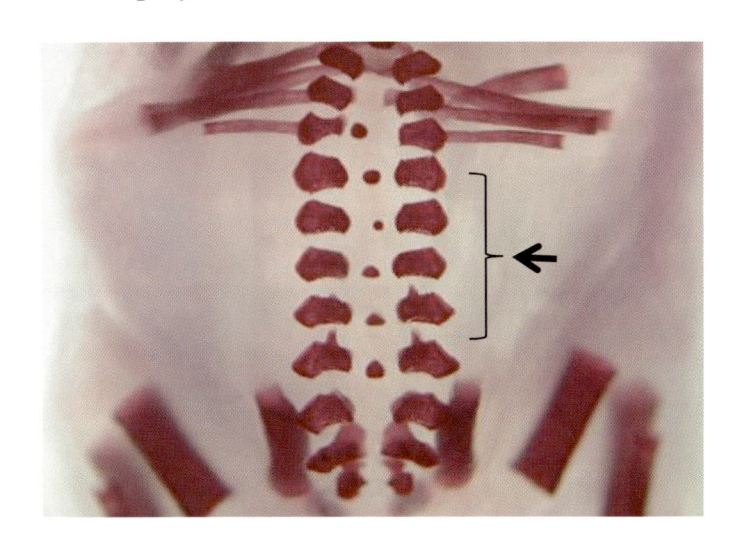

Species	Rat
Memo	Splayed lumbar vertebral arch: The lumbar arches diverge at the dorsal site (arrow), and lumbar centra are small and misaligned. This fetus may be considered to have "Spina bifida (10120)" in external examination or "Spinal bifida occulta (10120)" covered with skin which cannot be confirmed sometime in external examination.
	腰椎弓放散：腰椎椎弓が背部側で開放し（離れ）ている（矢印）。椎体も小さく、配列がずれている。外表観察では、二分脊椎（10120）と思われる。また、外表では判断できない場合もある「潜在性二分脊椎」かもしれないので留意する。

10-4 Supernumerary site in lumbar vertebral arch   腰椎弓過剰部位   (New)

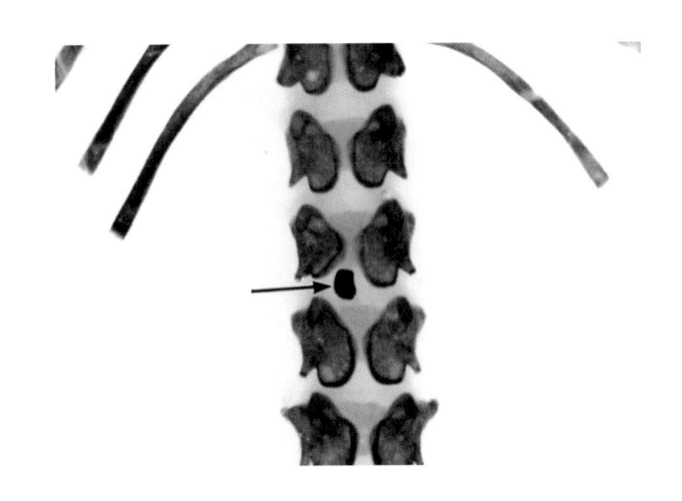

Species	Rabbit
Memo	Supernumerary site in lumbar vertebral arch: Isolated ossification site is observed (arrow).
	腰椎弓過剰部位：椎弓に分離した過剰な化骨部位がある（矢印）。

10-5 Increased ossification of the lumbar vertebral arch　　腰椎弓骨化亢進　(New)

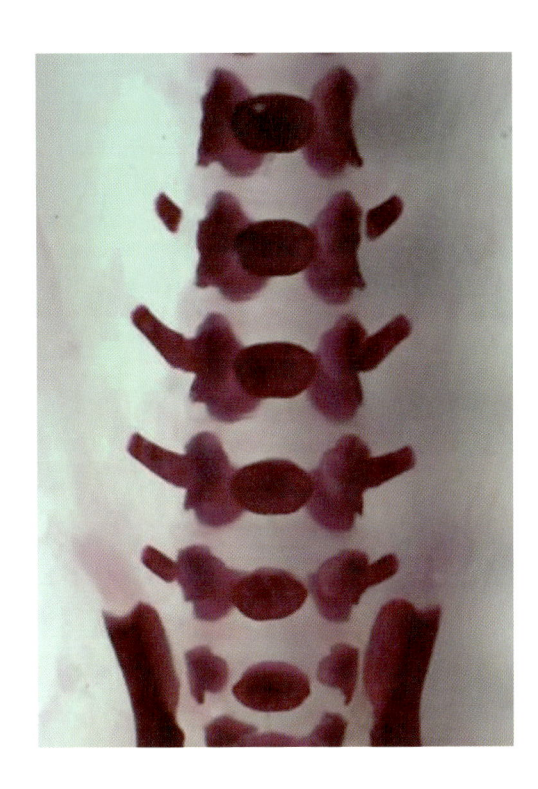

Species	Rabbit
Memo	Increased ossification of the lumbar vertebral arch: Transverse processes of lumbar vertebrae are clear compared with normal fetuses on same day of gestation..
	腰椎弓骨化亢進：同一胎齢の胎児と比較し、横突起が明確である。

10-6　Fused lumbar vertebral centra　　腰椎体癒合　(10711)

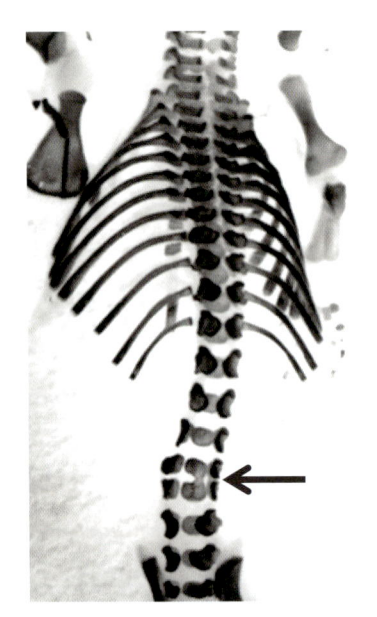

Species	Rabbit
Memo	Fused lumbar vertebral centra (arrow)
	腰椎体癒合（矢印）

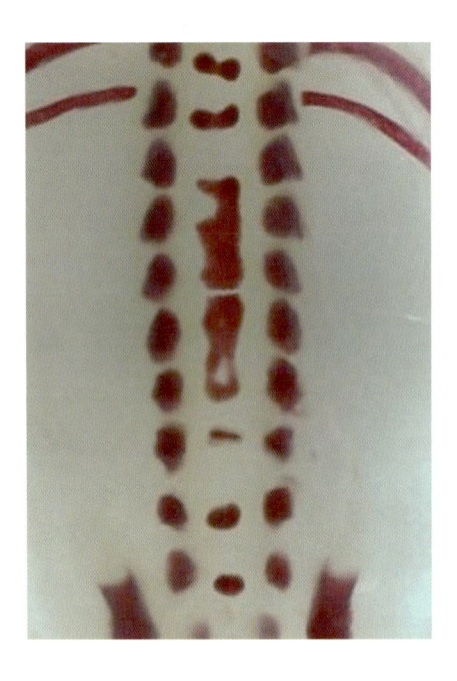

Species	Rat
Memo	Fused lumbar vertebral centra
	腰椎体癒合

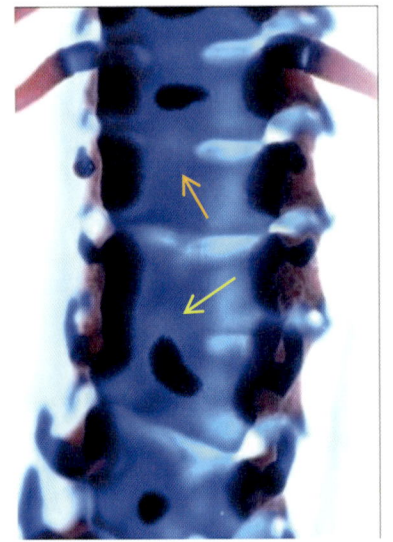

Species	Rat
Memo	Fused lumbar vertebral centra with Fused lumbar vertebral arches (10699): This is a double-stained specimen. Unossified area of the lumbar vertebral centra fused (arrow) and ossified centrum is abnormally shaped.
	腰椎体癒合：二重染色標本。未骨化部位が癒合している（矢印）。椎弓の癒合（10699）を伴う。

10-7　Misaligned lumbar vertebral centra　腰椎体配列異常　(10715)

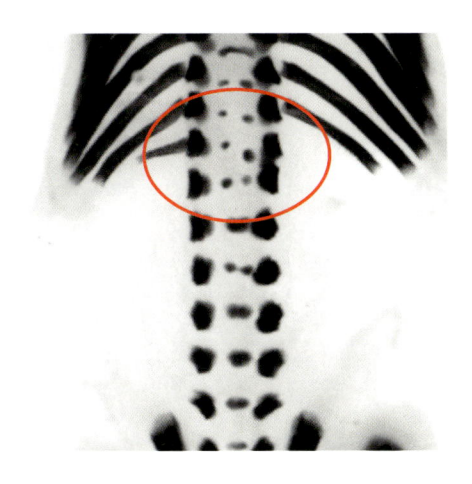

Species	Rat
Memo	Misaligned lumbar vertebral centra (circle) with Fused lumbar vertebral arches (10699) and Bipartite ossification of lumbar vertebral centra (10708):
	腰椎体配列異常（円）：腰椎弓癒合（10699）及び腰椎体二分骨化（10708）を伴う。本所見は腰椎弓癒合を伴う変化である。

10-8　**Bipartite ossification of lumbar vertebral centra**　　腰椎体二分骨化　(10708)

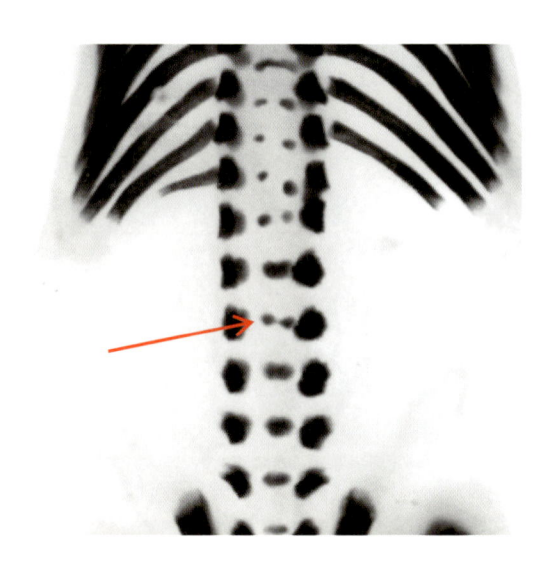

Species	Rat
Memo	Bipartite ossification of lumbar vertebral centra with Fused lumbar vertebral arches (10699), Misaligned lumbar vertebral centra (10715), and Full thoracolumbar supernumerary rib (left, 10628)
	腰椎体二分骨化：腰椎弓癒合（10699）、腰椎体配列異常（10715）及び完全過剰肋骨（腰肋、10628）を伴う。

10-9　Absent lumbar vertebra　　腰椎欠損　(10721)

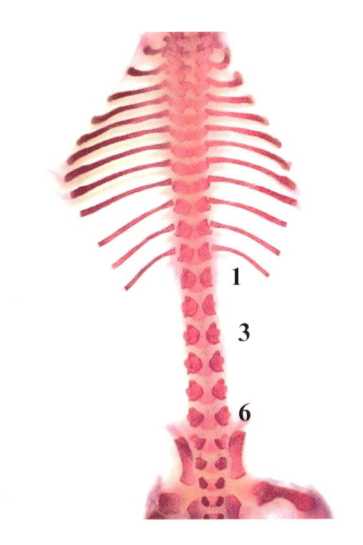

Species	Rabbit
Memo	Absent lumbar vertebra or reduced number of lumbar vertebrae: The number of lumbar vertebrae is reduced to 6 although there are usually 7 lumbar vertebrae in rabbits. This may be considered as Decreased number of lumbar vertebrae.
	腰椎欠損：左右６対の椎弓と６個の椎体（ウサギの正常は７）腰椎数減少でも良い。

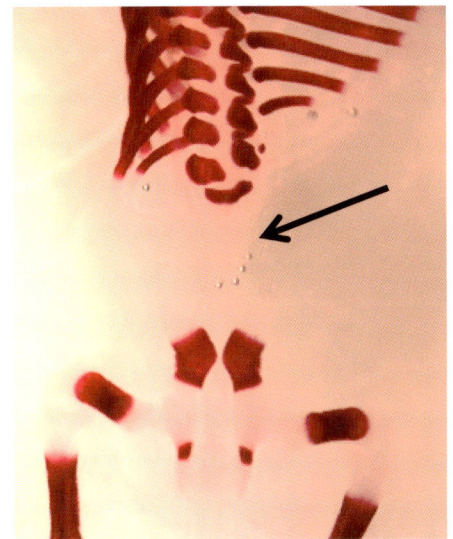

Species	Rat
Memo	Absent lumbar vertebrae (arrow) with Absent sacral vertebrae (10748) and Absent caudal vertebrae (10769)
	腰椎欠損（矢印）：仙椎欠損（10748）及び尾椎欠損（10769）を伴う。

10-9 Continued

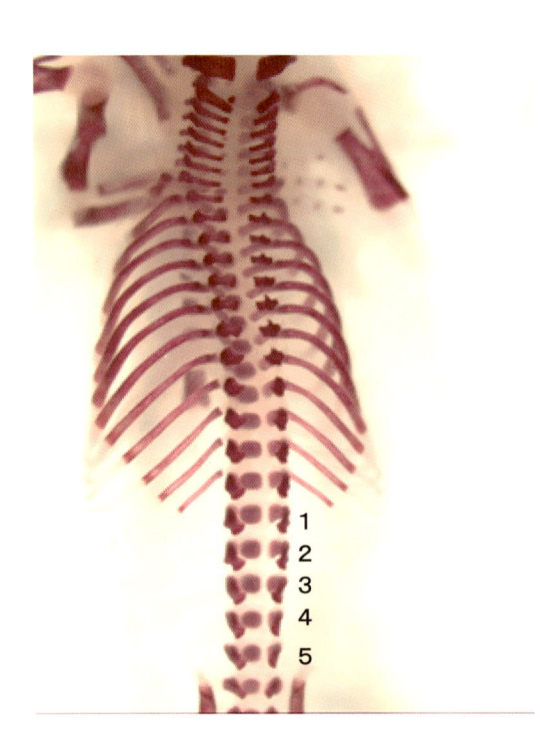

Species	Rat
Memo	Absent lumbar vertebrae or Reduced number of lumbar vertebrae: The number of lumbar vertebrae in this fetus is 5 although there are usually 6 lumbar vertebrae in rats. This may be considered as Decreased number of lumbar vertebrae.
	腰椎数減少、腰椎欠損：腰椎が5個（通常は6個）腰椎数減少でも良い。

10-10   Lumbar hemivertebra   腰椎半椎   (10722)

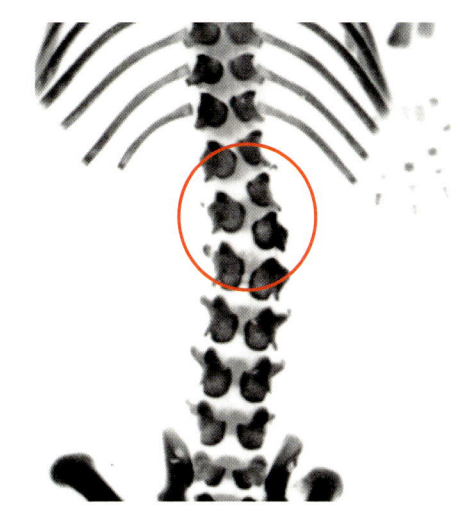

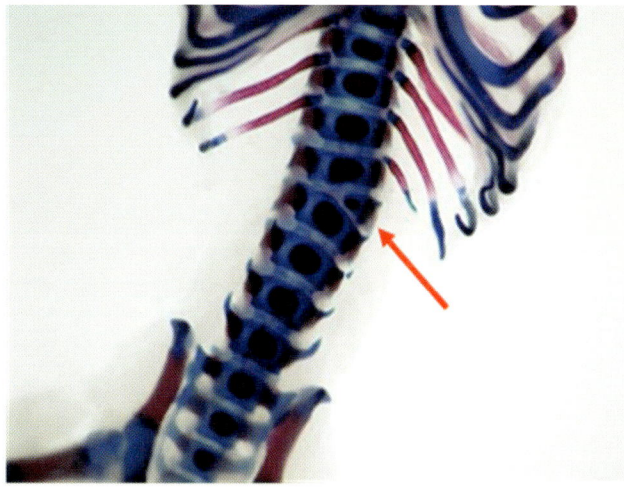

Species	Rabbit
Memo	Lumbar hemivertebra (circle or arrow)
	腰椎半椎（円あるいは矢印）

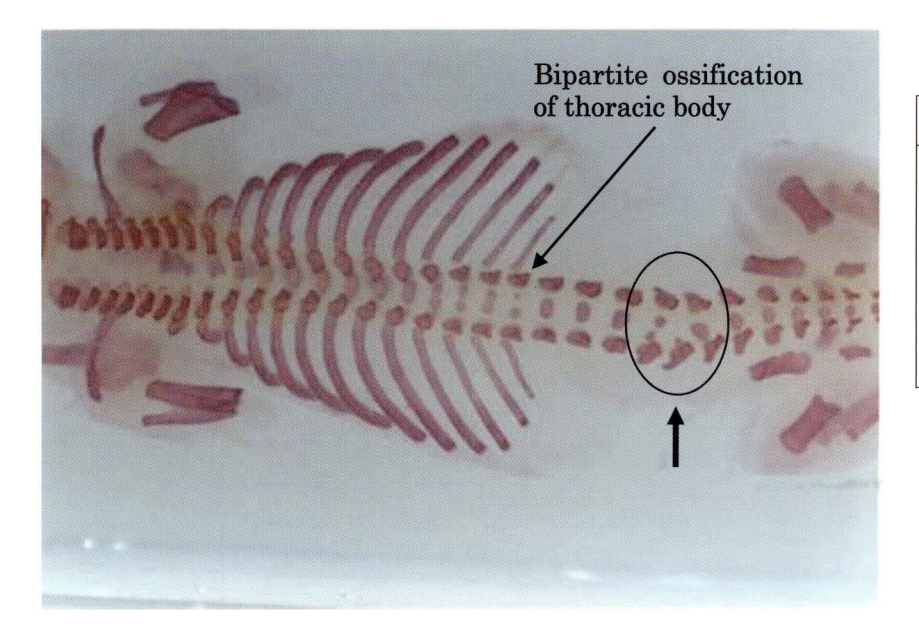

Bipartite ossification of thoracic body

Species	Rat、SD
Memo	Lumbar hemivertebra (circle) with Increased number of lumbar vertebrae (10724) and Bipartite ossification of thoracic vertebral centrum (10681).
	腰椎半椎（円）：腰椎過剰（10724）及び胸椎体二分骨化（10681）を伴う。

10-11　Supernumerary lumbar vertebrae　　腰椎過剰　(10724)

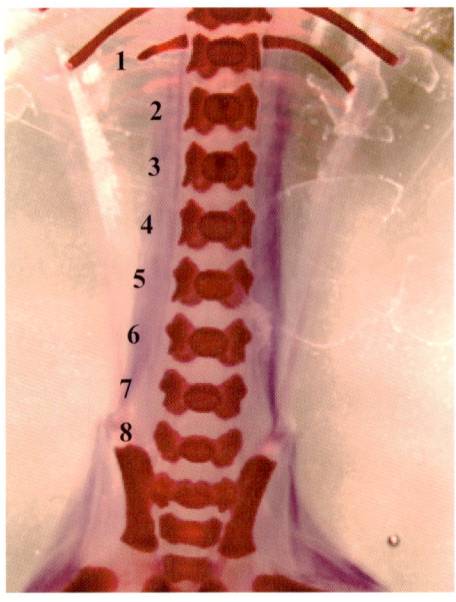

Species	Rabbit
Memo	Supernumerary lumbar vertebrae or Increased number of lumbar vertebrae with Full supernumerary thoracolumbar rib (10628)
	腰椎数過剰：完全過剰肋骨（胸腰部、10628）を伴う。

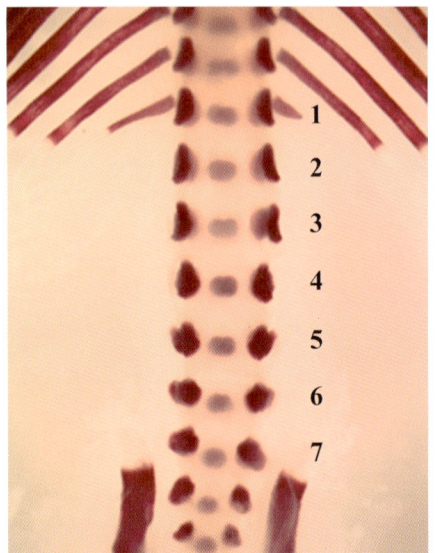

Species	Rat
Memo	Supernumerary lumbar vertebrae or Increased number of lumbar vertebrae with Full supernumerary thoracolumbar rib (left; 10628) and Short supernumerary thoracolumbar rib (right; 10638)
	腰椎数過剰：過剰肋骨（胸腰部肋骨、完全；10628、短小；10638）を伴う。

10-11 Continued

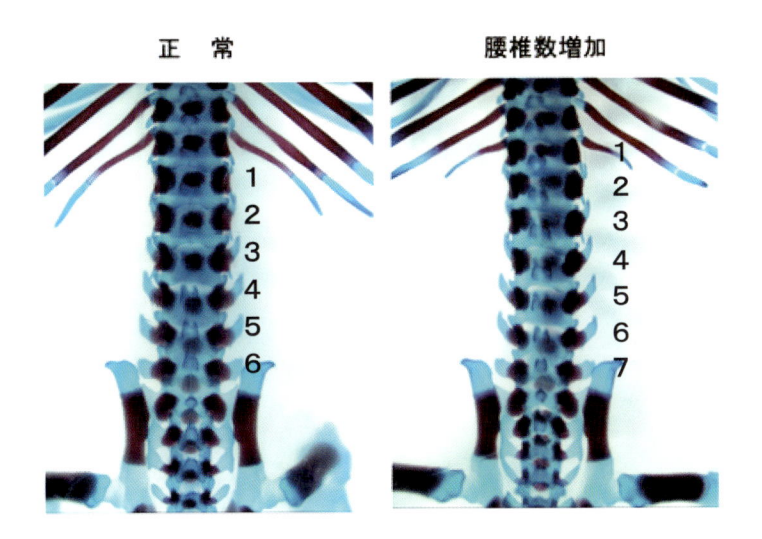

Species	Rat
Memo	Supernumerary lumbar vertebrae or Increased number of lumbar vertebrae with Full supernumerary thoracolumbar rib (10628) (Right photograph). The left photograph shows normal features.
	腰椎数増加、腰椎数過剰（右写真）:腰肋骨（10628）も伴う。左写真は正常。

Photographs of Skeletal Anomalies

11. Sacral and Caudal vertebrae

11-1 Fused sacral vertebral arches 仙椎弓癒合 (10726)

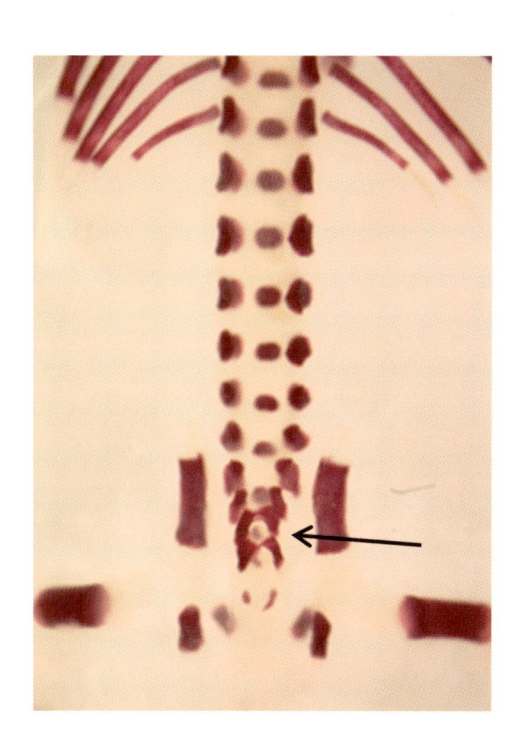

Species	Rat
Memo	Fused sacral vertebral arches (arrow) with Absent caudal vertebrae (10769)
	仙椎弓癒合（矢印）：尾椎欠損（10769）を伴う。

11-2　Misshapen sacral vertebral arch　　仙椎弓形態異常　(10730)

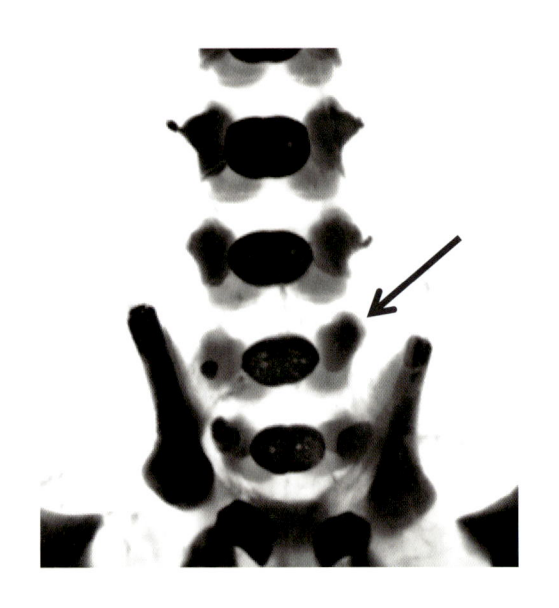

Species	Rabbit
Memo	Misshapen sacral vertebral arch or Lumbarization of the 1st sacral vertebra: The left process of the 1st sacral arch transforms as same as the process of lumbar vertebral arch.
	仙椎弓形態異常、仙椎腰椎化：片側性で仙椎弓の突起が腰椎の様になっている。

Species	Rabbit
Memo	Misshapen sacral vertebral arch or Lumbarization of the 1st sacral vertebra: The right 1st sacral vertebral arch (S1) resembles sacral vertebra, and its left arch resembles lumbar vertebra. Malpositioned caudal unilateral pelvic girdle (New) is also observed because left pelvic girdle shifts caudally direct (note broken line).
	仙椎弓形態異常（腰椎化）：S1の椎弓は、左側は腰椎型であるが、右側は仙椎型であり、仙椎の腰椎化と考える。左側の後肢体が尾方向にずれているので、後肢体片側性尾方位置異常（New）を伴っている（破線に注目）。

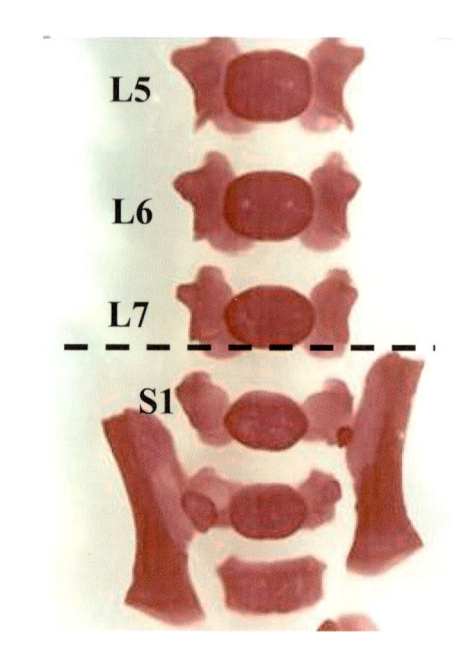

11-3 Sacral vertebral arch not fused 　　仙椎弓未癒合　(New)

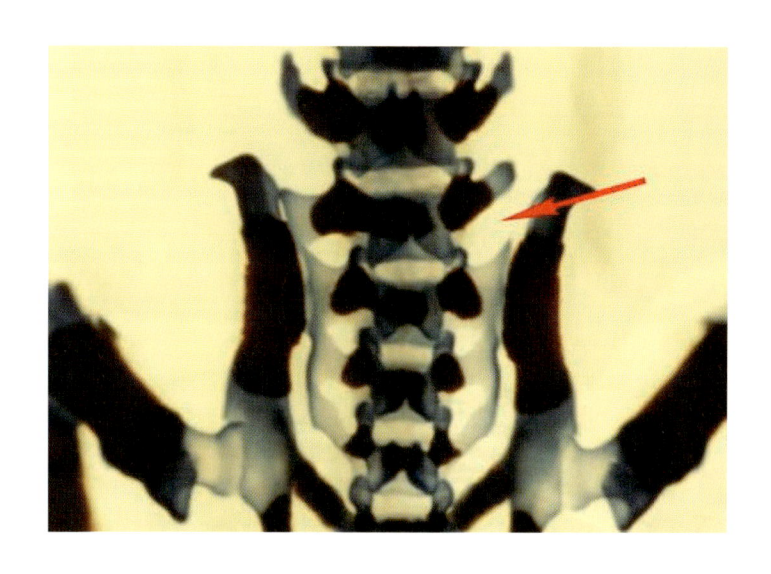

Species	Rat
Memo	Sacral vertebral arch not fused (red arrow): This fetus was double-stained for bone and cartilage. If it is single-stained for ossified bone, the abnormal shape of the right sacral vertebral arch would be considered as "Misshapen sacral vertebral arch or Lumbarization of the 1st sacral vertebra (10730)".
	仙椎弓未癒合（矢印）：単染色の場合、右第1仙椎はその形態から「仙椎弓形態異常（仙椎腰椎化、10730）」であると考えられる。

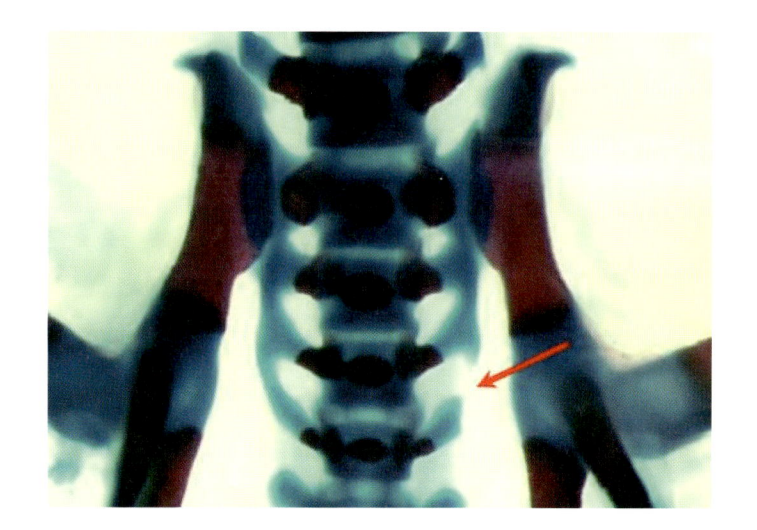

Species	Rat
Memo	Sacral vertebral arch not fused (red arrow)
	仙椎弓未癒合（矢印）

11-4　Absent sacral vertebrae　　仙椎欠損　　(10748)

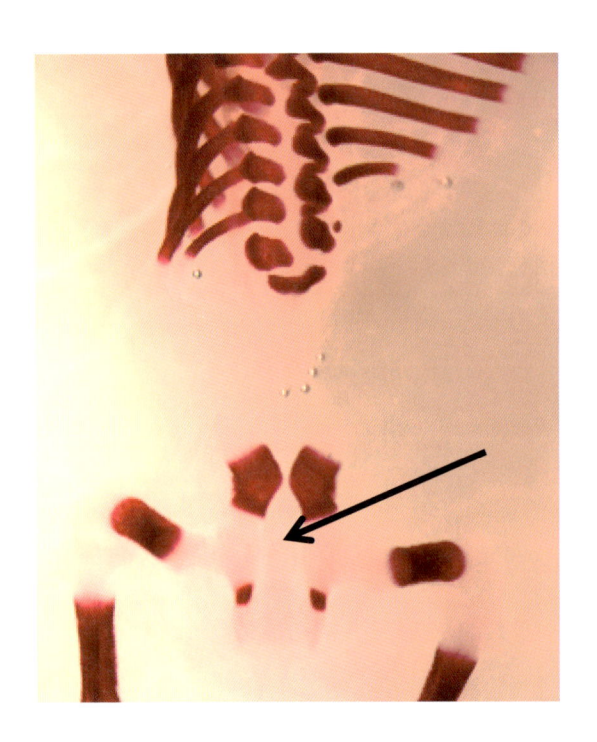

Species	Rat
Memo	Absent sacral vertebrae (arrow) with Absent lumbar vertebrae (10721) and Absent caudal vertebrae (10769)
	仙椎欠損（矢印）：腰椎欠損（10721）及び尾椎欠損（10769）を伴う。

11-5 Fused caudal vertebral centra　　尾椎体癒合　(10763)

Species	Rabbit
Memo	Fused caudal vertebral centra (arrow)
	尾椎体癒合（矢印）

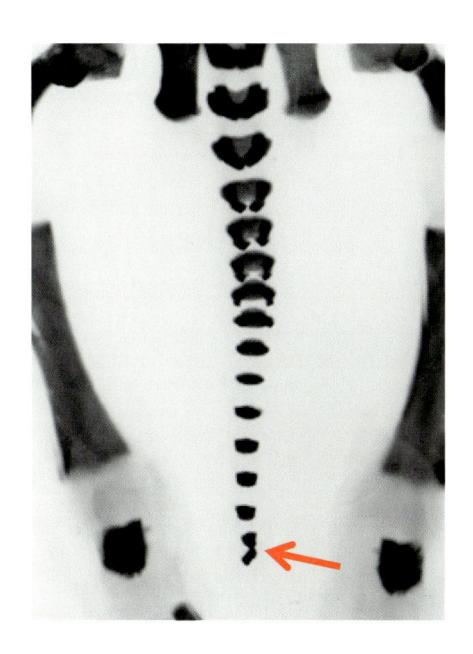

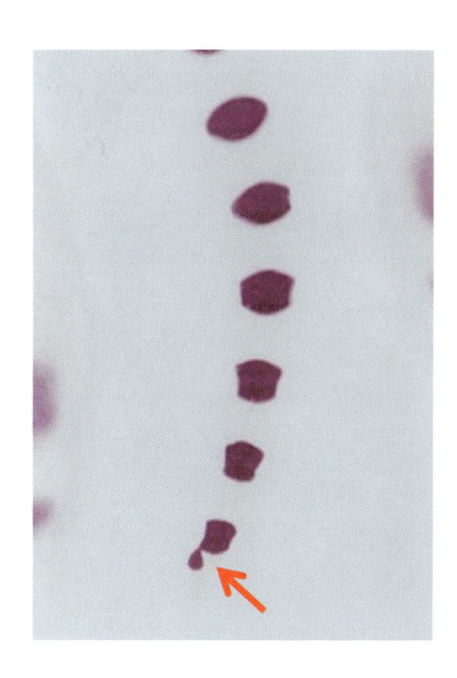

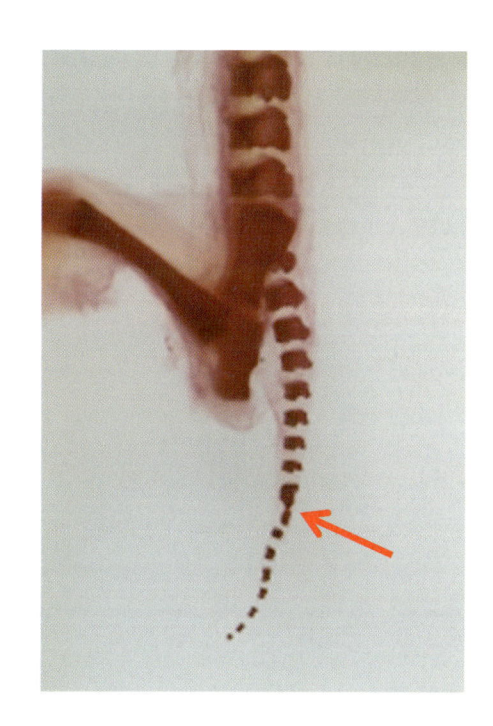

11-5 Continued

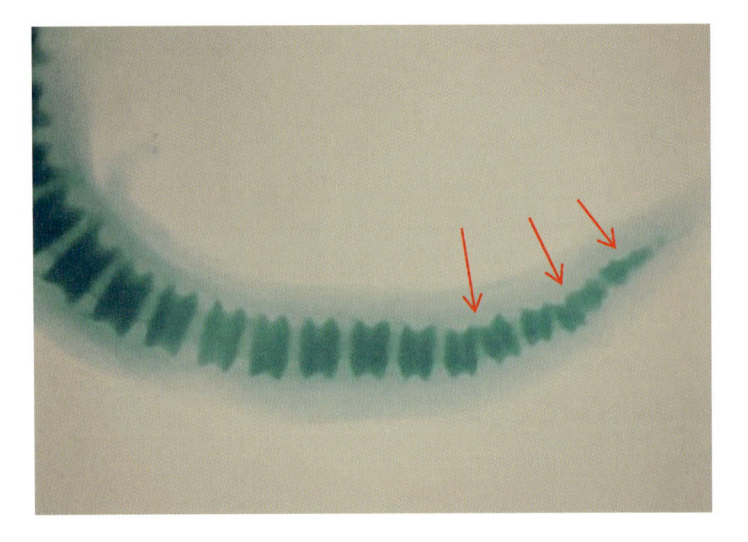

Species	Rat
Memo	Fused caudal vertebral centra (arrow)
	尾椎体癒合（矢印）

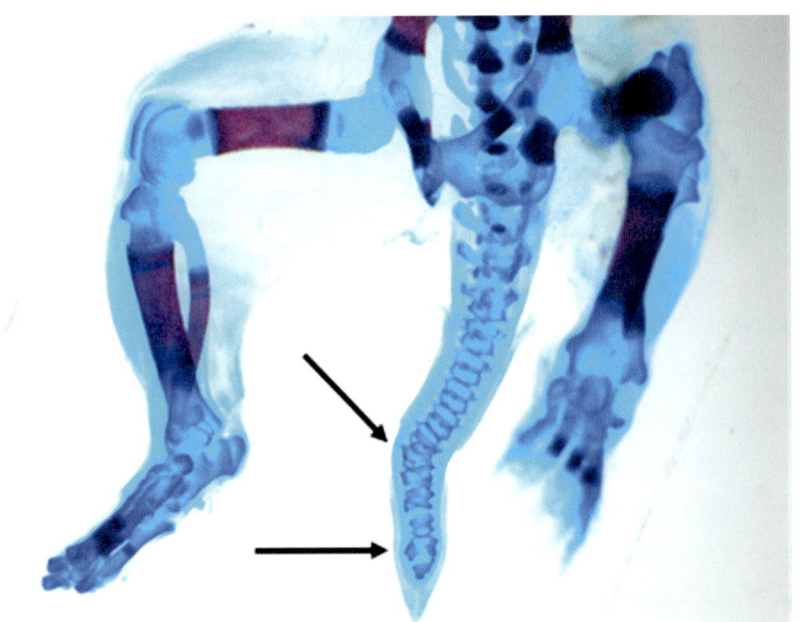

Species	Rat
Memo	Fused caudal vertebral centra: Fusion of caudal vertebrae at the bent point and the tip of the tail (arrow). This specimen is stained by double-staining method.
	尾椎（体）癒合：尾屈曲が見られる部分及び先端に癒合がある（矢印）。

11-6　Misaligned caudal vertebral centrum　尾椎体配列異常　(10766)

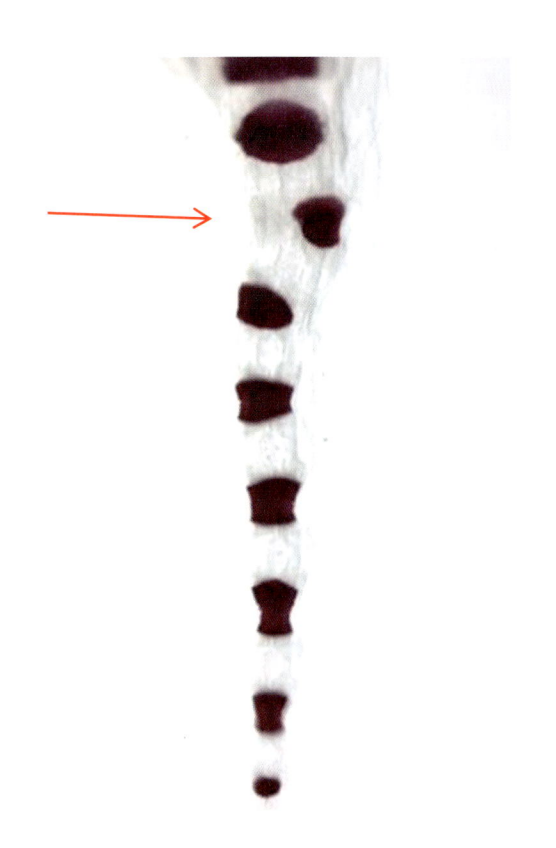

Species	Rabbit
Memo	Misaligned caudal vertebral centrum (arrow)
	尾椎体配列異常（矢印）

11-7　Incomplete ossification of caudal vertebral centra　　尾椎体不完全骨化　(10765)

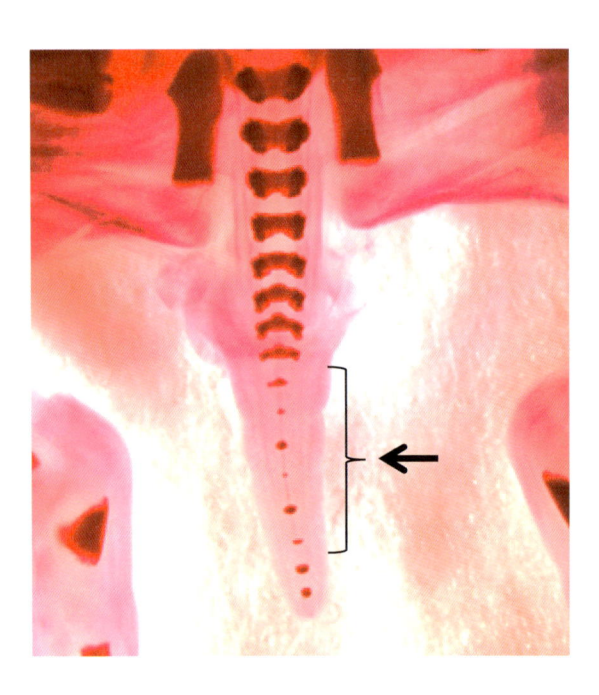

Species	Rabbit
Memo	Incomplete ossification of caudal vertebral centra (arrow)
	尾椎体不完全骨化（矢印）

11-8 Unossified caudal vertebral centra   尾椎体未骨化   (10768)

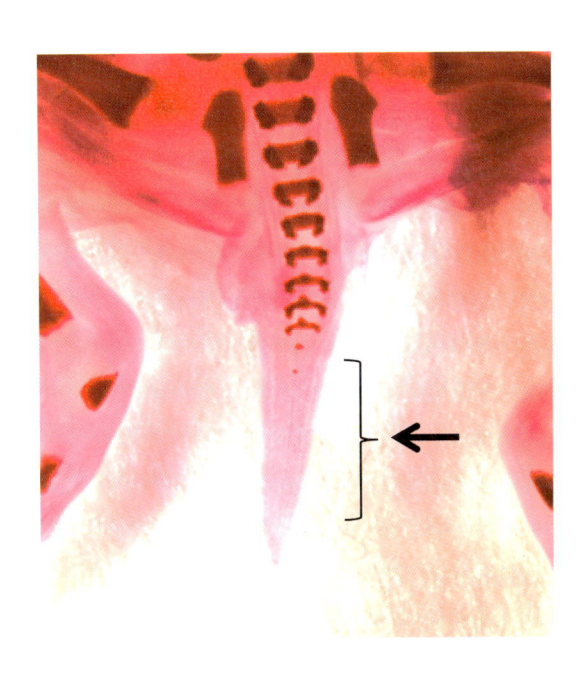

Species	Rabbit
Memo	Unossified caudal vertebral centra (arrow): If cartilage is not confirmed to be present, this would be considered as "Absent caudal vertebra".
	尾椎（体）未骨化（矢印）：軟骨が確認できる場合。軟骨が確認できなければ、「尾椎欠損」が妥当。

11-9 Absent caudal vertebrae　尾椎欠損　(10769)

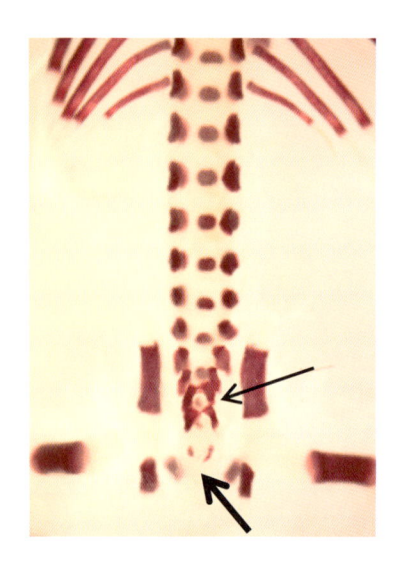

Species	Rat
Memo	Absent caudal vertebrae (thick arrow) with Fused sacral vertebral arches (thin arrow, 10726)
	尾椎欠損（太矢印）：仙椎弓癒合（細矢印、10726）を伴う。

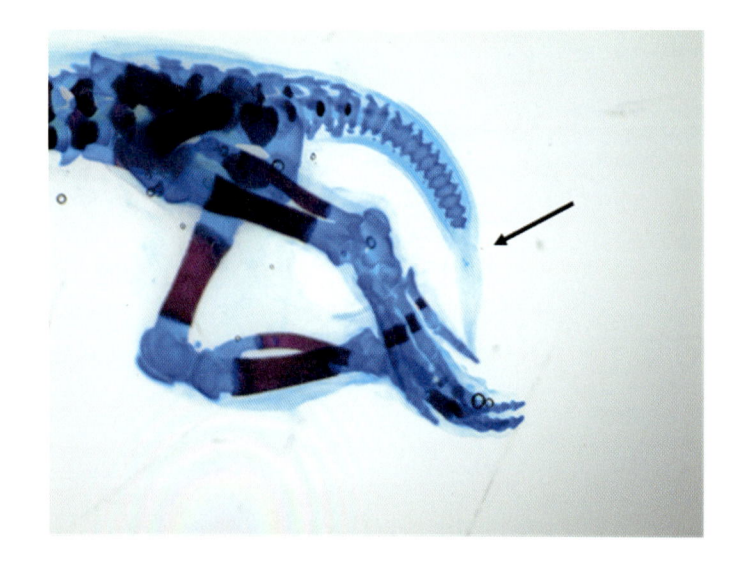

Species	Rat
Memo	Absent caudal vertebrae: Caudal vertebrae beginning from narrowed point are absent (arrow). This specimen is stained by double-staining method.
	尾椎欠損（矢印）：尾狭窄部位以降の尾椎が欠損している。二重染色標本

11-9 Continued

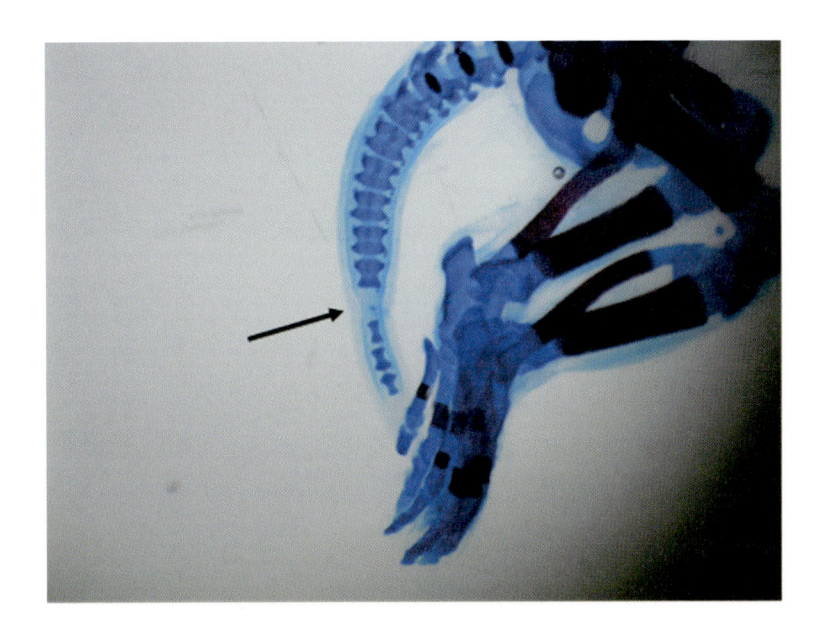

Species	Rat
Memo	Absent caudal vertebrae: Caudal vertebrae at the narrowed point are absent (arrow). This specimen is stained by double-staining method.
	尾椎欠損：尾狭窄が見られる部分の尾椎が欠損している。二重染色標本

11-10 Caudal hemivertebra 尾椎半椎 (10770)

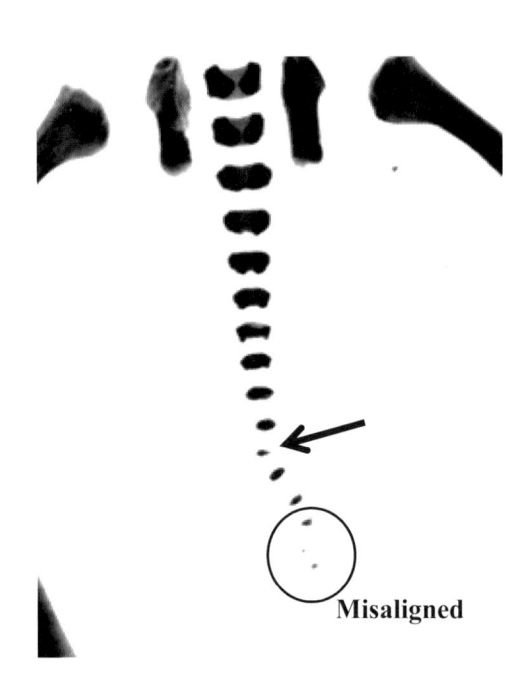

Species	Rabbit
Memo	Caudal hemivertebra (arrow) with Misaligned caudal vertebrae (circle, New)
	尾椎半椎（矢印）：配列異常（円、New）も伴う。

Misaligned

11-11   Misaligned caudal vertebrae   尾椎配列異常   (New)

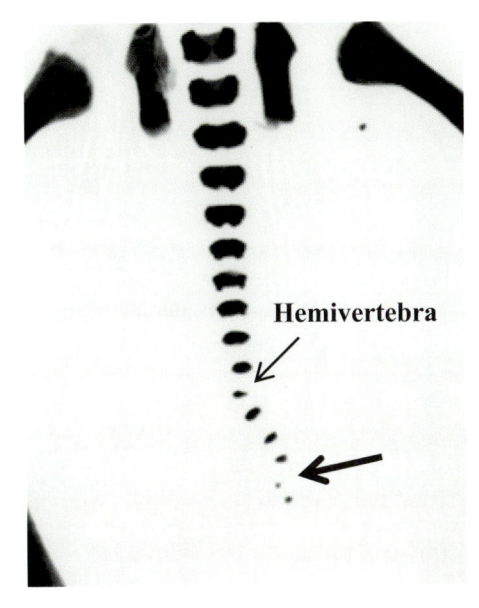

Species	Rabbit
Memo	Misaligned caudal vertebrae (thick arrow) with Caudal hemivertebra (thin arrow, 10770)
	尾椎配列異常（太矢印）：尾椎半椎（細矢印、10770）も伴う。

Species	Rabbit
Memo	Misaligned caudal vertebrae (arrow or circle): This finding is considered to be "Misaligned" because of its continuous feature although Small caudal vertebra is also observed.
	尾椎配列異常（矢印／円）：尾椎小型化も含まれるが、連続性があり、配列異常とする。

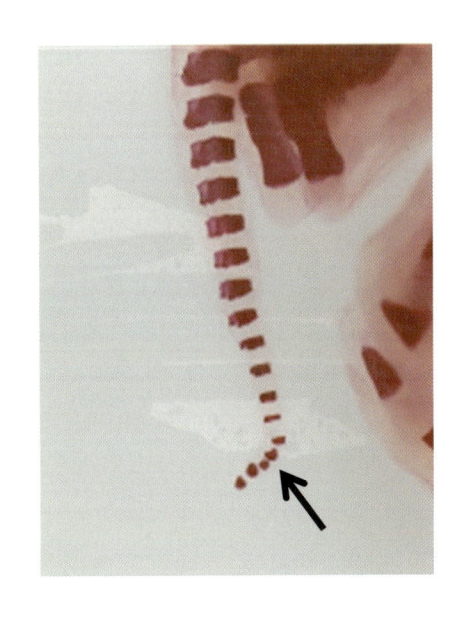

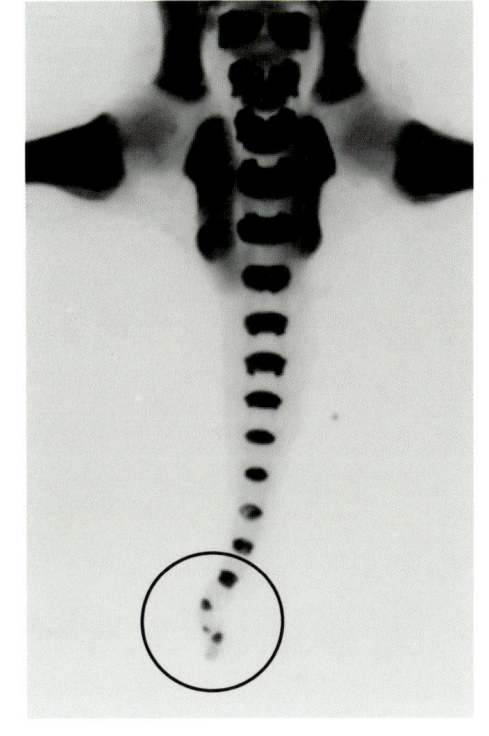

11-11　Continued

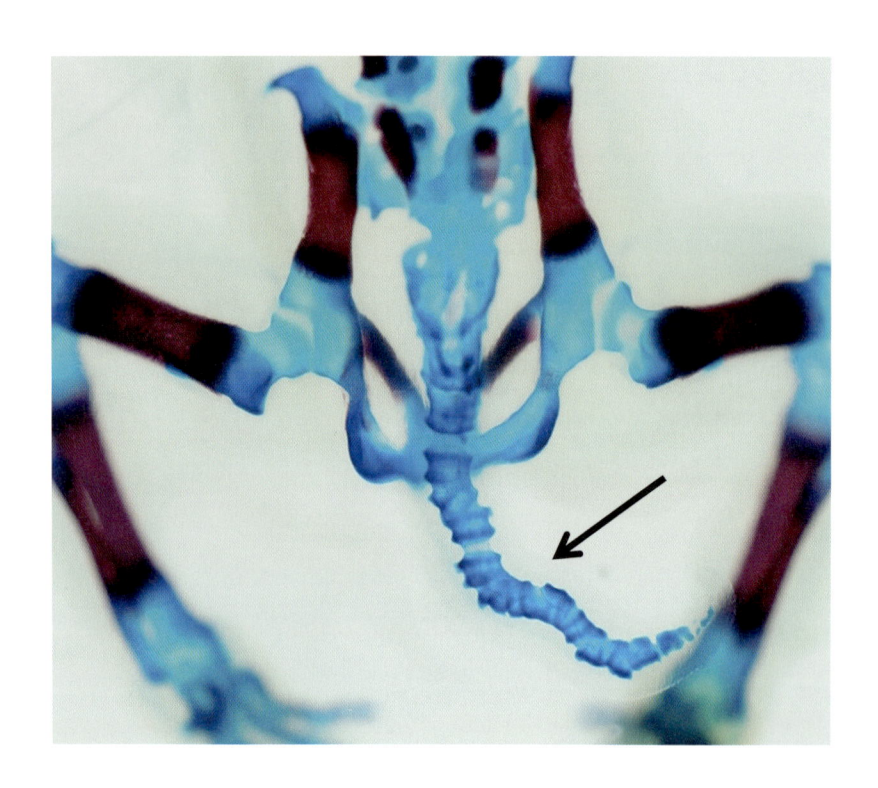

Species	Rat
Memo	Misaligned caudal vertebrae (arrow) with Fused sacral vertebral arch and centrum (10726 and 10738, respectively) and Misshapen sacral vertebral arch and centrum (10730 and 10743, respectively): This fetus has complex anomalies such as Fused caudal vertebral arch and centrum (10753 and 10763, respectively) and Misshapen caudal vertebral arch and centrum (10757 and 10767, respectively). This fetus may be considered as "Bent tail (10094)" in external observation.
	尾椎配列異常（矢印）：本例は尾椎（椎弓、椎体）の癒合（10753 と 10763）と形態異常（10757 と 10767）を伴う複合異常である。仙椎の癒合・形態異常（10726、10730、10738、10743）を伴う。外表観察では尾屈曲（10094）と思われる。

Photographs of Skeletal Anomalies

12. Pelvic girdle

12-1 Malpositioned pelvic girdle (cranial, bilateral)　後肢帯両側性頭方位置異常　(New)

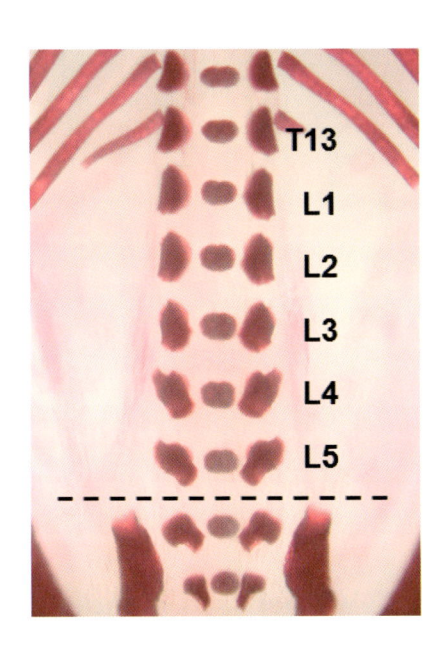

Species	Rat
Memo	Malpositioned pelvic girdle (cranial, bilateral) with Absent lumbar vertebra or Reduced number of lumbar vertebrae (10721) and Short rib (10637): bilateral cranial shift of the pelvic girdle.
	後肢体両側性頭方位置異常：両側の後肢体が頭方に移動している。腰椎欠損（腰椎数減少、10721）及び肋骨短小（右第13肋骨、10637）を伴う。

12-2 Malpositioned caudal unilateral pelvic girdle　　後肢帯片側性尾方位置異常　(New)

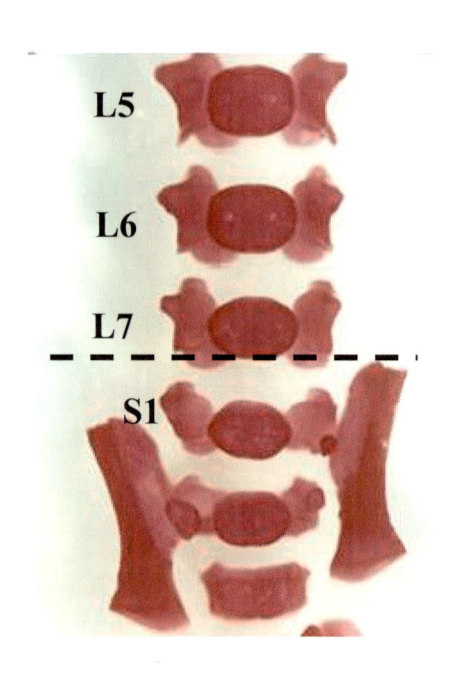

Species	Rabbit
Memo	Malpositioned caudal unilateral pelvic girdle: Left pelvic girdle shifts caudally (note broken line). The right arch of S1 resembles sacral vertebra, and its left arch resembles lumbar vertebra. So this is considered to be Misshapen sacral vertebral arch (10730) or Lumbarization of sacral vertebra.
	後肢体片側性尾方位置異常：左側の後肢体が尾方向にずれている。S1の椎弓は左側は腰椎型であるが、右側は仙椎型であり、仙椎の形態異常（腰椎化）と考える。

Atlas of Developmental Anomalies in Experimental Animals
実験動物発生異常アトラス

Skeletal Anomalies
骨格異常

2015 年 10 月 20 日　第 1 刷発行

編集　日本先天異常学会用語委員会
Edited by Project of the Terminology Committee of the Japanese Teratology Society

発行　株式会社 薬事日報社　YAKUJI NIPPO, LTD.
http://www.yakuji.co.jp
本社　東京都千代田区神田和泉町 1
電話　（03）3862-2141
支社　大阪市中央区道修町 2-1-10
電話　（06）6203-4191

印刷・製本　昭和情報プロセス株式会社

落丁本・乱丁本はお取り替えいたします。本書の無断複製を禁じます。